THE BIOLOGICAL ACTIVITY OF THYMIC HORMONES

THE BIOLOGICAL ACTIVITY OF THYMIC HORMONES
International Workshop and Symposium

Organized by:
Professor Dr. D. W. van Bekkum, Radiobiological Institute TNO, The Netherlands
and
Dr. Ada M. Kruisbeek, Institute for Experimental Gerontology TNO, The Netherlands

and the groups of:
Professor Dr. N. Trainin, Weizmann Institute of Science, Israel
Professor Dr. J.-F. Bach, Hôpital Necker, France
Professor Dr. A. L. Goldstein, University of Texas, U.S.A.

Held at the REP-Institutes of the Organization for Health Research TNO, Rijswijk, The Netherlands, from 12-27 November 1974

THE BIOLOGICAL ACTIVITY OF THYMIC HORMONES

edited by

D. W. VAN BEKKUM

KOOYKER SCIENTIFIC PUBLICATIONS
Rotterdam-The Netherlands

HALSTED PRESS DIVISION
JOHN WILEY & SONS
New York – London – Sydney – Toronto

KOOYKER SYMPOSIUM SERIES No. 001

LIBRARY OF CONGRESS
CATALOGING IN PUBLICATION DATA

Main entry under title:

The Biological activity of thymic hormones.

1. Thymic hormones–Congresses. 2. T cells–Congresses.
I. Bekkum, Dirk Willem van, 1925- II. Kruisbeek, Ada M.
QP572.T46B56 574.1'927 75-17617
ISBN 0-470-89835-6

Distributed solely by Halsted Press,
a Division of John Wiley & Sons, Inc.,
New York

ISBN 90-6212-001-6

Cover: Rein Wentink/Leiderdorp
Printed by: B.V. Boekdrukkerij F.E. MacDonald, Nijmegen, The Netherlands

CONTENTS

PART ONE, PROCEEDINGS OF THE SYMPOSIUM INCLUDING THE RESULTS OF THE WORKSHOP

PART ONE

Proceedings of the Symposium,
including the Results of the Workshop

Biological Activity of Thymic Hormones

THYMOLOGY IN THE RADIOBIOLOGICAL INSTITUTE - T.N.O.

Introducing the hosts, the setting, and the participating teams

D. W. VAN BEKKUM

Why do scientists undertake certain studies and not others? A general answer to this question can perhaps not be given but one of the determining factors seems to be the field of interest of the group in which the individual investigator operates, if we ignore the lone investigator who has become increasingly rare with the development of teamwork in research.

One of the long-term interests of a changing group of investigators in the Radiobiological Institute has been the development of a clinically useful procedure for bone marrow transplantation. The studies were originally aimed at the protection against the effects of lethal whole body exposure to ionizing radiation, later directed at the treatment of bone marrow aplasia and leukemia, and, more recently, the treatment of combined immune deficiency disease (CID).

There were several properties of the thymus which made it a favorite organ at our Institute, the first being its content of a highly radiosensitive population of lymphocytes (1); the second, its role in radiation leukemogenesis (2) as discovered by H. S. Kaplan (3) and extended by Haren-Ghera and others. But the most persistently fascinating aspects of the thymus were those concerned with the central role of this organ in immunological responses, now generally described as the cellular immunity. Following the pioneering work of J. F. A. P. Miller and R. Good on thymectomized animals which revealed the decisive role of the thymus in the development of the immune capacities and perhaps of immunological tolerance, our group invested much effort in thymus research, with the hope that it would provide us with clues for the prevention of certain complications of allogeneic bone marrow grafting which were identified by the early sixties as being due to an immunological graft versus host (GvH) reaction. We studied the process of immunological reconstitution in thymectomized radiation chimaeras and observed a partial recovery starting three months after bone marrow transplantation with the establishment of the tolerance of the donor type cell towards the host (4). Thus, it appeared that a thymus-like function is provided by other (unidentified) sources and that the development of specific tolerance is not exclusively dependent on the thymus. A similar interest in immunological tolerance - this

Radiobiological Institute-T.N.O., Rijswijk (Z.H.), The Netherlands

time with regard to self - lead de Vries & Hijmans to study the cellular composition of the thymus of New Zealand Black mice at different ages. They observed, among other abnormalities, an early decline in the number of epithelial cells in the NZB thymus, a decline which occurs in nonautoimmune strains only with advanced age (5).

A different but parallel line of investigation at that time focused on neonatally thymectomized mice. We found ourselves unable to reproduce the finding of Miller, Law and others, that a high incidence of wasting and mortality occurs in these animals. After excluding the possibility of inadequate surgical techniques and of genetic differences, we had to conclude that the high viability of our neonatally thymectomized mice was due to the absence of pathogenic microorganisms in our SPF mouse colony. This allowed us to follow these thymectomized mice for prolonged periods of time and to pick up lesions (mostly non-fatal) which were strikingly reminiscent of the histopathological changes that we were by then familiar with in GvH disease. In addition, typical wire loop lesions were observed in the kidneys and this led us to propose the hypothesis that, under proper protective conditions, the removal of the thymus immediately after birth may lead to an autoimmune syndrome (6) thus strengthening the idea that the thymus is involved in preventing immunological reactivity against self, as was subsequently confirmed by Yunis *et al.* (7, 8), Monier *et al.* (9) and others.

These observations resulted in two separate lines of work. One was concerned with the phenomenon termed isologous secondary disease: the occurrence of a wasting syndrome in mice exposed to high supralethal doses of whole body irradiation and rescued with isologous bone marrow. The histopathological changes observed in these animals were again strikingly similar to those seen in GvH disease following allogeneic bone marrow transplantation - though less severe. Since the syngeneic bone marrow graft could not possibly elicit a GvH reaction, we were forced to think in terms of autoimmunity and thus to focus our attention on the thymus. A systematic investigation of the thymus in these isologous chimaeras revealed a striking decrease in the number of epithelial cells in the thymuses of animals exposed to doses of over 800 rad (10). Furthermore, the mortality from isologous secondary disease could be significantly diminished by implanting three new born thymuses under the renal capsule (11). Thus, a very high dose of irradiation seems to irreversibly damage the thymus epithelium and thereby to disturb the function of the thymus. Lower doses of irradiation in the range of 300-400 rad (high dose rate exposure) do not seem to cause significant damage, since such irradiated thymus grafts still have the capacity to reconstitute nude mice (12, 13).

The other line of investigation emerging from our early adventures with the post-thymectomy and other autoimmunity syndromes and with GvH disease, was more clinically orientated. It was concerned with various immune deficiencies in children, in particular those with Swiss-type agammaglobulinemia (CID). At that time, the pathogenesis of that disease was thought to reside in the thymus, but numerous attempts to reconstitute these patients with thymus implants had uniformly failed. On the basis of certain analogies between the pathological changes in CID patients and experimental animals, de Vries developed a "completely new pathogenic theory for the Swiss type of agammaglobulinemia" (Quotation - R. Good, see ref. 14 [p 188] 1968) (14) which led our group to propose and attempt the transplantation of small numbers of bone marrow cells from normal compatible siblings for the treatment of CID. This resulted in successful reconstitutions simultaneously in Minneapolis (15) and in Leiden (16) and bone marrow transplantation is by now an accepted and rewarding therapy for CID, provided that a histocompatible donor can be found.

Our more recent interest in the thymus has been focused on the thymic hormone(s), mainly because of its obvious function in the treatment of other immune deficiencies and because it might provide a remedy for the late immune deficiency state which develops in monkeys and man following successful abrogation of both the acute and the delayed type of GvH disease by means of donor selection, grafting of purified stem cell concentrates, bacteriological decontamination and isolation of the recipients, and so forth (17). The isolation of the active principle of the thymus poses formidable technical difficulties, because a simple and reproduceable assay for monitoring the purification of the hormone was, until recently, not available. Some of the most attractive assays for this purpose such as the rosette inhibition assay of Jean-Francois Bach and the *in vitro* GvH assay developed by the Trainin group were found to be extremely costly in terms of man hours involved and many groups including ours, had problems in establishing these tests in a routine fashion. Also, in those cases when a series of reproduceable results were obtained, they did not seem to fit in completely with the findings and the theories of the initiators of those assays. For instance, our group found that the Goldstein preparation and not the Trainin principle induced a positive GvH response *in vitro* when nude spleen cells were employed as the effector cells (18). In addition the results reported by the three main groups of investigators, those of Bach, Trainin, and Goldstein which were engaged in the isolation of the thymic hormone, deviated in several aspects from each other. Therefore, by the beginning of 1974 it seemed timely to get these three teams together for a thorough intercomparison of the various hormone preparations in as many assays as were operational within each of the groups. We were fortunate to have available some of the experience necessary to understand at least what was going on, the facilities to house several teams of workers simultaneously and to allow them to perform, and finally to receive the financial support from a variety of sponsors to pay for this expensive operation*. But facilities and

* The J. A. Cohen Institute
The Ministry of Education and Science
The Ministry of Public Health and Environmental Hygiene
The Netherlands Kidney Foundation
The Queen Wilhelmina Fund
Biomed-Benelux bv
The Netherlands Society of Gerontology

logistics alone are not sufficient; the most important requirement for the undertaking of such a workshop is the presence of a number of motivated staff and technicians to carry the burden of providing the tools and the help required for such a large-scale concentrated technical operation. It was gratifying to find that such people and such enthusiasm existed within the Radiobiological Institute and the Institute for Experimental Gerontology T.N.O. But we are even more grateful for finding that the three thymus hormone teams found our setting an adequate environment to perform the intercomparison and to entrust us with the delicate task of coding and decoding their precious preparations and of acting as "neutral observers", interpreters and, last but not least, as editors of the Proceedings of this Workshop, its results, and the ensuing Symposium.

We hope that our guests were as satisfied as we were with the experience. Considering the fact that fourteen different assays were performed (many of them repeatedly) with three different hormone preparations and their appropriate controls, and that the conditions in Rijswijk (especially the hydrobiological ones) were obviously different from those in the respective home laboratories, it is amazing that ten of these assays yielded useful results. The data obtained clearly established the biological activity of all three hormone preparations, so that any possible doubt about the reality of the thymus hormone or hormones has now been removed. This will obviously provide a strong stimulus for the large-scale production of purified thymic hormones and thereby allow the biologist to study the activity of the hormone in a number of *in vivo* situations in both animals and human patients, studies which could not be performed so far for lack of active substance. As indicated by Dr. Kruisinga, the President of the Dutch Society of Gerontology who was kind enough to deliver an introductory speech on the day of the symposium, we all look forward to the information which may now soon be provided as to the influence of thymic hormones on immune deficiencies, cancer, and immunological derangements associated with ageing.

REFERENCES

1. Van Bekkum, D. W., de Vries, M. J. & Klouwen, H. M. (1965) *Int. J. Rad. Biol.* **9**, 449.
2. Van Bekkum, D. W. & Balner, H. (1973) In: Unifying concepts of leukemia, *Bibl. Haemat.* no. 39. Ed. by: R. M. Dutcher and L. Chieco-Bianchi, Karger, Basel, 677.
3. Kaplan, H. S. (1957) In: BEGG Proc. 2nd Canadian Cancer Research Conference, 1956, vol. 2, Academic Press, New York, 127.
4. Van Bekkum, D. W. (1965) La greffe des cellules hématopoiétiques allogéniques, Paris, 7-9 sept. 1964. Editions du Centre Nat. de la Recherche Scientifique, 1965, p. 381-390, CNRS.
5. De Vries, M. J. & Hijmans, W. (1967) *Immunol.* **12**, 179.
6. De Vries, M. J., van Putten, L. M., Balner, H. & van Bekkum, D. W. (1964) *Rev. Franc. Etudes Clin. et Biol.* **9**, 381.
7. Yunis, E. J., Teague, P. O., Stutman, O. & Good, R. A. (1969) *Laboratory Investigation* **20**, 46.
8. Yunis, E. J., Hong, R., Gerwe, M. A., Martinez, C., Cornelius, E. & Good, R. A. (1967) *J. Exp. Med.* **125**, 947.

9. Monier, J. C., Thivolet, J. & Sepetjian, M. (1969) *Rev. Franç. Etudes Clin. et Biol.* **14**, 185.
10. Van Bekkum, D. W. (1967) In: *Brookhaven Symposia in Biology* no. 20. Recovery and repair mechanisms in radiobiology 190.
11. Van Bekkum, D. W. (1969) In: Comparative Cellular and Species Radiosensitivity, Igaku Shoin, Tokyo, 175.
12. Nieuwerkerk, H. T. M., Löwenberg, B. & van Bekkum, D. W. (1974) In: Proc. of the First Int. Workshop on Nude Mice, Aarhus, Oct. 11-13, 1973, Gustav Fischer Verlag, Stuttgart, 175.
13. Blankwater, M. J. & Lina, P. H. C. (1974) In: Proc. of The First Int. Workshop on Nude Mice, Aarhus, Oct. 11-13, 1973, Gustav Fischer Verlag, Stuttgart, 167.
14. De Vries, M. J., Dooren, L. J. & Cleton, F. J. (1968) Birth Defects IV, orig. art. series, Immunologic Deficiency Diseases in Man, 173.
15. Gatti, R. A., Allen, H. D., Meuwissen, H. J., Hong, R. & Good, R. A. (1968) *Lancet* **II**, 1366.
16. De Koning, J., van Bekkum, D. W., Dicke, K. A., Dooren, L. J., van Rood, J. J. & Rádl, J. (1969) *Lancet* **I**, 1223.
17. Van Bekkum (1974) *Transplant. Proc.* (in press).
18. Löwenberg, B., Nieuwerkerk, H. T. M. & van Bekkum, D. W. (1972) *Annual Report* 1972 REPGO TNO, 105.

Biological Activity of Thymic Hormones

THYMUS HORMONES: A NEW FIELD IN ENDOCRINOLOGY AND ITS SIGNIFICANCE FOR HOST IMMUNOLOGICAL COMPETENCE

ABRAHAM WHITE

The evidence that a given anatomical structure in mammals is an endocrine gland includes the demonstration that extirpation of the tissue or organ results in physiological or biochemical aberrations or deficiencies in the operated animal. This approach has been utilized since 1845 in studies of the thymus gland. During the subsequent seventy year period, studies of thymectomy in a wide variety of animal species yielded both dramatic and contradictory results. The reasons for this are, in retrospect, rather clear: a) the slow development of successful operative procedures for total thymectomy; b) the failure to consider species variations in the anatomy of the thymus; c) the lack of adequate knowledge of the variation among species in the state of development and function of lymphoid tissue at birth and in the postnatal years; and d) inadequate facilities for housing operated animals resulting in frequent recording of early deaths from apparent infections (see (1) for review).

The simultaneous observations in 1961 by Miller (2) and by Archer & Pierce (3) that neonatal thymectomy in the mouse and in the rabbit, respectively, results in failure of normal postnatal growth, lymphoid tissue development and maturation, and development of parameters of immunological competence initiated a resurgence of interest in the thymus gland. The dramatic effects of neonatal thymectomy added significance to our earlier observations (4), in collaboration with Dr. Sidney Roberts, that cell-free extracts of calf and rat thymic tissue specifically produced a lymphocytosis and lymphoid tissue hypertrophy when administered to normal rats. Confirmation of the presence of a lymphocytopoietic factor in thymic extracts by Gregoire & Duchateau (5) and by Metcalf (6), and the subsequent demonstrations of the immunological impairment resulting from neonatal thymectomy in a variety of species (7, 8), also aided significantly in the interpretation of the possible role of normal thymic function in the human being (9).

The foregoing data and the rapidly accumulated experimental observations made during the past decade permit, at the present time, the following conclusions:

1. The thymus *is* an endocrine gland that has at least three regulatory roles in the growth and maturation of host immunological competence. These roles

Syntex Research, Palo Alto, California 94304 and the Department of Biochemistry, Stanford University School of Medicine, Stanford, California 94305, U.S.A.

are: a) the production and export to the peripheral tissues, notably to the spleen and lymph nodes, of specific lymphoid cells, termed T cells, that under appropriate hormonal influences provide the basis for host immunological competence; b) the synthesis and secretion by the thymic reticuloepithelial cells of one or more polypeptide hormones; and c) the provision of an intrathymic microenvironment that contributes to the expression of specific parameters of host immunological competence.

2. The purification and characterization of the first thymic polypeptide hormone was achieved in our laboratory in collaboration with Dr. Allan Goldstein and Dr. Arabinda Guha in 1972 (10). We had earlier named this principle thymosin (11).

3. Thymosin may exert its influence both in the thymus and in extrathymic loci (12-16).

4. Thymosin has been demonstrated to function by acting on progenitor cells (predetermined T cells or T_0 cells) promoting their maturation to T_1 cells and accelerating the progress of the latter to T_2 cells (16-18).

5. The T_1 cells that mature under the influence of thymosin may function in at least three ways: a) in cell-mediated immunological phenomena; b) in cooperative reactions with B cells to promote antibody synthesis; and c) as cells with specialized functions, *e.g.*, as suppressor T cells (16-19).

TABLE I

BIOLOGICAL ACTIVITIES OF THYMOSIN IN *in vitro* MODELS

Conversion of precursor cells to immunologically competent lymphocytes in the following systems:
- Rosette assay
- Cytotoxicity assay: expression of θ and TL antigens
- Responsivity to mitogens
- Mixed lymphocyte interaction
- Secondary antibody response
- Conversion of bone marrow cells *in vitro* into cells reactive in the graft vs host *in vivo* assay
- T and B cell cooperation (*in vitro*→ *in vivo*)

The above roles of thymosin in the development and maturation of lymphoid cells and their contributions to host immunological competence have been indicated in a wide variety of *in vitro* and *in vivo* model systems. These are summarized in Tables I and II.

All of our own data, and most of the literature from other laboratories that have established the thymus as an endocrine gland whose secretory activity is fundamental for host immunological competence, have derived from experiments utilizing preparations from earlier stages of purification. In our own, as well as in other laboratories, these studies are being repeated with more highly purified preparations and, ultimately, will require exploration with a physical-chemically homogeneous product. This last approach is essential for

TABLE II

BIOLOGICAL ACTIVITIES OF THYMOSIN IN *in vivo* MODELS

Normal Mice:
- Lymphocytopoiesis
- Enhanced rate of allograft rejection
- Enhanced resistance to progressive growth of Moloney virus induced sarcoma
- Enhanced mixed lymphocyte reaction (*in vivo*→ *in vitro*)
- Enhanced lymphoid cell response to mitogens (*in vivo*→ *in vitro*)

Germ Free Mice:
- Lymphocytopoiesis

Adrenalectomized Mice:
- Enhanced lymphocytopoiesis

Neonatally Thymectomized Mice:
- Increased survival and rate of growth
- Lymphocytopoiesis
- Restoration of ability to reject skin allograft
- Enhancement of mixed lymphocyte interaction

Athymic "Nude" Mice:
- Lymphocytopoiesis
- Restoration of response of lymphoid cells to mitogen
- Reduction of allogeneic and xenogeneic tumor growth rate

Immunosuppressed Mice:
- Enhancement of ability to reject skin allograft

NZB Mice:
- Delay of appearance of abnormal thymocyte differentiation, with loss of suppressor function

answers to the question of the possible multiplicity of products synthesized and secreted by the thymus gland, a topic that may next be discussed.

First and paramount consideration must be given to establishment of the physical and chemical homogeneity of each thymic preparation. To the present time, some seven different products have been isolated from calf thymus, each with a significant degree of purity and influencing one or more immunological parameters and with reported molecular weights ranging from 500 to 70,000. In addition, Dr. Bach and his colleagues, following their demonstration of thymosin-like activity in the blood of the human being and in selected species of mice, have succeeded in the preparation and characterization of this activity from pig blood (17, 18, 20).

Are the larger biologically active preparations precursors or prohormones of the molecules of lower molecular weight? What are the products synthesized by the thymic epithelium and are they identical with the hormones entering the blood and identifiable in the circulation? Do the divergent physical and chemical properties reported for the different products reflect, in part, artifacts of the preparative procedures? Factors that could contribute to artifactual results are aggregation phenomena, possible protein-protein interactions, and the electrostatic and hydrophobic interactions of proteins and polypeptides with other molecules present in thymic tissue as well as in the blood.

In our own experience with calf thymus as starting material, and depending upon the nature of the purification steps, we can obtain an active thymosin fraction of molecular weight 12,500, similar in size to that described from our laboratory in 1972 (10). However, we can also obtain an active thymosin preparation of molecular weight approximately 70,000 by lyophilization of thymosin preparations in the presence of a trace of phosphate buffer. This phenomenon has been well-documented (21-22). Moreover, in our own experience, alterations in the ionic strength of the initial medium used for extraction of thymus glands may markedly influence the yield, activity, and behavior of the active fractions obtained during subsequent purification steps.

In view of the later papers in this symposium volume, further consideration will not be given here to the chemistry of thymosin or the chemical nature of other recently characterized thymic factors. Three of these, namely, thymosin and one additional thymic preparation, which has been termed thymic humoral factor by Dr. Trainin, and Dr. Bach's preparation from pig serum that he has designated as serum TA or serum thymic activity, are described later. Rather, the subsequent comments will focus on some aspects of the possible significance of the addition of the newest member, the thymus, to the family of endocrine glands and on certain of the interrelationships already established between the thymus and other endocrine structures.

It may have been anticipated that the evidence that the thymus is an endocrine gland would add significance to the already established interrelationships of thymic structure and function to the secretory activity of other endocrine glands. Indeed we reported a number of years ago (23) that, of the lymphoid structures studied, the thymus gland is the most sensitive to the involutionary effects of the hypophyseal-adrenal cortical hormonal axis. Of particular relevance for more recent studies of the endocrine role of the thymus was the observation that, due to hormonal treatment, the disappearance of numerous lymphocytes ordinarily present in the medulla of the thymus left the endodermal reticular cells more exposed, thus giving the impression that an increase in these cells had occurred. These and subsequent studies have indicated that these reticular cells, the probable site of hormone synthesis, are relatively hydrocortisone-resistant (24).

The involution of the thymus and other lymphoid structures resulting from augmented adrenocorticotropic-adrenal cortical secretion can be mimicked by a wide variety of nonspecific stimuli, *viz.*, physical, chemical, and neural, that increase the activity of this endocrine axis (25). Thus, alterations in the physical environment, such as heat or cold, endogenously produced hormones (*e.g.*, epinephrine), drugs, and psychogenic factors all have a common relationship at this level, thus providing partial explanation for the reports of depressed immunological responsiveness resulting from such stimuli. Androgenic hormones have similar effects on thymic structure and function, whereas the estrogenic hormones have a proliferative action on lymphoid tissue (26). Such observations assume added significance in considerations of sex differences in immunological responsiveness, as well as related phenomena such as a possible causal relationship between immunological competence and the aging process (27).

Of interest for considerations of the growth and maturation of immunological competence as influenced by the thymus are the reported interrelationships of the latter structure to somatotropin, or growth hormone, and to thyrotropin. The proliferative actions of these last two hormones on lymphoid tissue are well-established from both experimental and clinical observations (26). The effects of these and other endocrine secretions are particularly marked on the thymus, which has long been recognized as having a significantly higher rate of cellular turnover and metabolic activity than other lymphoid structures.

More recently, Baroni and Pierpaoli and their colleagues (28-30) succeeded, by administration of somatotropin together with thyroxine, in reconstituting 19 S antibody production in the genetically hypopituitary Snell-Bagg dwarf mouse, which is immunologically deficient and has lymphoid tissue abnormalities characteristic of the neonatally thymectomized mouse.

Contributions to the interrelationships of the thymus and other endocrine glands have also stemmed from studies of Comsa and his associates (31) and from those of Talwar and his colleagues (32-34). The collective data demonstrate a probable synergistic action of the endocrine role of the thymus with that of growth hormone and the thyrotropic-thyroid axis, and an antagonist interrelationship between the thymus and adrenocorticotropic-adrenal cortical activity.

My own interpretation of the present state of the art of thymic hormones is based upon the published results from several laboratories including our own. It may be postulated that the thymus gland produces a family of several hormones, each of which may alter the extent of expression of one or more, but perhaps not all, of the immunological parameters thought to reflect a role for the thymus in the regulation of host immunological competence. This hypothesis can be experimentally tested and ultimate analysis of its validity should be based primarily on data obtained from *in vivo* studies with physical-chemically homogeneous products in animals deprived of sources of endogenous thymic factors. This reservation is suggested because it represents the more stringent of experimental approaches and may circumvent possible artifacts of unknown nature that may enter into *in vitro* assays. This is not meant to denigrate the utility of *in vitro* assays for initial evaluation of preparative procedures, for establishing probable quantities of fractions required for *in vivo* studies, or for the dissection of the mechanism of action of thymic factors.

In the studies of thymic hormones conducted *in vivo*, it may also be suggested that some consideration be given to variable factors that are becoming delineated in both the thymectomized animal and in the absence of one or another endocrine gland, based upon the interplay of the endocrine roles of the thymus with those of other glands of internal secretion. This is of particular significance in studies of host immunological competence, inasmuch as the overwhelming majority of stimuli, both hormonal and nonhormonal, that alter the numbers, structure, or functions of lymphoid cells are influencing the response of a major cell that contributes to both humoral and cell-mediated immunological phenomena.

In concluding, the potential practical significance of thymosin and other described thymic factors may be briefly indicated. With the increasing degree of understanding of the biological roles of the thymus gland, the retrospective and current evaluations of clinical syndromes related to thymic function have ranged from immunological deficiency syndromes, including thymic aplasias and dysplasias, to autoimmune diseases, to malignancies (9). The potential practical utility of purified thymic factors is suggestively significant based on three types of evidence. First, the encouraging therapeutic benefit obtained in clinical studies utilizing transplants of whole thymus glands (17). Second, initial reports from several laboratories that assessment *in vitro* of specific paramaters of cell-mediated immunity indicates that lymphoid cell populations from peripheral blood of patients may be lower than normal in thymic aplasias and dysplasias, as well as in a variety of malignancies, and that these parameters may be increased by incubation of such lymphoid cells with thymosin (35-37). Third, suggestive evidence derived both from the rosette assay and a radioimmunological assay that circulating levels of blood thymosin in the human being are abnormally low, in comparison with individuals of the same age, in both the congenitally athymic or post-thymectomized human being, and in patients with specific types of malignancies (27, 38, 39).

Indeed, two clinical groups have reported preliminary trials with calf thymosin preparations. Drs. Wara and Amman, utilizing a partially purified thymosin fraction prepared in Dr. Allan Goldstein's laboratory, have reported (37) clinical improvement in a single case of a five and one-half-year-old girl with thymic hypoplasia, deficient immunoglobulin synthesis, and evidence of diminished cell-mediated immunological competence.

A second clinical study with thymosin was reported at the International Congress of Immunology held in Brighton, England (1974). Dr. Aleksander Skotnicki, spokesman for a group at the Hematology Clinic of the Institute of Medicine in Krakow, Poland, described results obtained in leukemia and cancer patients with a thymosin preparation made in his country by our published procedure. (Their report appears elsewhere in this volume).

Thus, the thymus has come of age as a member of the endocrine family. To achieve this status, data have been obtained fulfilling five of the six postulates essential for designation of a tissue or structure as an endocrine gland. These are: 1) extirpation or absence of the gland in early neonatal life does result in serious deficiencies for the host; 2) successful replacement therapy has been achieved by both transplantation and the administration of cell-free extracts; 3) administration of excessive amounts of suitable preparations has yielded evidence of exaggeration of phenomena normally regulated by the gland; 4) isolation and chemical characterization of one or more of the biologically active principles in cell-free extracts has been achieved; and 5) it has been demonstrated that the isolated principle or principles when administered can substitue effectively for the functions normally dependent on its presence in the absence of the thymus.

It may be anticipated that the sixth and final essential postulate, the chemical synthesis in the laboratory of one or more of the postulated thymic hormones, will be achieved, with the subsequent demonstration that the synthetic product has the chemical and physiological properties of the hormonal product isolated from the thymus gland.

REFERENCES

1. White, A. & Goldstein, A. L. (1968) *Perspectives in Biol. and Med.* **11**, 475.
2. Miller, J. F. A. P. (1961) *Lancet* **ii**, 748.
3. Archer, O. K. & Pierce, J. E. (1961) *Fed. Proc. Am. Soc. Exp. Biol.* **20**, 26.
4. Roberts, S. & White, A. (1949) *J. Biol. Chem.* **178**, 159.
5. Gregoire, C. & Duchateau, G. (1956) *Arch. Biol.* (Liege) **67**, 269.
6. Metcalf, D. (1956) *Brit. J. Cancer* **10**, 442.
7. Miller, J. F. A. P. & Osoba, D. (1967) *Physiol. Revs.* **47**, 137.
8. Trainin, N. (1974) *Physiol. Revs.* **54**, 272.
9. Good, R. A. & Gabrielsen, A. E., eds. (1964) *The Thymus in Immunobiology. Structure, Function and Role in Disease*, Hoeber Medical Division, Harper & Row, New York, N.Y.
10. Goldstein, A. L., Guha, A., Zatz, M. M., Hardy, M. A. & White, A. (1972) *Proc. Natl. Acad. Sci., U.S.A.* **69**, 1800.
11. Goldstein, A. L., Slater, F. D. & White, A. (1966) *Proc. Natl. Acad. Sci., U.S.A.* **56**, 1010.
12. White, A. & Goldstein, A. L. (1970) In *Control Processes in Multicellular Organisms*, eds. G. E. W. Wolstenholme & J. Knight, Churchill, London, pp. 210-237.
13. White, A. & Goldstein, A. L. (1970) In *Hormones and the Immune Response*, eds. G. E. W. Wolstenholme & J. Knight, Churchill, London pp. 3-23.
14. Goldstein, A. & White, A. (1971) *Adv. Metabolic Dis.* **5**, 149.
15. Goldstein, A. & White, A. (1971) *Current Topics in Exptl. Endocrinol.* **1**, 121.
16. Goldstein, A. & White, A. (1973) *Contemporary Topics in Immunobiol.* **2**, 239.
17. White, A. & Goldstein, A. L. (In press) Adv. Metabolic Dis. **8**, Nobel Symposium 28.
18. White, A. (In press) *Ann. N-Y. Acad. Sci.*
19. Dauphinee, M., Talal, N., Goldstein, A. L. & White, A. (1974) *Proc. Natl. Acad. Sci. U.S.A.* **71**, 2637.
20. Bach, J.-F., Dardenne, M. & Bach, M.-A. (In press) *Ann. N-Y. Acad. Sci.*
21. Chilson, O. P., Costello, L. A. & Kaplan, N. O. (1965) *Biochemistry* **4**, 271.
22. Everse, J. & Stolzenbach, F. E. (1971) In *Methods in Enzymology*, ed. W. B. Jakoby, vol. XXII, Academic Press, Inc., New York pp. 33-38.
23. Dougherty, T. F. & White, A. (1945) *Am. J. Anat.* **77**, 81.
24. Metcalf, D. (1964) In *The Thymus in Immunobiology. Structure, Function, and Role in Disease*, eds., R. A. Gorch & A. E. Gabrielsen, Hoeber Medical Division, Harper & Row Publishers, New York, N.Y. pp. 150-182.
25. Dougherty, T. F. & White, A. (1947) *J. Lab. & Clin. Med.* **32**, 584.
26. White, A. & Goldstein, A. L. (1972) In *Immunogenicity: Physical, Chemical and Biological Aspects*, ed., F. Borek, North-Holland, Amsterdam pp. 334-364.
27. Goldstein, A. L., Hooper, J. A., Schulof, R. S., Cohen, G. H., Thurman, G. B., McDaniel, M. C., White, A. & Dardenne, M. (1974) *Fed. Proceed.* **33**, 2053.
28. Baroni, C., Fabris, N. & Bertoli, G. (1969) *Immunol.* **11**, 303.
29. Pierpaoli, W., Baroni, C., Fabris, N. & Sorkin, E. (1969) *Immunol.* **16**, 217.
30. Pierpaoli, W. & Sorkin, E. (1969) In *The Immune Response and Its Suppression*, ed. E. Sorkin, Karger, New York pp. 124-134.
31. Comsa, J. (1973) In *Thymic Hormones*, ed. T. D. Luckey, University Park Press, Baltimore, Maryland pp. 59-96.
32. Pandian, M. R. & Talwar, G. P. (1971) *J. Exp. Med.* **134**, 1095.
33. Talwar, G. P. (1972) *Intl. J. Biochem.* **3**, 39.
34. Talwar, G. P. (In press) *Recent Progr. Hor. Res.*
35. Hooper, J. A., McDaniel M. C., Thurman, G. B., Cohen, G. H., Schulof, R. S. & Goldstein, A. L. (In press) *Ann. N-Y. Acad. Sci.*
36. Wara, D. W., Goldstein, A. L., Doyle, N. & Ammann, A. J. (1975) *New Engl. J. Med.* **292**, 10.
37. Wara, D. W. & Ammann, A. J. (In press) *Ann. N-Y. Acad. Sci.*
38. Schulof, R. S. (1972) *Texas Rpts. Biol. Med.* **30**, 195.
39. Schulof, R. S., Hooper, J. A., White, A. & Goldstein, A. L. (1973) *Fed. Proc. Am. Soc. Exptl. Biol.* **32**, 962.

Biological Activity of Thymic Hormones

THYMOCYTE DIFFERENTIATION *IN VITRO* AFTER INCUBATION WITH AUTOLOGOUS THYMIC TISSUE

JAN G. VAN DEN TWEEL, PIETER F. GROLLÉ, EUGENIE H. VAN MEERBEKE, DIËNNE ELFERINK, LIDA VAN WOESIK & CHRIS J. MEIJER

INTRODUCTION

When the response of lymphocytes of different lymphoid organs of inbred and outbred guinea pigs is studied after stimulation with the mitogens Phytohaemagglutinin (PHA), Pokeweed mitogen (PWM), and Concanavalin A (Con A), it appears that lymphocytes obtained from lymph nodes, spleen, and Peyer's patches are good responders to these mitogens (unpublished observations). The response of thymocytes, however, is negative under varying tissue culture conditions. In this study, we investigated the conversion of mitogen nonresponsive thymocytes to mitogen-responsive cells under the influence of autologous thymic tissue. Furthermore, we studied the antigen-independent interaction of thymocytes with autologous and allogeneic peritoneal macrophages, their ability to form spontaneous (E) rosettes with rabbit red blood cells, and the formation of C_3 (EAC) rosettes. These were combined with studies on surface Ig.

MATERIALS AND METHODS

Thymocyte suspensions

Thymocyte suspensions were prepared by pressing thymus fragments through a wire screen. The single cell suspensions obtained were incubated with fragments of autologous thymus tissue (<1 mm^3) in microtiter trays (Linbro Chemical Co.) for 24 h in a humidified incubator (37°C, 95 per cent air, 5 per cent CO_2) at a concentration of 0.5×10^6 cells per well. The culture medium was RPMI 1640 (Flow Laboratories) supplemented with L-glutamine (0.06 mMol), penicillin (40 U/ml), streptomycin (40 μg/ml), and 20 per cent heat-inactivated fetal bovine serum (Flow Laboratories). As controls, cultures with heart tissue fragments or medium with no additional tissue were used. After incubation,

Department of Immunohaematology, University Hospital and Institute of Pathology, State University, Leiden, The Netherlands
This work was supported in part by the Dutch Organization for Medical Research (FUNGO) which is subsidized by the Dutch Organization for the Advancement of Pure Research (ZWO); the Koningin Wilhelmina Fonds (KWF); and the J. A. Cohen Institute for Radiopathology and Radiation Protection (IRS).

the organ fragments were removed, the cells were washed two times in Hank's balanced salt solution, and resuspended in supplemented RPMI; 0.5×10^6 cells were cultured in microtiter trays with optimal concentrations of the mitogens (PHA, Wellcome Reagents Ltd., Beckenham, England, 20 μl stock solution/ml medium; Con A, Calbiochem, San Diego, Calif., 5 μg/ml medium; PWM, Grand Island Biological Co., Grand Island, New York, 20 μl stock solution/ml medium). After 48 h, 2 μCi ^{3}H-Thymidine (The Radiochemical Centre, Amersham) was added to each well. Cells were harvested 18 hours later and the radioactivity was counted in a Packard liquid scintillation spectrometer.

Thymocyte receptors

a. Rosette formation. Rosettes were prepared as described by Zeylemaker *et al.* (1).

b. Macrophage-thymocyte interaction was studied according to a modified method as described by Lipsky & Rosenthal (2).

RESULTS

The negative response of guinea pig thymocytes (Table I) to various mitogens becomes positive after incubation with autologous thymus tissue. There is a great increase in the PHA and Con A responses but only a slight increase in the response to PWM.

TABLE I

BEHAVIOUR OF GUINEA PIG THYMOCYTES BEFORE AND AFTER INCUBATION WITH AUTOLOGOUS THYMIC TISSUE

Mitogen response[a]	*after incubation with non-thymic tissue*[b]	*after incubation with thymic tissue*
PHA	196 (34)	11380 (10)
Con A	155 (13)	7233 (14)
PWM	162 (12)	1217 (7)
Medium only	137 (20)	460 (32)
Receptor studies[c]		
% thymocytes forming E rosettes	89 (5)	88 (5)
% thymocytes forming EAC rosettes	<0.1	<0.1
% thymocytes with surface Ig	<0.1	<0.1
Binding to autologous macrophages:		
% MØ[d] with thymocytes	83 (7)	28 (54)
number of thymocytes per 100 MØ	244 (29)	33 (58)
Binding to allogeneic macrophages:		
% MØ with thymocytes	36 (29)	48 (11)
number of thymocytes per 100 MØ	56 (42)	89 (16)

a) results are of one representative experiment
b) c.p.m.; in parenthesis coefficient of variation (also in receptor studies)
c) results are the mean of three representative experiments
d) MØ – macrophages

The number of thymocytes forming spontaneous E rosettes (89 per cent) and the number of cells forming EAC rosettes (<0.1 per cent) do not change during incubation with autologous thymic tissue. No surface-Ig-bearing cells are present in the system (<0.1 per cent). When autologous peritoneal macrophages are incubated with thymocytes, there is a significant decrease in the autologous thymocyte-macrophage interaction after incubation of the thymocytes with thymic tissue. The macrophage-thymocyte interaction after incubation is in the same range as the macrophage-lymphocyte interaction (Table II).

TABLE II

INTERACTION OF LYMPH NODE CELLS (LNC) AND MACROPHAGES

	autologous system	*allogeneic system*
% MØ with LNC	24 (22)	34 (57)
Number of LNC per 100 MØ	42 (17)	52 (45)

DISCUSSION

The response of lymphocytes to PHA, Con A, and PWM is a property of a mature lymphocyte population. The negative thymocyte response to these mitogens can therefore be interpreted as being the result of the fact that mainly immature lymphocytes are present in the guinea pig thymus. This is in contrast with our (unpublished) observations that human thymocytes respond very well to PHA and Con A. The positive response of thymocytes after incubation with autologous thymic tissue is probably the result of differentiation to a more mature T cell population. Although we have no direct evidence in this system, it is likely that thymus tissue *in vitro* produces a humoral factor (a thymic hormone) which induces the differentiation of thymocytes to more mature T cells. This differentiation is accompanied by a decreased autologous macrophage-thymocyte interaction. This might indicate that we are dealing with a loss of receptors for autologous macrophages with maturation. This fits in with the observation that peripheral lymphoid cells show less binding to macrophages than do thymocytes. This interaction is a property of autologous cells (2). In contrast to the decrease in the number of thymocyte receptors for macrophages, there is no change in the number of thymocytes which bind erythrocytes. The fact that the number of E rosettes remains constant before and after incubation with thymic tissue indicates that immature thymocytes already have that particular receptor on their cell surface; further differentiation does not influence these receptor sites. These observations suggest that thymocytes have different receptors for both RBCs and macrophages.

From the results presented in Table I, it is also clear that there is no B cell switch during the incubation period. The response to PWM remains negative and there are no changes in the numbers of cells forming EAC rosettes or those bearing surface Ig.

REFERENCES

1. Zeylemaker, W. P., Roos, M. Th. L., Meyer, C. J. L. M., Schellekens, P. Th. A. & Eijsvoogel, V. P. (1974) *Cellular Immunology* **14**, 346.
2. Lipsky, P. E. & Rosenthal, A. S. (1973) *J. Exp. Med.* **138**, 900.

Biological Activity of Thymic Hormones

ADENYL CYCLASE ACTIVATION AND EXPRESSION OF THETA ANTIGEN ON FOETAL THYMOCYTES

UPENDRA SINGH

The initial differentiation of stem cells (prethymic cells) within the thymus is accompanied by the expression of the surface alloantigens TL and Thy-1 (θ) (1). It has been shown recently that a subpopulation of cells within foetal liver and adult spleen (including spleen of "nude mice") may be activated to express the TL and Thy-1 (θ) alloantigens by a variety of agents which stimulate adenyl cyclase and thus increase levels of intracellular cyclic AMP (3′ 5′ adenosine mono phosphate) (2). It is not clear whether such changes can be induced in stem cells which have entered the thymus or thymic microenvironment, but which have yet not expressed T cell alloantigens. This communication deals with the changes which occur in expression of Thy-1 antigen on the surface of stem cells obtained from the 14-day mouse embryo thymus after incubation with agents which increase cyclic AMP levels.

Thymic stem cells were teased from thymic rudiments of 14-day-old BALB/c mouse embryos. Cell suspension was made in serum-free medium (RPMI 1640) at a concentration of 3×10^6/ml. Cells were then incubated for 90 minutes at 37°C in an atmosphere of 5 per cent CO_2 in air. Complement-dependent cytotoxicity tests using Trypan blue were carried out and cell counts were performed with the haemocytometer.

The proportion of 14-day thymic stem cells that are Thy-1 positive is low and remains low even after incubation with either RPMI 1640 or antitheta serum or complement alone. However, after incubation in RPMI 1640 containing cyclic AMP, Prostaglandin E1, Prolactin, and supernatant of 7-day-old thymus cultures, the proportion of Thy-1 positive cells is much higher (Table I).

These results indicate that thymic stem cells (14 days) can be induced to enter accelerated T cell differentiation by treatment with agents which increase intracellular cyclic AMP levels. *In vivo* and *in vitro*, under organ culture conditions without such agents, it takes a few more days before a large proportion of cells show Thy-1 antigen (θ) (1). Furthermore, these experiments provide an excellent model for studying the effects of various agents on differentiation of stem cells in the thymus without having to use a small subpopulation of cells separated by density centrifugation on bovine serum albumin. It remains

Department of Anatomy, The Medical School, The University of Newcastle-upon-Tyne, Newcastle-upon-Tyne, England.

TABLE I

% OF THY-1 (θ) POSITIVE CELLS IN 14 DAY OLD FOETAL THYMUS, AS DETERMINED IN A CYTOTOYICITY TEST (DYE EXCLUSION)

Agents used & doses.	*incubation without agents*	*incubation with agents.*
cAMP 1 mM	10 ± 3	44 ± 6
PGE1 25 μg/ml.	13 ± 2.5	38 ± 2.5
Prolactin 20 m.I.U.	16 ± 4.5	55 ± 5.7
Thymus culture supernatant. 0.1 ml/ml	16 ± 4.5	67 ± 7
Insulin 80 m.I.U.	12 ± 2.5	14 ± 3.5

The cells were incubated in RPMI 1640 (serum-free) for 90 minutes at 37°C ; the per cent of dead cells after incubation in either of the agents alone (without treatment with antisera and complement) was 4.5% for cAMP, 3.8% for PGE, 4% for Prolactin and 7% for complement and the agents. ±SD of 3 experiments.

to be seen, however, if the cells so induced to enter accelerated differentiation by using the aforesaid agents are immunocompetent and, if so, whether they can participate in cell-mediated immune reactions.

REFERENCES

1. Owen, J. J. T. & Raff, M. C. (1970) *J. Exp. Med.* **132**, 1216.
2. Scheid, M. P., Hoffman, M. K., Komuro, K., Hammerling, U., Abborr, J., Boyse, E. A., Cohen, G. H., Hooper, J. A., Schulof, R. S. & Goldstein, A. L. (1973) *J. Exp. Med.* **138**, 1027.

Biological Activity of Thymic Hormones

THYMIC FACTORS AND HUMAN T LYMPHOCYTE DIFFERENTIATION

J. L. TOURAINE*, F. TOURAINE, G. S. INCEFY, A. L. GOLDSTEIN & R. A. GOOD

Introduction

The *in vivo* maturation of stem cells to immunocompetent thymus-dependent (T) lymphocytes is a complex process that involves the migration of hematopoietic T lymphocyte precursors to the thymus, the acquisition of surface characteristics and development of functional properties in the thymus, followed by migration to peripheral lymphoid organs where additional properties are acquired. *In vitro* experiments in the mouse (Bach *et al.* 1971, Komuro & Boyse 1973) and in man (Touraine *et al.* 1974a) have established that certain T lymphocyte characteristics are expressed by predetermined T lymphocyte precursors from the bone marrow or the spleen after a short incubation with thymic extracts. We present here evidence that a) *in vitro* differentiation can be used in the analysis of various immunodeficiency diseases, and b) some further stages in T lymphocyte maturation can also be induced *in vitro* by thymic factors.

Acquisition of human T lymphocyte antigens (HTLA) by normal bone marrow cells

Incubation of Ficoll-Hypaque-separated human bone marrow (BM) cells with thymic extracts did not appear to lead to a significant increase in the percentage of $HTLA^+$ cells (i.e., cells killed by a specific anti-HTLA serum [Touraine *et al.* 1974b] in the presence of rabbit complement). However, when nucleated bone marrow cells were fractionated into five layers of various densities on a discontinuous albumin gradient (Dicke *et al.* 1970), some fractions of BM cells appeared to be enriched in T lymphocyte precursors. The incubation of only these fractions with thymic extracts for 2 h yielded observable conversion to the $HTLA^+$ phenotype (Touraine *et al.* 1974a).

Such an induction of $HTLA^+$ phenotype was consistently observed in layers

Université Claude Bernard, Lyon, Memorial Sloan-Kettering Cancer Center, New York, and University of Texas Medical Branch, Galveston
* Present address and correspondence: Dr. J. L. Touraine, Transplantation and Immunobiology Unit, Clinic of Nephrology, Pav P., Hôpital Edouard Herriot, 69374 Lyon Cedex 2, France.

TABLE I

DIFFERENTIATION OF HUMAN BONE MARROW CELLS INTO $HTLA^+$ T LYMPHOCYTES AFTER 2-HOUR INCUBATION WITH THYMIC EXTRACTS

	Cytotoxic index ($\%HTLA^+$ cells) in bone marrow layer				
Extracts	*I*	*II*	*III*	*IV*	*V*
Human thymus (fraction 3)	7	15	26	8	5
Calf thymus (fraction 3)	9	17	24	6	7
Human spleen (fraction 3)	6	8	10	7	6
Transfer factor	5	3	4	7	5
RPMI-1640 medium (control)	4	5	4	6	5

III and/or II of normal BM cells and Table I presents the mean of results obtained with cells from 3 normal donors after incubation with thymic extract fraction 3 (Goldstein *et al.* 1972) at a concentration of 1 mg/ml. Human and calf thymus extracts were both effective.

Spleen extracts at the same concentration only slightly increased the proportion of $HTLA^+$ cells in BM layer III. A more purified thymosin fraction 5 (Hooper *et al.* 1975) was effective in a dose range of 20-400 μg/ml but the number of BM cells converted to $HTLA^+$ phenotype was somewhat lower than that obtained when fraction 3 of thymus extracts was used.

By absorption experiments, the tissue extracts were shown to lack free HTLA and thus the conversion to $HTLA^+$ phenotype could not be attributed to mere fixation of antigens at the cell surface.

Incubation of layer III BM cells with thymic extracts also resulted in a slight increase in the numbers of E-rosette forming cells, especially when the incubation was extended to 18 h.

This induction of the first stage of T lymphocyte differentiation is an active phenomenon requiring RNA and protein synthesis, since it can be inhibited by actinomycin D, α-amanitin, and puromycin (Incefy *et al.* 1974). How the thymic factors exert their effect on the precursor cells remains to be determined. Results from other laboratories indicate that cyclic AMP and prostaglandins may play a role (Bach & Bach 1972, and Hadden, personal communication).

In vitro *T lymphocyte differentiation of BM cells from patients with immunodeficiency diseases (Table II)*

The above-described model not only provides a means for the investigation of the *in vitro* action of thymic factors, but also allows the study of early T lymphocyte differentiation in patients with immunodeficiency diseases (Touraine *et al.* 1975).

In contrast to our findings in normal individuals, we could not detect T cell precursors capable of acquiring surface characteristics of T lymphocytes

TABLE II

BONE MARROW T LYMPHOCYTE PRECURSORS AND *in vitro* T LYMPHOCYTE DIFFERENTIATION IN IMMUNODEFICIENCY DISEASES

Group	*Number studied*	*Number with T cell differentiation of BM cells*
Normal	12	12
SCID autosomal recessive form	3	0
SCID with ADA deficiency	2	0
Partial DiGeorge syndrome	2	2
X-linked agammaglobulinemia	1	1
Common variable immunodeficiency	1	1

in five infants with a severe combined immunodeficiency disease (SCID), including two cases associated with a deficiency in adenosine deaminase activity (later reconstituted by a BM transplant from an "identical sibling"). In patients with other forms of immunodeficiency, the *in vitro* T lymphocyte differentiation of BM cells could be induced, thus establishing the presence of precursors sensitive to the action of thymic factors. This was the case in two infants with partial DiGeorge syndrome, one of whom later received a fetal thymus transplant that resulted in a significant increase in peripheral T cell numbers.

This new methodology therefore provides an approach to the investigation of BM T lymphocyte precursors in patients with immunodeficiency and may be of value in determining which patients with T cell deficiencies may require a transplant of precursor cells or which patients might be expected to respond either to transplant of thymic epithelium or possible treatment with extracts or defined inducers from the thymus.

Enhancement of mitogen responsiveness

When unfractionated marrow nucleated cells from normal donors were incubated with thymosin for 18 h, washed, and then cultured for 3 days, the following results were obtained: increased spontaneous proliferation, a slight and inconsistent increase in the response to phytohemagglutinin (PHA), a more consistent and pronounced enhancement of the response to concanavalin A (Con A). After separation of BM cells on a discontinuous albumin density gradient and incubation with thymosin, a significantly increased index of stimulation by Con A was demonstrated in layers II and III, and less so in layer I.

The effect of thymosin on the proliferative response of human thymus cells to mitogens and to allogeneic cells was also investigated. Fragments of thymus obtained from children undergoing cardiac surgery were minced and thymocytes separated on a Ficoll-Hypaque gradient; 3×10^6 thymocytes were incubated with 500 μg of thymosin fraction 5 in 2 ml of RPMI-1640 culture medium for 18 h. They were then washed and recultured for 3 days in microtiter plates. After being treated with thymic extracts, these cells were markedly more responsive to Con A (Fig. 1). Incubation with 50 μg of thymosin fraction 5 (per 2 ml) led to increased spontaneous proliferation only without a further increase in stimulation when Con A was added. The two effects, elevated background and enhanced response to Con A, can then apparently be dissociated.

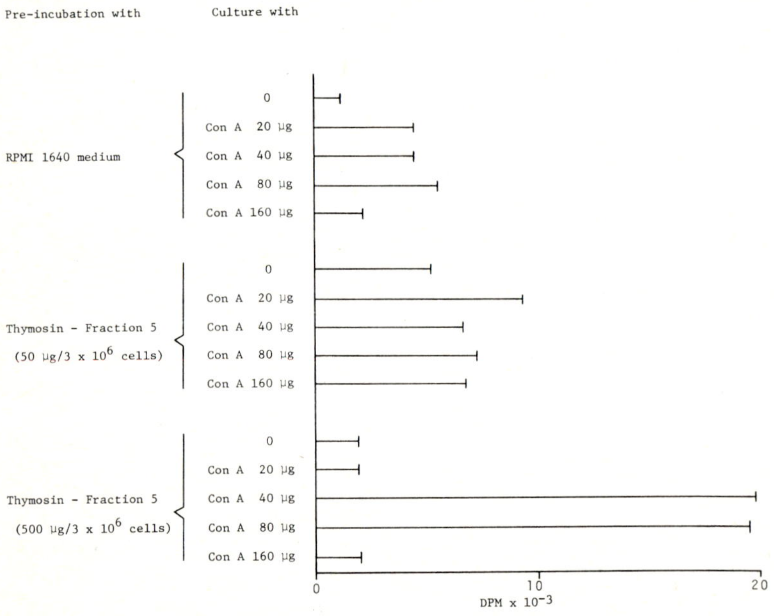

Fig. 1. Proliferative response of human lymphocytes to concanavalin A after *in vitro* incubation with thymosin.

Some degree of stimulation of human thymocytes can be induced by mitomycin-treated allogeneic lymphocytes (one-way mixed leukocyte culture). This response to allogeneic cells was also increased by prior incubation of the thymocytes with thymosin (500 μg/3×10^6 cells in 2 ml). A slight but still noticeable effect of thymosin on the response of thymocytes to PHA or pokeweed mitogen (PWM) was also usually observed. When thymocytes were initially unresponsive to PHA and PWM, some stimulation could be demonstrated after an 18-hour incubation *in vitro* in the presence of thymosin. When they were slightly responsive to these two mitogens, the degree of stimulation after incubation was even greater.

The augmentation of response of human thymocytes to Con A, PWM, PHA, or allogeneic cells after thymosin treatment *in vitro* required an 18-hour incubation (3 h was insufficient). To show this effect, the thymosin had to be removed from the medium before culture with the stimulating mitogen or allogeneic cells. Fraction 3 was also effective in eliciting this responsiveness, but somewhat less so than fraction 5. Spleen extracts had comparatively little effect on stimulation by Con A.

From these experiments, it appears that thymosin may act on cells in various stages of maturation. At least two target cells, cells at different stages in a continuum of differentiation, can thus be defined: a) the marrow-derived T lymphocyte precursor which can acquire *in vitro* the surface characteristics of T cells under the influence of thymic factors; and b) the T lymphocyte present in the thymus cortex and undergoing early stages of differentiation.

ACKNOWLEDGMENTS

We are indebted to Dr. G. Champsaur for providing fragments of human thymus, to Mrs Odette de Bouteiller for excellent technical assistance, and to Dr. J. W. Hadden for assistance with the manuscript. We also acknowledge support by the Institut National de la Santé et de la Recherche Médicale (ATP 11.74.32), the Délégation Générale à la Recherche Scientifique et Technique, the National Cancer Institute (U.S.A.) (CA 08748, CA 14108, CA 15081 and CA 15419), the National Foundation March of Dimes, (U.S.A.) and the John Hartford Foundation (U.S.A.).

REFERENCES

Bach, J.-F., Dardenne, M., Goldstein, A. L., Guha, A. & White, A. (1971) *Proc. Nat. Acad. Sci. Wash.)* **68**, 2734.

Bach, M. A., Bach, J.-F. (1972) *C.R. Acad. Sci. (Paris)* **275**, 2783.

Dicke, K. A., Lina, P. H. C. & van Bekkum, D. W. (1970) *Rev. Europ. Etudes Clin. et Biol.* **15**, 305

Goldstein, A. L., Guha, A., Katz, M. M., Hardy, M. A. & White, A. (1972) *Proc. Nat. Acad. Sci. Wash.)* **69**, 1800.

Hooper, J. A., McDaniel, M., Thurman, G. B., Cohen, G. H., Schulof, R. S. & Goldstein, A. L. (1975) *Ann. N-Y. Acad. Sci.* (in press).

Incefy, G. S., Touraine, J. L. & Good, R. A. (1974) *Fed. Proc.* **33**, 736 (abstr.).

Komuro, K. & Boyse, E. A. (1973) *Lancet* **1**, 740.

Touraine, J. L., Incefy, G. S., Touraine, F., Rho, Y. M. & Good, R. A. (1974a) *Clin. Exp. Immunol.* **17**, 151.

Touraine, J. L., Touraine, F., Kiszkiss, D. F., Choi, Y. S. & Good, R. A. (1974b) *Clin. Exp. Immunol.* **16**, 503.

Touraine, J. L., Touraine, F., Incefy, G. S. & Good, R. A. (1975) *Ann. N.Y. Acad. Sci.* (in press).

Biological Activity of Thymic Hormones

EFFECTS OF THE THYMUS EXTRACT ON CONGENITAL HYPOGAMMAGLOBULINAEMIA AND IMMUNOLOGICAL DEFICIENCY ACCOMPANYING THE PROLIFERATIVE AND APLASTIC HAEMATOLOGICAL DISEASES

J. ALEKSANDROWICZ, J. BLICHARSKI, M. CZYZEWSKA-WAZEWSKA, K. JANICKI, J. LISIEWICZ, A. B. SKOTNICKI, B. SLIWCZYŃSKA, G. TOROWSKI & Z. SZMIGIEL

Transplantation of human foetal thymus in patients with congenital immunodeficiency diseases and malignancy of the lymphoid system results in partial recovery of their immunological activity (1, 2). Similar results have been noted by us after transplantation of thymus tissue originating from patients with myasthenia gravis into patients with leukaemia or Hodgkin's disease (3). Thymus extracts have not been used so far in the treatment of immune defects in man. The purpose of this paper is to present the results of the therapeutic use of calf thymus extract in human immunological deficiencies.

MATERIALS AND METHODS

Subjects

The following groups of patients were investigated: 1) eight previously untreated patients with chronic lymphocytic leukaemia (CLL); 2) three patients with chronic granulocytic leukaemia (CGL); 3) one case of acute leukaemia; 4) three cases of bone marrow hypoplasia with pancytopenia; and 5) three cases of inborn and acquired immune defects of the hypogammaglobulinemia type.

The thymus extract (TE)

The aqueous extract of thymus tissue (TE) was prepared according to the method described by Goldstein *et al.* (4) from fresh thymuses obtained from young calves aged 5 to 7 weeks. The original method was modified in some minor details which will be published separately (Czarnecki *et al.* - Pharmaceutical Firm "Polfa" in Jelenia Góra, Poland). Sterile solution of TE was ampouled in a concentration of 10 mg of protein per ml of normal saline.

Presented by A. B. Skotnicki
The Haematological Department of the Institute of Internal Medicine, Cracow Academy of Medicine, Cracow Poland

Mode of administration

TE was administered to patients intracutaneously. In patients with leukaemia, 0.5 ml of TE preparation was injected at 7-day intervals; 4 to 30 injections were given per individual. In other patients, 4 to 8 injections of 0.2 ml were administered.

RESULTS

In the majority of *patients with CLL*, the TE injections resulted in a decrease in the lymphocyte count, an increase in the reticulocytes, and the appearance of a positive tuberculin skin test in previously tuberculin-negative subjects.

In all cases with *CGL and acute leukaemia*, an increase in the lymphocyte count as well as in the total leukocyte count was observed. The number of immature cells of the granulocytic series increased. No significant changes were noted in erythrocyte count. Two patients were tuberculin-positive before treatment. One patient became positive after 7 injections of TE. In the patient with acute leukaemia, the long term administration (8 months) of TE resulted in an improvement in the clinical state, a gradual increase of gammaglobulins, and the appearance of a positive skin test after 3 months of therapy. A rise in the platelet count from 6,000 to 30,000 was also noted. During the last 6 months, the patient received no other treatment.

The patients with *bone marrow aplasia* received only 3 injections of TE. In one patient, a marked elevation of erythrocyte, leukocyte, and platelet counts was seen (from 2,100,000 to 2,700,000; from 2,500 to 5,000; and from 12,000 to 60,000, respectively). In the other patients, the results of treatment with TE were less significant and transient. In two cases, a bone marrow biopsy was repeated after 15 days from the start of the TE administration and an increased percentage of lymphocytes as well as of erythrocyte precursors was observed in the myelogram.

In the first patient with *congenital hypogammaglobulinemia* accompanied by thrombocytopenia, the four injections of TE resulted in a striking elevation of the absolute lymphocyte count (from 1428 to 3016) and of the content of gammaglobulins in the serum (222 mg per cent to 770 mg per cent). During TE administration, the number of T lymphocytes in the rosette test increased from 18 to 30 per cent. A moderate increase in the platelet count was also noted. It is worth mentioning that this patient has been treated during the last 12 years with various agents, including gammaglobulin injections, and no comparable improvement has been noted. In recent times, no infectious complications have been noted in the patient, despite the numerous recurrent infections in the past. In another patient with Louis-Bar syndrome (Ataxia telengiectasia), three injections of TE caused an increase in T cell rosettes from 5 to 20 per cent. In the third patient with an acquired hypogammaglobulinemia, eight injections of TE resulted in a rise in immunoglobulin level (from 57 mg per cent to 250 mg per cent) and in the lymphocyte count (from 785 to 2,620 per μl). Simultaneously, the PHA response of his peripheral blood lymphocytes increased from nearly O to 28 per cent.

The administration of TE in *one healthy subject* (one of us) resulted in only slight variation in the leukocyte count (4,400 and 5,000 per μl before therapy and 5,400 to 5,900 after two injections of 0.2 ml of TE). It is of special interest that the lymphocyte percentage in the differential cell count did not change. However, it is worth mentioning that the injection of TE resulted in the disruption of lysosomal granules containing acid phosphatase in the lymphocyte cytoplasm and the appearance of numerous lymphocytes with a diffuse reaction type (staining according to the Barka and Anderson method). A slight decrease in the number of T lymphocytes was observed.

DISCUSSION

The results of our studies indicate that our calf thymus extract induces similar results as thymus transplantation. The partial recovery of immunologic responses was noted after repeated administration of TE, both in patients suffering from CLL and bone marrow aplasia, and in patients with a non-malignant form of hypogammaglobulinemia. In the light of our investigation, further studies of this nature seem to be justified, as the clinical usefulness of TE still remains to be established.

REFERENCES

1. Kay, H. E. M. (1971) Foetal thymus transplants in man. Ontogeny of Acquired Immunity. Ed.: ASP, Amsterdam p. 249
2. Marcolongo, R. & Di Paolo, N. (1973) *Blood* **41**, 625.
3. Rzepecki, W. M., Lukasiewicz, M., Aleksandrowicz, J., Szmigiel, Z., Skotnicki, A. & Lisiewicz, J. (1974) *Lancet* **1**, 990.
4. Goldstein, A. L., Guha, A., Zatz, M. M. & Hardy, H. A. (1972) *Proc. Natl. Acad. Sci. US.* **69**, 1800.

Biological Activity of Thymic Hormones

THE FIRST THYMUS EXTRACT ADMINISTRATION TO A PATIENT WITH ADVANCED CANCER

GABRIEL J. TUROWSKI, LECH CYBULSKI & ANNA URBAN

Extract from calf thymuses as a Thymus Factor X (TFX) preparation (1) was administered on December 13, 1973 to a patient suffering from advanced rectal cancer with hepatic metastases and diffuse peritonitis due to perforation of the bowel at the cancer site.

The postoperative course was very serious with circulatory and respiratory complications with an extremely low absolute number of lymphocytes (468×10^3) and a high DLT (direct lymphocytotoxic test) value (2, 3). To the nearly agonizing patient, we administered a small amount of TFX (0.1 mg subcut.). The injections were continued 2-4 times per month.

A progressive improvement in the general condition of the patient occurred, as well as significant changes in the immunological status as confirmed by such tests as DLT, skin reaction (PPD, PHA), Ig level, WBC count, and differential count.

Specimens of the tumour taken by rectal biopsy were examined histologically.

Fibroblastic proliferation with disseminated ossified plaques and massive tumour necrosis (4) were observed in the tumour area for the first time in July 1974, that is, 6 months after onset of the TFX administration. Two following specimens, taken at intervals of about two months, showed similar histology.

Comparing this patient with similar cases quoted in the literature (according to the world statistics, the maximum time of the survival is 6 months), we are tempted to ascribe the beneficial course of the disease to the treatment with TFX.

REFERENCES

1. Aleksandrowicz, J., Turowski, G., Czarnecki, J., Szmigiel, Z., Cybulski, L. & Skotnicki, A. (1974) *Second Inter. Congress Immunol.*, Brighton.
2. Cybulski, L., Turowski, G. & Zubel, M. (In press) *Pol. Przegl. Chir.*
3. Turowski, G., Cybulski, L. & Skotnicki, A. (1974) *Second Intern. Congress Immunol.*, Brighton.
4. Turowski, G., Urban, A., Cybulski, L., Turaszwili, T. & Zubel, M. (In press) *Patol. Pol.*

Presented by L. Cybulski
The third Department of Surgery and Immunological Transplantation Unit and Department of Pathomorphology, Institute of Pathology, Copernicus Medical Academy, Cracow, Poland

Biological Activity of Thymic Hormones

ENHANCEMENT OF T LYMPHOCYTE DIFFERENTIATION *IN VITRO* BY THYMIC EXTRACTS AFTER BONE MARROW TRANSPLANTATION IN SEVERE COMBINED IMMUNODEFICIENCIES

G. S. INCEFY, L. BOUMSELL, J. L. TOURAINE, P. L'ESPÉRANCE, E. SMITHWICK, R. O'REILLY & R. A. GOOD

We have found that children with severe combined immunodeficiency (SCID), who are thought to lack lymphoid stem cells capable of developing into either the B or T lymphocyte populations, do not possess cells in their marrow which can be induced by partially purified thymic extracts to differentiate into T lymphocytes *in vitro*. The initial observations were made with marrow cells

TABLE I

PERCENTAGE OF T LYMPHOCYTES (HTLA-POSITIVE CELLS) DETECTED AFTER INCUBATION WITH THYMIC EXTRACTS IN MARROW OF PATIENT WITH SEVERE COMBINED IMMUNODEFICIENCY *before* BONE MARROW TRANSPLANTATION

Additions to marrow cells	*Cytotoxic Index (%HTLA⁺ cells) in gradient[c] layers of*									
	Patient #1					*Normal*				
Gradient[c] layer	I	II	III	IV	V	I	II	III	IV	V
Medium	3	4	5	3	4	6	4	4	6	4
Human thymic extract-7-F3[a]	4	4	6	3	6	10	9	30	8	4
Calf thymic extract-7-F3	–	4	5	2	3	7	8	27	7	3
	% cells induced[b]									
Human thymic extract-7-F3	1	0	1	0	2	4	5	27	2	–
Calf thymic extract-7-F3	–	0	0	–	–	1	4	24	1	–

[a] Marrow cells were incubated for 2 h in the presence of thymic extracts; F3 = fraction 3, according to A. L. Goldstein *et al.* (*Proc. Nat. Acad. Sci.* **69** (1972) 1800).
[b] Calculation: 100 (b−a/100−a), where a = % HTLA positive cells after incubation with medium, b = % HTLA positive cells after incubation with human or calf thymic extracts.
[c] BSA density gradient according to Dicke and van Bekkum (rev. Europ. Et. Clin. et Biol. 17 (1972) 645–649).

from three untreated infants with SCID under the same conditions which revealed clear evidence of induced differentiation in normal individuals (Table I).

Marrow cells from two of these children were studied again after bone

Memorial Sloan-Kettering Cancer Center, New York, N.Y. 10021, U.S.A.
This investigation was supported by the National Foundation - March of Dimes, The National Cancer Institute CA-08748-09 and CA-05826-13, and the National Institute of Allergy and Infectious Diseases AI-11843-02.

TABLE II

PERCENTAGE OF T LYMPHOCYTES (HTLA+ AND RFC) DETECTED AFTER INCUBATION WITH THYMIC EXTRACTS IN MARROW OF PATIENT WITH SEVERE COMBINED IMMUNODEFICIENCY *after* BONE MARROW TRANSPLANTATION

Additions to marrow cells (Patient #1)	*Cytotoxic Index (% HTLA+ cells) in gradient layers*					*E-Rosette (% Large R[a]) in gradient layers*				
Gradient layer	I	II	III	IV	V	I	II	III	IV	V
Medium	2	10	17	38	9	11	6	0.7	0.3	12
Human thymic extract-20-F2[b]	6	14	40	4	6	0.5	5	0.3	4	27
Calf thymic extract-7-F3	9	6	25	17	8	0.5	3	2	0.8	10
	% cells induced[c]									
Human thymic extract-20-F2	4	4	28	–	–	–	–	–	4	17
Calf thymic extract-7-F3	7	–	10	–	–	–	–	1	–	–

[a] R = large rosette, four or more SRBC adhering to a lymphocyte.
[b] Marrow cells were incubated for 2 h in the presence of thymic extracts; F2 = fraction 2.
[c] See Table I for calculation.

marrow transplantation (BMT). Clear indication of precursor cells was obtained in marrow after successful transplantation. The newly acquired precursors could be differentiated *in vitro* into T lymphocytes under the influence of thymic extracts. T cell characteristics were established both with a specific anti-human T cell serum (ATCS) and by the E rosette technique using sheep red blood cells (SRBC) (Table II).

This approach reveals a new means of dissecting the immunodeficiency diseases before BMT and a method for assessing cellular reconstitution following marrow transplantation.

Biological Activity of Thymic Hormones

DISCUSSION

DICKE, Rijswijk

Dr. White, with regard to the experiments in the NZB animals in which you found a proliferative effect on the thymus cells which are going into the spleen: Do you think that it is just a matter of switching on these thymocytes or is it a matter of homing of these thymocytes in the spleen?

WHITE, Stanford

The working hypothesis at the present time is that thymosin in this system is either delaying the disappearance of suppressor T cells or the somewhat unlikely possibility that T cells which have become aberrant in the presence of thymosin are being reconverted into suppressor T cells.

WARREN-JOHNSON, Copenhagen

My question is directed to Dr. Touraine. I noticed in his first slide that he incubated his bone marrow fractions with transfer factor but I did not see the results.

TOURAINE, Lyon

There was no differentiation at all when bone marrow cells were incubated with transfer factor. We have also tested thymosin plus transfer factor in the mitogen-induced proliferation assay and we don't have any more effect than with thymosin alone.

WHITE, Stanford

Since the burning question is: are there multiple thymic factors, may I ask Dr. Incefy what thymic fraction she used?

INCEFY, New York

This was prepared in our own lab using Allan Goldstein's procedure.

GOLDSTEIN, Galveston

I have a comment on Dr. Touraine's very elegant report. Very recently, Dr.

D. Wara and Dr. A. Amman at the University of California Medical Center have similarly completed experiments with human fetal thymocytes. They have found that fetal thymocytes before the age of 14 week's gestation do not respond in a MLR *in vitro*, but after 14 weeks gestation they do. Drs. Wara and Amman have found that addition of thymosin fraction 5 to the thymocytes of less than 14-weeks-old fetuses induces a normal MLR response. Their results would be in agreement with your findings Dr. Touraine.

STUTMAN, New York

One question to Dr. White: In the NZB experiments, do you use anything besides BSA in the assay as control for thymosin?

WHITE, Stanford

Yes, spleen and liver extracts.

LÖWENBERG, Rijswijk

I would like to comment on the observations of Dr. Incefy concerning the stimulation of haemopoietic graft proliferation by thymic extract. In this context, I would like to mention the results of experiments which were performed

TABLE I

EFFECT OF *adult* THYMOCYTES ON SPLEEN COLONY FORMATION BY FETAL LIVER AND BONE MARROW CELLS IN *syngeneic* HOSTS
C57BL→C57BL

	number of CFU-S per 10^5 fetal liver cells injected								*% of control without thymocytes*
	exp. 1	*exp. 2*	*exp. 3*	*exp. 4*	*exp. 5*	*exp. 6*	*exp. 7*	*exp. 8*	*Mean ±SE*
−thymocytes (control)	6.1	6.6	8.0	6.9	8.0	7.3	10.0	7.5	100
$+30\times10^6$ thymocytes	11.4			13.1	11.0	7.2	14.4	9.4	139±15
$+100\times10^6$ thymocytes		16.0	14.0	17.2	11.5	8.8	12.0		175±24

100×10^6 thymus cells alone: 0.6±0.2 CFU-S

by our group in Rijswijk on the enhancement of the spleencolony-forming ability of haemopoietic cells by high numbers of thymus cells. The number of spleen colonies produced by fetal liver cells was nearly doubled by the additional injection of thymocytes (Table I). The effect of the thymus cells was also exerted when they had been exposed to a high dose of irradiation in vitro prior to their inoculation (Table II). However, when the fetal liver cells were irradiated, no colonies were observed. These data show that the additional colonies which were produced under the influence of the thymus cells were neither of endogenous origin nor thymus-cell-derived. Although we do not have

TABLE II

EFFECT OF ADULT THYMOCYTES ON THE ABILITY OF FETAL LIVER CELLS TO FORM SPLEEN COLONIES IN SYNGENEIC HOSTS
C57BL→C57BL

Nr. of cells injected		*CFU-S per 10^5 fetal liver cells*	
fetal liver	*thymus*	*exp. 1*	*exp. 2*
2×10^5	–	6.3	8.5
1×10^5	50×10^6	9.5	14.3
1×10^5	50×10^6 (2000 rad γ)	12.0	12.9
2×10^5 (2000 rad γ)	50×10^6	0	0

data on the effect of thymic factors, our findings with irradiated thymus cells seem in good agreement with the observations on the promoting effect of thymic extracts on haemopoiesis and seem to be possible further evidence in support of a relationship between the thymus and haemopoietic proliferation.

Biological Activity of Thymic Hormones

THE POSSIBLE CONTRIBUTION OF THE THYMUS LYMPHOCYTE TO THYMUS HUMORAL FUNCTION

MARIA DE SOUSA* & GENEVIEVE INCEFY

Some years ago, to gratify the repeated visits of a publisher representative I had to outline the potential chapters of an atlas of the lymphoid system. When I got round to the chapter on the thymus I decided that an appropriate title would be 'the thymus, cet inconnu' paraphrasing Carrell's famous title about man. The atlas project never reached completion, but my conviction that the thymus is an organ that has kept well the secret of its identity to itself remains unchanged.

It is therefore for me a privilege to be here, amongst people who have done so much to unravel the thymus secret (1, 2, 3). By a rather fortunate coincidence a week after Dr. van Bekkum asked me to come I joined Dr. Good's lab where a lot has been done recently on the role of human thymus extracts on differentiation of human bone marrow (4, 5, 6, 7, 8). All I had to do was to walk round the next bay in the lab and ask newcomer questions to Genevieve Incefy: had people prepared extracts from thymus epithelium? They hadn't we thought, before we read Pike & Gelfand's paper (9), so we did. Had supernatants from thymus lymphocytes been tried as inducers of T cell differentiation? To the best of our knowledge they hadn't and they haven't. So we did it also.

The background reasons for my asking these questions were twofold:

1. From the work of others (10, 11, 12, 13) and my own work (14, 15, 16) on the morphology of the mouse thymus, its susceptibility to cortisone treatment and irradiation (Figs. 1, 2, 3) it is clear that the epithelial component with the medullary lymphocyte constitute the equivalent to a 'constant region' of the thymus architecture, and that the cortical lymphocyte corresponds, as it were, to the 'variable region'. In the 'variable region' in the absence of lymphocytes, plasma cells are frequently seen after cortisone treatment and irradiation; in the late stages of pregnancy in the mouse, Maroni and I (16) have also observed loss of the cortico-medullary boundaries (Fig. 4) with large numbers of plasma cells present. However, recovery to a fully developed

Memorial Sloan-Kettering Cancer Center, New York, N.Y. 10021, U.S.A.
* Visiting Investigator at the Sloan-Kettering Institute
Permanent Address: Department of Bacteriology and Immunology Glasgow University, United Kingdom

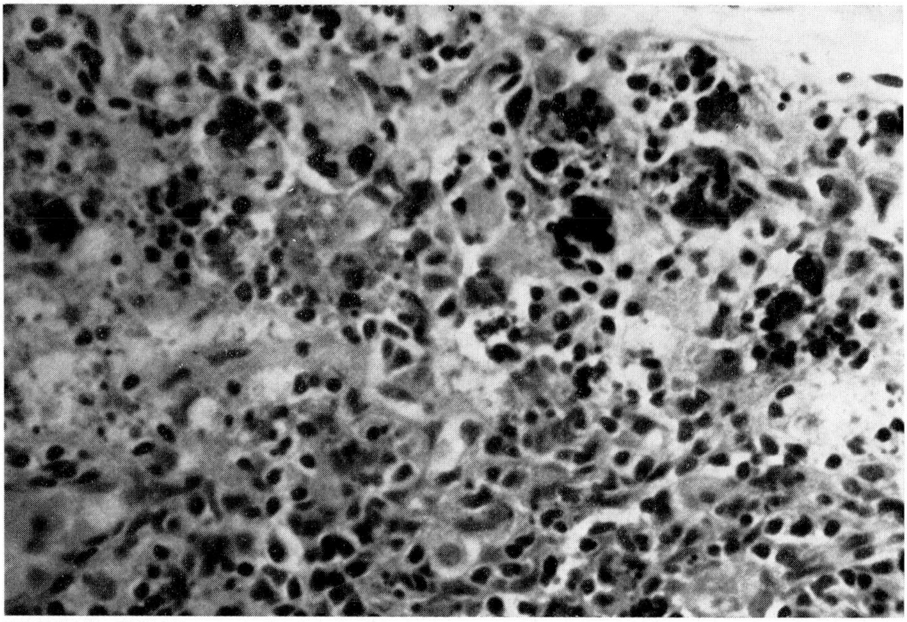

Fig. 1. Section of mouse thymus removed at 24 h after a subcutaneous injection of cortisone acetate (Adreson, Organon Laboratories, Surrey, England), dose: 40 mg/100 g body weight. Note the presence of small lymphocytes in the medulla (bottom half), the narrow lymphocyte depleted cortex with pockets of necrotic material.

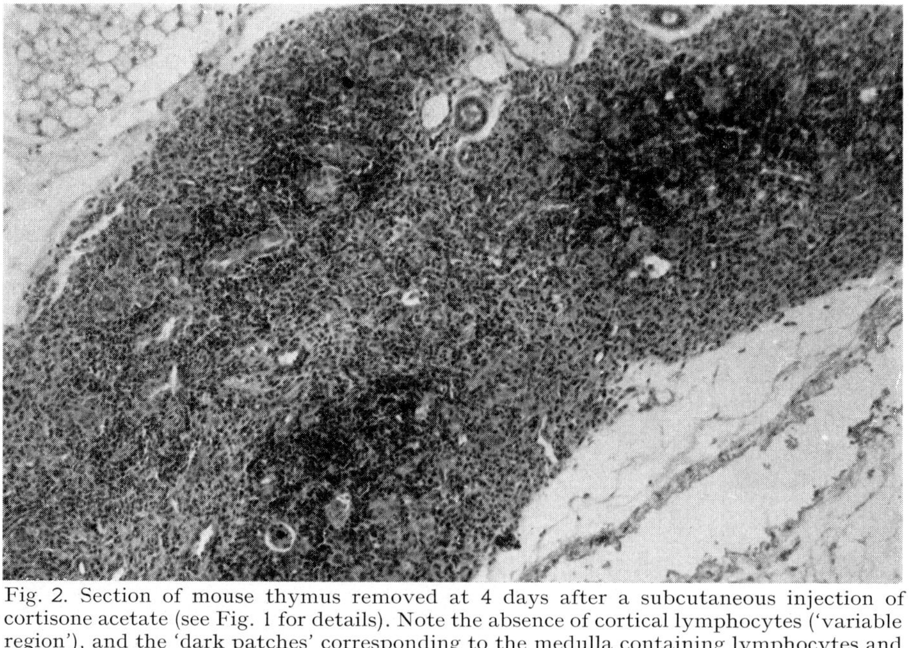

Fig. 2. Section of mouse thymus removed at 4 days after a subcutaneous injection of cortisone acetate (see Fig. 1 for details). Note the absence of cortical lymphocytes ('variable region'), and the 'dark patches' corresponding to the medulla containing lymphocytes and epithelial cells ('constant region').

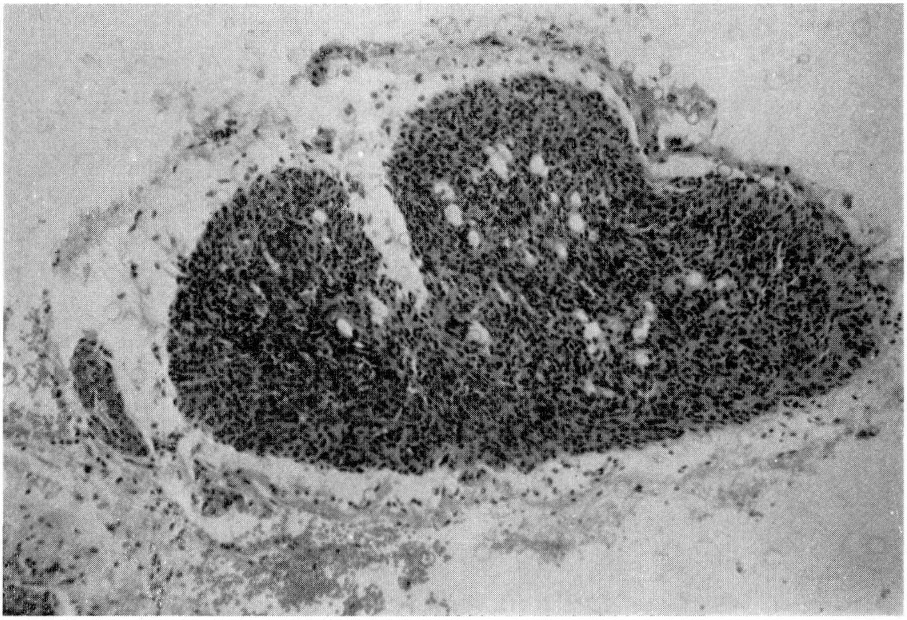

Fig. 3. Section of mouse thymus removed at 5 days after whole body x-irradiation (850R). Note the complete loss of definition between cortex and medulla and the persistence of the epithelial framework plus some lymphocytes ('constant region').

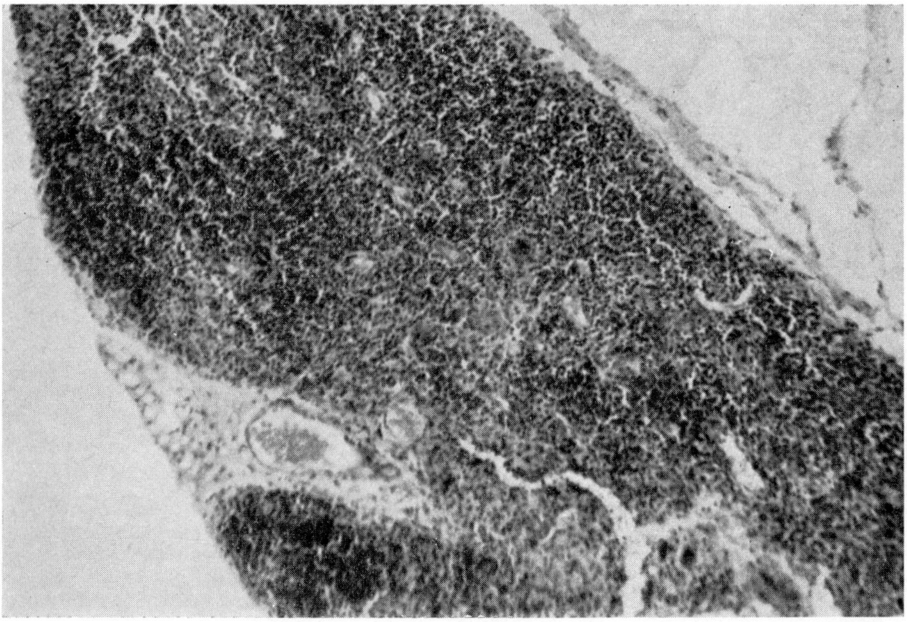

Fig. 4. Section of thymus removed after parturition from BALB/C female mated to C3H/Bi male. Note the absence of clear-cut demarcation between cortex and medulla.

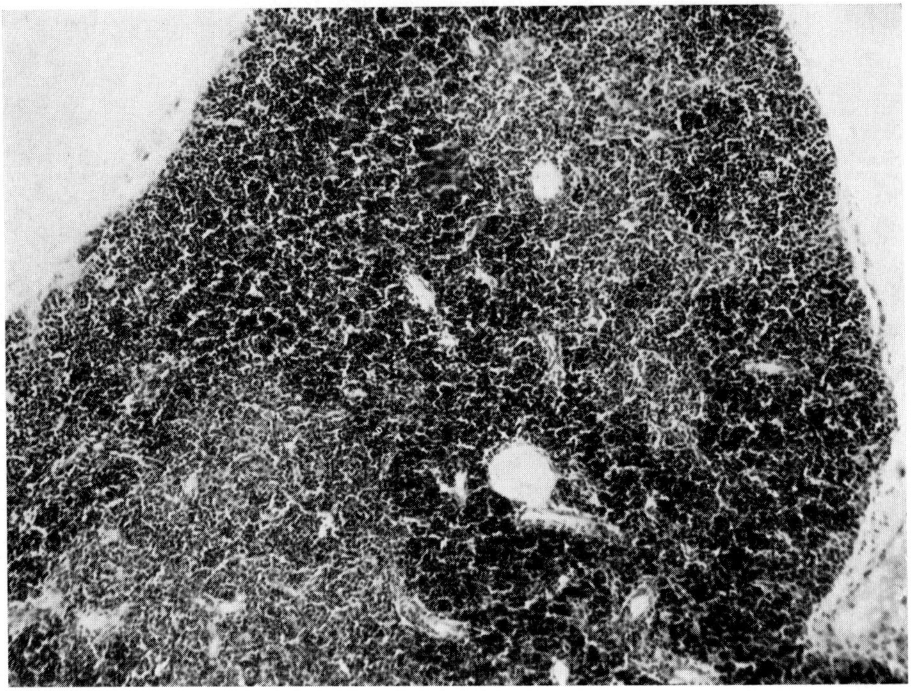

Fig. 5. Section of mouse thymus removed at 3 weeks after the subcutaneous injection of cortisone acetate. Compare with Fig. 2 and note the presence of a clear demarcation between cortex and medulla, with a much more heavily lymphocyte populated cortex than medulla.

lymphoid organ takes place after irradiation or cortisone treatment, (Fig. 5) and this must happen under the influence of the persisting constant region.

2. The other reason why I wanted to test the action of the thymus lymphocyte both in its interaction with the epithelial extract and on its own, was based on the results of my recent experiments with Curtis (17) on the adhesive interactions between thymus and peripheral B lymph node cells. We found that there is in the supernatant of thymus or peripheral T cells a factor or factors that diminish the adhesion of the B cells. Using his method of measure of cell adhesion Curtis (18) has also been able to distinguish between normal and nude mouse serum when given coded samples, thus indicating that there must be factors released by the thymus cell which circulate and play a role in the interaction of T cells with B cells in the periphery.

The present paper is a summary of preliminary experiments of Incefy and myself, designed to ask two main questions:

1. Can inducing extracts be prepared from thymus epithelium?

2. Does the thymus lymphocyte contribute to induction or regulation of T cell induction?

Preliminary results should always be viewed with caution, but if of interest, they should also be shared, to be pursued by others.

MATERIALS AND METHODS

Preparation of thymus 'epithelium'. Human thymus obtained during thoracic surgery from two children aged 11 and 24 months were used. The majority of the lymphoid component was removed by extensive teasing of the organ with a fine pair of forceps and fine scalpel and kept separately for preparation of the supernatant (see below). The tissue was then passed through a sterile fine wire mesh; the remaining material consisted mainly of epithelial cells although histologically some obvious medullary lymphocytes were present in association with Hassall's corpuscles.

Preparation of the extract. The extract was prepared from pooled human 'thymus epithelium' (weight: 13.06 g) using the method described by A. Goldstein and his co-workers (19). The fractions used in the experiments were fractions 2 and 3 from which 5.25 mg protein/g tissue and 7.12 mg protein/g tissue were obtained respectively.

Preparation of the supernatant. The lymphoid thymus cells were spun three times for 10 min at 1600 rpm and the supernatants from all washes pooled and kept at $-20°C$. The lability of the supernatant was tested by bringing the temperature to 80°C stirring continuously following the same procedure used in the preparation of the thymus extract.

Target cells and incubation with thymus extract. Due to the scarce availability of human bone marrow and having prior knowledge that it is possible to differentiate cells in the peripheral blood (8), we used as target cells for T cell differentiation, peripheral blood cells. The white blood cells were first separated in a Ficoll-hypaque gradient and subsequently fractionated in a discontinuous BSA gradient slightly modified from the method originally described by Dicke *et al.* (20); details of the gradient preparation and cell separation have been published elsewhere (7). The unfractionated and fractionated peripheral blood cells were washed twice in RPMI and the final suspensions adjusted to a concentration of 1.6×10^6/ml. Duplicate or triplicate samples were incubated for 2 h at 37°C in a CO_2 incubator with the extract (100 μl cells: 100 μl extract). Additional groups were set adding to the cells supernatant alone or supernatant and extract simultaneously. The cell concentration at incubation was kept constant in all experiments: $0.8\text{-}1.0 \times 10^5$ cells in 100 μl.

Indicator. The indicator adopted for detection of the presence of T cells was the formation of E rosettes. After incubation the cells were washed once with RPMI, and 100 μl of RPMI and 100 μl of a 0.5 per cent suspension of SRBC added to the pellet. The cells were incubated for 5 min at 37°C, spun at 400 rpm for 5 min and incubated overnight at 4°C. The following day, the cells were suspended gently and counted in a hemacytometer chamber. Four or 5 separate 100 cell counts were done from each tube and the number of erythrocytes per rosette (1, 2, 3, 4 or more erythrocytes) recorded. The results are expressed as %rosettes in a total of at least 400 cells counted from each tube, representing a total of 800 or 1200 cells counted per experimental sample. In one experiment, the numbers of EAC rosettes were also estimated, the cell concentrations were similar to those used for the E rosettes, sensitized SRBC were added to the cells, incubated for 30 mins at 37°C. The EAC rosettes were counted immediately after incubation.

RESULTS

Effect of 'thymus epithelium' extract on unfractionated and fractionated peripheral blood cells. The percentage of E rosette forming cells (with 4 or more sheep

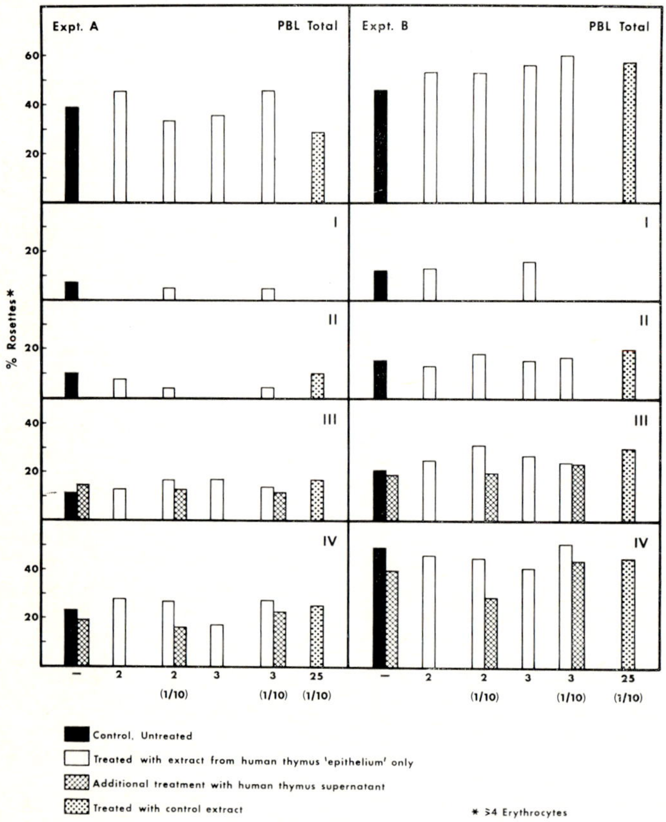

Fig. 6. Summary of the results of two experiments (A, B) on the effect of incubation of unfractionated and fractionated peripheral blood cells with human thymus extract prepared from thymus epithelium on the % of E rosette forming cells. Control extract (25) was prepared from whole thymus. Note that the addition of the thymus cell supernatant seems to counteract the inducing effect of the extract, in particular of F_2 (1/10). Each bar represents the mean values of duplicate or triplicate samples from which at least 8 separate 100 cell counts were made. I, II, III, IV: cell fractions. 2, 3: extract fractions.

erythrocytes) varied slightly from blood sample to blood sample. The average percentage found in the samples routinely collected from the blood center was 54.9 (±3.29) in one sample of freshly drawn blood from one of us, the percentage was higher (81.75 per cent). We observed, however, that the relative distribution of T cells in the gradient was very similar in both experiments, low T cell numbers were found in fractions I and II (6.88 per cent and 9.8 per cent in Exp. A and 11.91 per cent and 15.45 per cent in Expt. B) fraction IV contained the highest concentrations (23.10 per cent and 49.45 per cent) and fraction III percentages of 14.51 and 21.1.

The two 'thymus epithelium' extract fractions were added to all cell fractions either neat or in a dilution of 1/10 (Fig. 6). No striking changes were observed in the percentage of E rosette forming cells in fractions I and II treated with the extract. If anything, there was some indication of a slight decrease induced by the addition of the neat fraction and a slight increase with the 1/10 dilution. The impression that the 1/10 diluted extract samples were more

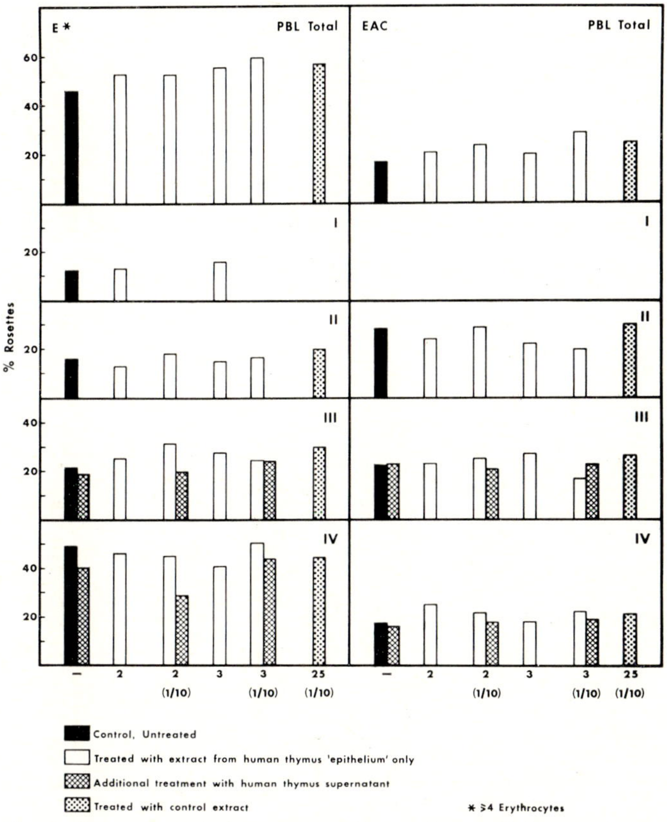

Fig. 7. Summary of the results of Experiment B in which both the % of the E and EAC rosette forming cells were estimated, before and after incubation with thymus epithelium extract. There is no striking change in the numbers of EAC rosette forming cells except in unfractionated PBL treated with F_3 (1/10 dilution).

effective in inducing the appearance of increased numbers of 'E' rosette forming cells than the neat samples was further substantiated by the results with cell fractions III and IV, and the unfractionated cells (Fig. 6). Increases of the order of 5 to 14 per cent were observed.

The highest concentration of EAC rosette forming cells was found in fraction II (28 per cent). Addition of neat and diluted extract fractions provoked minor increases in the numbers of EAC rosettes found in fractions II and III (1-4 per cent) and slightly higher (6-11 per cent) increase in the unfractionated pool and in fraction IV (Fig. 7).

Effect of thymus supernatant on fractionated peripheral blood cells. Thymus cell supernatant was either added alone or combined with the extract to the cells from fractions III and IV of the BSA gradient. The results of experiment A indicated that the addition of the supernatant was counteracting the stimulatory action of the thymus extract regarding the numbers of E rossette forming cells (Fig. 6). For example, in fraction IV addition of F_2 (1/10) of the thymus extract increased the percentage of T cells by 5 per cent, the further addition of the supernatant completely abolished this effect. In experiment B, this finding was confirmed (Fig. 6), addition of F_2 (1/10) to cell fraction III provoked a 10 per cent increase (21.27 to 31.17), further addition of the supernatant neutralized this effect (31.17 to 20.48). The neutralizing effect of the supernatant was most clearcut in combination with F_2 (1/10 dilution) although in experiment A a similar effect was observed with F_3 (1/10 dilution). Incubation of the fractionated cells with the supernatant alone did not result in any marked or consistent changes. Addition of the supernatant alone had no effect on the numbers of EAC rosette forming cells; addition of the supernatant to the thymus extract appeared to neutralize whatever little increase the extract induced in the numbers of EAC rosettes (Fig. 7).

Effect of short exposure of peripheral blood cells to supernatant. To investigate the possibility that addition of the supernatant could on its own affect in some way E rosette formation, we did one experiment adding either supernatant or extract or both to unfractionated peripheral blood cells for 5 to 10 minutes at room temperature, studying the numbers of E rosette forming cells after treatment. As can be seen from Fig. 8, no changes were induced by this short term treatment.

Effect of incubation of unfractionated peripheral blood cells with normal or heat inactivated supernatant. Incubation of unfractionated cells with untreated thymus supernatant was done in two experiments. Addition of the supernatant increased the numbers of E rosette forming cells (Figs. 8, 9). Based on the results of the neutralizing action of the supernatant on F_2 of the extract, we tested the action of this fraction on the unfractionated cells; addition of the extract alone did not change the numbers of T cells, however, addition of the extract clearly neutralized the supernantant effect.

One final point we wanted to clarify was the heat stability of the supernatant accordingly we compared the action of heat inactivated supernatant (at 80°C) with normal supernantant. As shown in Fig. 9, heat inactivation abolished the E rosette enhancing action of the supernatant.

DISCUSSION

We have set out to answer two questions regarding the functional dissection of the two main thymus cellular components, the epithelial and the lymphoid. The questions were: 1) can thymus cell differentiation be induced by extracts prepared from thymus epithelium? 2) does the lymphoid component play a role in differentiation or in regulation of differentiation?

We have observed that extracts prepared from 'thymus epithelium' (which, on subsequent histological examination were seen to contain medulary lymphocytes) can induce an increase in peripheral blood cell fractions obtained after separation in a BSA discontinuous gradient. Moreover, comparison of the estimated amount of protein obtained per gram of tissue (F_2: 5.25 mgP/g, F_3:

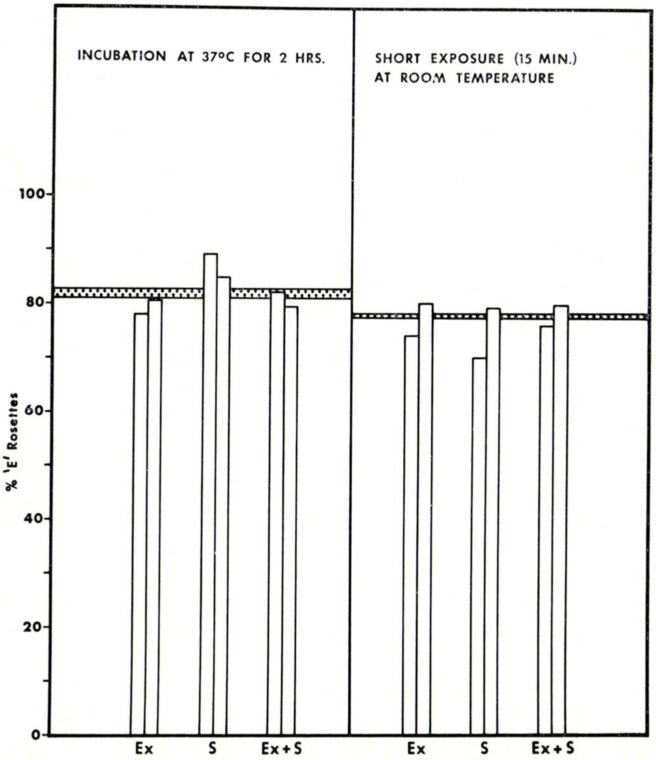

Fig. 8. Effect on the % of E rosettes of short exposure at room temperature or 2 hr incubation of human peripheral blood cells with human thymus epithelium extract F^2 (1/10) (Ex), thymus cell supernatant (S) or combined extract (F^2-1/10) and supernatant (Ex+S) the horizontal shaded area represents the range of values obtained with the control untreated samples. The identity of each sample was coded and unknown to the reader of the results.

7.12 mgP/g) with the amounts usually obtained from whole thymus (Incefy, unpublished data) indicated that much more protein was obtained from thymus epithelium only.

This finding was to be expected from the evidence accumulated over the years since the early experiments of Metcalf (21, 22) showing the importance of the medullary epithelial component for the effectiveness of thymus transplants and the production of LSF (lymphocytosis stimulating factor), to the more recent observations of Clark (23) of active synthesis of some sulphated mucopolysaccharide in the epithelial cells, the *in vivo* action of epithelium grafts in diffusion chambers (24) and the definitive experiments of Pike & Gelfland (9), who induced an increase in the numbers of 'E' rosette forming cells in human bone marrow treated *in vitro* with conditioned media from human thymus epithelium.

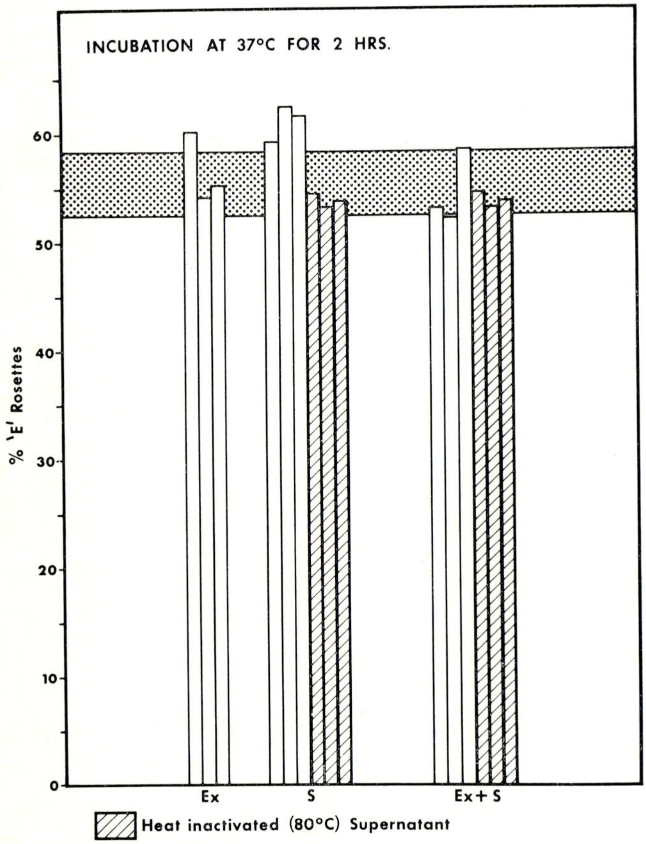

Fig. 9. Comparison between the effect of incubation with thymus epitheljum extract F2 (1/10) (Ex), normal or heated thymus cell supernatant (S) or combined extract and normal or heated supernatant on the % of E rosette forming cells in unfractionated peripheral blood cells. Shaded horizontal area represents the range of values of control untreated samples. The identity of each sample was coded and unknown to the reader of the results.

In addition to the expected positive induction activity of the extract prepared from the thymus epithelium, we have found some evidence for a neutralizing factor in supernatants of thymus lymphoid cells. This neutralizing effect was particularly striking in relation to F_2 (1/10 dilution). This finding can be greatly significant to the understanding of a regulatory mechanism of T cell induction within the thymus itself. The existence of an inhibitory effect associated with the presence of the thymus lymphocyte could for instance explain the observation of Pike & Gelfland (9) that in their experiments "the most effective conditioned media were obtained when thymic lymphocytes were no longer present in the cultures". If regulation of thymus cell differentiation was conditioned by the attained levels of produced thymus cells, the actual equilibrium of induction-production would be a self-contained process independent of other external influences. This proposal is in line with the results of the elegant experiments of Metcalf (25) on multiple thymus grafting, in which he conclusively showed that multiple thymus grafting or the recipient's age did not influence the development of each individual grafted thymus.

Our final observation was that the addition of supernatant to unfractionated peripheral blood cells also increased the numbers of 'E' rosette forming cells. One is tempted to speculate that this finding is a reflection of binding of some thymus cell membrane product to Stutman's immunoincompetent post-thymic cell (26). This effect was abolished by heat inactivation of the supernatant at 80 °C and it is of interest to stress that heating to 80 °C is an essential step in the preparation of thymosin (19), this could be associated with the inactivation of some inhibitor otherwise present in the extract.

Another separate observation, based in a much larger number of experiments than the ones presented in this paper, of relevance to the peripheral action of products released by the thymus cell is the finding of Curtis & de Sousa (17, 18) that supernatants prepared from mouse or rat thymus cells diminish the adhesion of peripheral B lymph node cells and that this activity is present in normal mouse serum but lacking in the serum of nude mice.

In conclusion, we should like to propose that the thymus lymphoid cell may contribute to thymus humoral function both by regulating the inductive action of epithelium derived thymus hormones and by influencing the maturation of post thymic cells and their interaction with other lymphoid cells in the periphery.

ADDENDUM

Recent experiments done since this work was first presented, using BSA fractionated human bone marrow cells as the target for differentiation, have further confirmed the existence of an inductive activity of the medullary thymus extract which can be inhibited by the addition of the supernatant obtained from thymus cortical lymphocytes.

ACKNOWLEDGMENTS

This work was done with the support of the Public Health Service Research Grant #CA 08748-09 and CA 05826-13 from the National Cancer Institute, The National Foundation-March of Dimes. We wish to gratefully acknowledge the technical assistance of Mrs. R. Aninipot and Mr. R. Chua, without whose contribution it would not have been possible to do these experiments, and we want to thank Dr. J. Ascensão and Mr. A. Glantz for helping us to set the double blind experiments with unfractionated peripheral blood cells.

REFERENCES

1. Goldstein, A. L. & White, A. (1973) *Contemporary Topics in Immunobiology* **2**, 339. ed. A. J. S. Davies & R. L. Carter, Plenum Press, New York.
2. Trainin, N. & Small, M. (1973) *Contemporary Topics in Immunobiology* **2**, 321. ed. A. J. S. Davies & R. L. Carter, Plenum Press, New York.
3. Bach, J.-F. (1973) *Contemporary Topics in Immunobiology* **2**, 159. ed. A. J. Davies & R. L. Carter, Plenum Press, New York.
4. Touraine, J. L., Incefy, G. S., Touraine, F., Rho, Y. M. & Good, R. A. (1974) *Clin. Exp. Immunol.* **17**, 151.
5. Incefy, G. S., Touraine, J. L. & Good, R. A. (1974) *Fed. Proc.* **33**, 629.
6. Incefy, G. S., Touraine, J. L., Touraine, F., L'Esperance, P., Siegal, F. & Good, R. A. (1974) *Trans. Ass. Am. Phys.* (in press).
7. Incefy, G. S., L'Esperance, P. & Good, R. A. (1975) *Clin. Exp. Immunol.* **19**.
8. Vogel, J. E., Incefy, G. S. & Good, R. A. (1974) *Proc. Nat. Acad. Sc. USA* (submitted for publication).
9. Pike, K. W. & Gelfland, E. W. (1974) *Nature*, **251**, 421.
10. Dougherty, T. F. & White, A. (1945) *Amer. J. Anatomy*, **77**, 81.
11. Ishidate, M. & Metcalf, D. (1963) *Austr. J. Exp. Biol. Med. Sci.* **41**, 637.
12. De Vries, M. J. & Hymans, W. (1966) *J. Path. Bact.* **91**, 487.
13. De Vries, M. J. & Hymans, W. (1967) *J. Immunol.* **12**, 197.
14. East, J., de Sousa, M. A. B. & Parrott, D. M. V. (1965) *Transp.* **3**, 711.
15. de Sousa, M. A. B. & Fachet, J. (1972) *Clin. Exp. Immunol.* **10**, 673.
16. Maroni, E. S. & de Sousa, M. A. B. (1973) *Clin. Exp. Immunol.* **13**, 107.
17. Curtis, A. S. G. & de Sousa, M. A. B. (1973) *Nature New Biol.* **244**, 45.
18. Curtis, A. S. G. & de Sousa, M. A. B. (1975) (in preparation).
19. Goldstein, A., Guha, A., Zatz, M. M., Hardy, M. A. & White, A. (1972) *Proc. Nat. Acad. Sci. USA*, **69**, 1800.
20. Dicke, K., Van Hooft, J. I. & Van Bekkum, D. W. (1968) *Transp.* **6**, 562.
21. Metcalf, D., Sparrow, N., Nakamura, K. & Ishidate, M. (1961) *Austr. J. Exp. Biol. Med. Sci.* **39**, 441.
22. Metcalf, D. (1956) *Brit. J. Cancer* **10**, 442.
23. Clark, S. J. (1966) The Thymus: 3, Ciba Foundation Symposium. ed. Wolstenholme, G. E. & Porter, R.
24. Dardenne, M., Papiernik, M., Bach, J. F. & Stutman, O. (1974) *Immunology*, **27**, 299.
25. Metcalf, D. (1966) The Thymus: Experimental and Clinical Studies, Ciba Foundation Symposium, 242. ed. Wolstenholme, G. E. & Porter, R.
26. Stutman, O. (1975) *Ann. Nat. Acad. Sci. USA*.

Biological Activity of Thymic Hormones

IMPAIRMENT OF THE THYMUS FUNCTION IN NZB MICE

LOUIS KATER

Experiments were performed in order to investigate the epithelial outgrowth *in vitro* of thymic explants derived from NZB mice, a strain prone to autoimmunity and malignancies of the lymphoreticular system. Thymuses taken from Swiss-, CBA- and C57BL-mice served as controls. Thymic tissue was obtained from mice over an age range of 15 days to 6 months. Cultures were fixed on the 7th day. Differences in morphology between the experimental and control group became apparent in thymus cultures from mice at the age of 1 month and were statistically significant from 2 months onward. Cultured thymuses from NZB mice showed reduction of the epithelial outgrowth and an increasing number of multinucleated giant cells. These observations correspond with results *in vivo* but can be demonstrated earlier *in vitro*.

From these data we conclude that changes in the thymus of NZB mice can already be shown in animals of 1 month old. These findings are in accordance with data which show a decrease of thymosin levels in sera from NZB mice between two and eight weeks of age (1). The other organs of the animals used in the culture studies were examined histopathologically (Chr. Zurcher, Organization for Health Research, REP-TNO, Rijswijk). Those animals showing lesions of kidney and lymph node have also aberrations in morphology of thymus culture. Two possible explanations can be given: 1) lesions in thymus, lymph node and kidney are the result of the same pathogenetic mechanism; 2) lesions in lymph node and kidney are a result of a dysfunction of the thymus.

REFERENCE

1. Goldstein, A. L. (1974) Personal communication.

Division of Immunopathology, Department Internal Medicine, University Hospital, Utrecht, The Netherlands

Biological Activity of Thymic Hormones

EPITHELIAL CELLS AND MACROPHAGES IN THE NORMAL THYMUS

ELISABETH CH. M. HOEFSMIT & J. A. M. GERVER

After Moore & Owen (1967) showed that the thymus lymphocytes originate from a bone-marrow-derived stem cell, less attention was paid to the non-lymphoid cells of the thymus. Testing the concept of the mononuclear phagocyte system (v. Furth *et al.*, 1972) in lymphoid organs, it has been shown that,

TABLE I

DIFFERENT NON-LYMPHOID CELLS OF THE THYMUS ACCORDING TO DIFFERENT AUTHORS

Classification	*Distinctive properties*	*Authors*
Epithelial reticular cells	Tonofilaments and desmosomes	Clark (1963, 1968, 1973)
	In the cortex: PAS—*	
	In the medulla: PAS+ secretory granules	Hoshino (1963)
	Acid phosphatase— Phagocytizing lymphocytes	Lundin *et al.* (1965), Mandel (1968) ,Weiss (1963), Klug (1965)
	Acid phosphatase+	Pfoch (1971)
Mesenchymal reticular cells	Phagocytizing lymphocytes in the cortex; PAS+ granules	Ishidate & Metcalf (1962) Metcalf & Ishidate (1963)
	Reutilyzing desintegrated lymphocytes	Hoshino (1963)
	Acid phosphatase+	Lundin *et al.* (1965)
Macrophages	Phagocytizing lymphocytes in the cortex	Mandel (1968), Pfoch (1971), Clark (1973)

* PAS: periodicacid-shiff reaction

in peripheral lymphoid organs, "reticular cells" are actually reticulum cells and differ from mononuclear phagocytes (i.e., bone-marrow-derived macrophages) in morphological as well as functional aspects (Hoefsmit 1974). At east a portion of the "reticular cells" in central lymphoid organs are epithelial

Department of Electron Microscopy, Free University, Amsterdam, The Netherlands
The authors wish to acknowledge the excellent technical assistance of Miss J. H. S. de Leeuw and the photographical assistance of A. F. J. van Ballegoy.

in origin. In the thymus, the reticular cells demonstrating tonofilaments and desmosomes are generally classified as epithelial cells (Table I). In the medulla, these epithelial cells show secretory granules containing a periodic acid-Shiff (PAS) positive substance (Hoshino 1963, Clark 1968). However, cells phagocytizing pycnotic lymphocytes are mainly described as mesenchymal reticular cells or macrophages.

We studied the thymus of the normal adolescent male rat and guinea pig. After a short prewash in saline, the thymus was fixed by arterial perfusion with phosphate buffered glutaraldehyde 1.5 per cent (pH=7.4). The thymus was sectioned into small tissue blocks, postfixed in 1 per cent OsO_4, and embedded in epon after dehydration. After perfusion, some larger tissue blocks were embedded in paraffin wax to perform the bicolour reaction developed by Van Duyn (1956) in which the Feulgen reaction on DNA is indicated in blue and the PAS reaction in red. Other small tissue blocks were not postfixed in OsO_4 but were prepared for the silver metheneamine reaction on glycoproteins according to Rambourg *et al.* (1969). The cortex and the medulla are easily recognized in light microscopic pictures of thick epon sections. In the cortex, the lymphocytes are densely packed; the medulla contains large, pale, cells and Hassall's corpuscles.

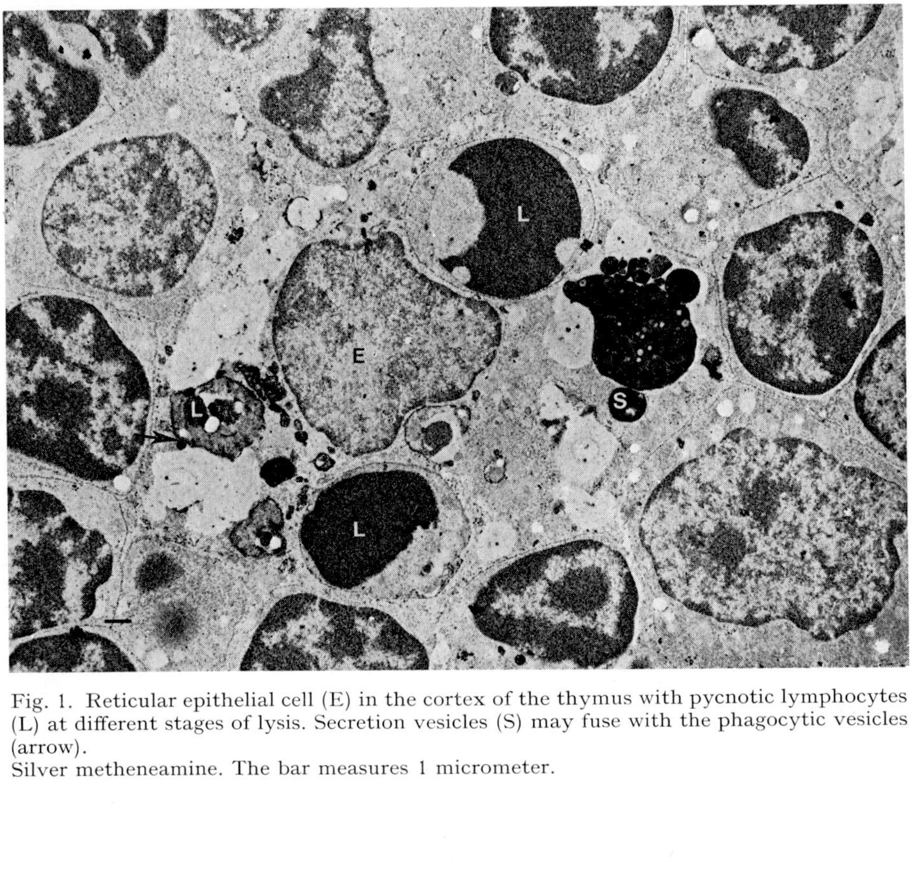

Fig. 1. Reticular epithelial cell (E) in the cortex of the thymus with pycnotic lymphocytes (L) at different stages of lysis. Secretion vesicles (S) may fuse with the phagocytic vesicles (arrow).
Silver metheneamine. The bar measures 1 micrometer.

The cortex

At the ultrastructural level, it appeared that the capsule and the capillaries were surrounded by epithelial cells demonstrating tonofilaments and desmosomes. In this way, the mesenchymal compartment and the epithelial compartment are completely separated in the cortex. We did not find mesenchymal reticular cells in the epithelial compartment. The epithelial reticular cells may also show vacuoles measuring 500-1000 nm in diameter and containing some small aggregates of amorphous dense material. The same cells may also contain some secretion granules which characteristically possess one or several microvilli. Some of these cells also contain pycnotic lymphocytes. In the paraffin sections stained according to Van Duyn, the same reticular cells which had ingested pycnotic lymphocytes demonstrated PAS positive granules (Fig. 1). The silver metheneamine reaction reveals glycoproteins in the secretiongranules at the ultrastructural level (Fig. 1). The secretion granules may fuse with the phagocytic vesicles.

The medulla

We also did not find mesenchymal reticular cells in the epithelial compartment

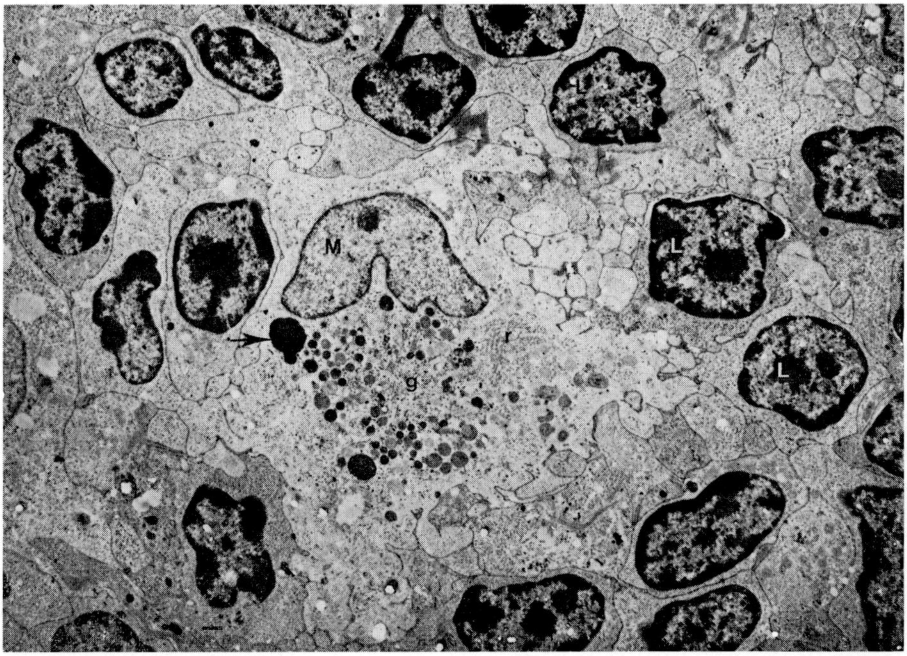

Fig. 2. Mononuclear phagocyte (M) of the medulla. Note the electron-lucent cytoplasm and the interdigitations with the surrounding lymphocytes (L). Some of the lysosomes (arrow) contain glycoproteins.
Silver metheneamine. The bar measures 1 micrometer, r: rough endoplasmic reticulum, g: Golgi area.

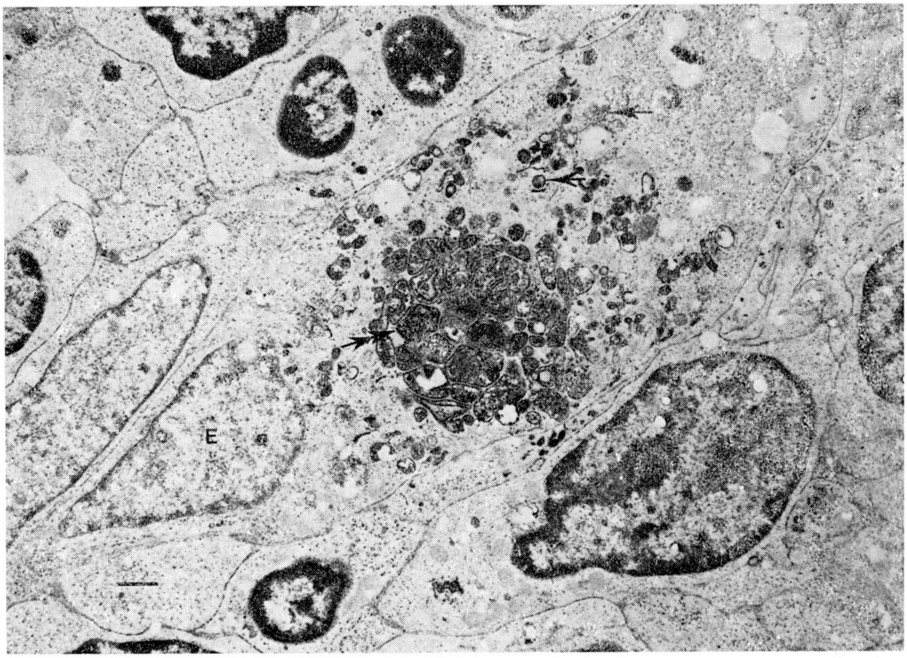

Fig. 3. Reticular epithelial cell (E) of the medulla. In the centre, secretion vacuoles (double arrow) containing microvilli and different amounts of glycoproteins are surrounded by secretion vesicles with microvilli (arrow) and Golgi apparatus (top-arrow).
Silver metheneamine. The bar measures 1 micrometer.

of the medulla. However, macrophages can be seen penetrating the epithelial border of the blood vessels. These mononuclear phagocytes are generally characterized by lysosomes and Golgi stacks surrounding a distinct cytocentre (Fig. 2). In the medulla, these macrophages present a specific pattern of the abundant and electron-lucent cytoplasm interdigitating with the surrounding lymphocytes. The silver metheneamine reaction shows positive Golgi stacks, many small vesicles, and tubules, and some of the lysosomes react intensely. Veldman (1970) described these types of cells as "interdigitatingcells"(IDC) in the paracortical area of the lymph node in the rabbit. We have found these cells also in the thymus-dependent areas of the spleen (Veerman 1974) and the other peripheral lymphoid organs (Hoefsmit 1974). Since the medulla of the thymus is also known to contain immunocompetent T cells (Leckband & Boyse 1971), we suggest that the "interdigitating cell" is the macrophage specifically related to the immunocompetent T cell.

There is less phagocytosis of pycnotic lymphocytes and more secretion of glycoproteins in the medulla. The silver metheneamine reaction shows glycoproteins in the Golgi stacks and in the secretion granules fusing with larger vacuoles with microvilli in the epithelial reticular cells (Fig. 3). Some of these vacuoles are densely packed with glycoproteins; others seem to be empty, especially the larger ones. Sometimes granulocytes may be found in these

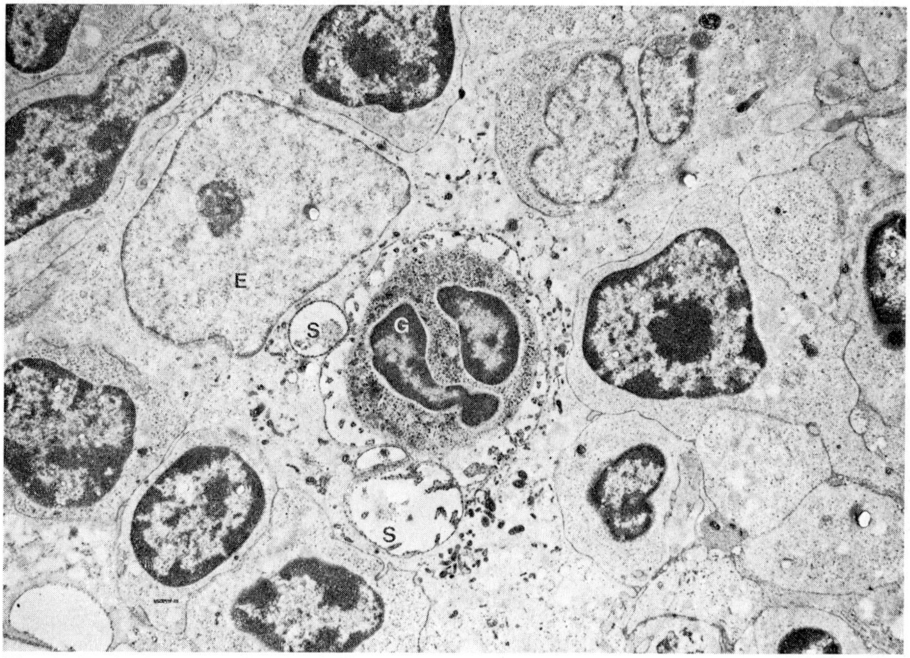

Fig. 4. Reticular epithelial cell of the medulla (E). Secretion vacuoles (S) in the cell centre, one of them containing a granulocyte (G).
Silver metheneamine. The bar measures 1 micrometer.

vacuoles, which apparently communicate with the intercellular space (Fig. 4). In the corpuscles of Hassall, degenerating granulocytes, lymphocytes, and degenerative epithelial cells are enclosed by epithelial cells with microvilli and secretion vesicles fuse with the cell membrane in the same way (Fig. 4).

TABLE II

DIFFERENT NON-LYMPHOID ELEMENTS OF THE THYMUS

Location	*Mesenchymal compartment*	*Epithelial compartment*
In the cortex	Endothelial cells Fibroblasts Collagenous fibres	Epithelial cells: Forming a cellular reticulum, bordering the mesenchymal compartment; Phagocytizing lymphocytes Secretion of glycoproteins *No* mononuclear phagocytes
In the medulla	Endothelial cells Fibroblasts Collagenous fibres	Epithelial cells: forming a cellular reticulum, bordering the mesenchymal compartment; Secretion of glycoproteins Forming Hassall's corpuscles Mononuclear phagocytes: mainly interdigitating cells

In conclusion (Table II): The thymus can be divided into a mesenchymal and an epithelial compartment. There are no mesenchymal reticular cells in the epithelial compartment of the cortex and medulla. The epithelial cells of the cortex demonstrate phagocytosis of pycnotic lymphocytes, probably stimulating secretion of glycoproteins. However, secretion of glycoproteins is more pronounced in the epithelial cells of the medulla and the Hassall's corpuscles. The mononuclear phagocytes are restricted to the medulla and have the same characteristics as they have in the thymus-dependent areas of the peripheral lymphoid organs.

REFERENCES

Clark, S. L. (1963) *Am. J. Anat.* **42**, 1.
Clark, S. L. (1968) *J. Exp. Med.* **128**, 927.
Clark, S. L. (1973) In: *Contemporary topics in immunobiology*, Vol. **2**. Ed. A. J. S. Davis & R. L. Carter, Plenum Press, New York - London.
Van Duyn, P. (1956) *J. Histochem. Cytochem.* **4**, 55.
Van Furth, R., Cohn, Z. A., Hirsch, J. G., Humphrey, J. H., Spector, W. G. & Langevoort, H. L. (1972) *Bull. Wld. Hlth. Org.* **46**, 845-852.
Hoefsmit, E. C. M. (1974) In: *Mononuclear phagocytes in immunity, infection and pathology.* Ed. R. Van Furth, Blackwell Scientific. Publ. Oxford.
Hoshino, F. (1963) *Z. Zellforsch.* **59**, 513.
Klug, H. (1965) *Z. Zellforsch.* **68**, 43.
Leckband, E. & Boyse, E. A. (1971) *Science* **172**, 1258.
Lundin, P. M. & Schelin, U. (1965) *Acta path. et microbiol. Scandinav.* **65**, 379.
Mandel, J. (1968) *Austr. J. Exp. Biol. Med. Sci.* **47**, 153.
Moore, M. A. S. & Owen, J. J. T. (1967) *J. Exp. Med.* **126**, 715.
Pfoch, M. (1971) *Z. Zellforsch.* **114**, 271.
Rambourg, A., Hermandez, W. & Leblond, C. P. (1969) *J. Cell Biol.* **40**, 395.
Veerman, A. J. P. (1974) *Cell Tiss. Res.* **148**, 247.
Veldman, J. E. (1970) Histophysiology and electron microscopy of the immune response. Dykstra and Niemeyer N.V. Groningen, The Netherlands.
Weiss, L. (1963) *Anat. Rec.* **145**, 413.

Biological Activity of Thymic Hormones

ULTRASTRUCTURE STUDIES ON CELLS CONTAINING SECRETORY GRANULES IN THE EARLY EMBRYONIC THYMUS

R. K. JORDAN

Lymphopoiesis commences in the thymus of foetal lamb at about 35 days of gestation (term = 150 days). The first sign of this lymphopoiesis is the appearance of large basophilic cells within the epithelial thymus. These probably represent stem cells which have already undergone "blast" transformation rather than the initial immigrant stem cells.

Ultrastructural studies have revealed within the epithelial thymus, immediately prior to the appearance of the large basophilic cells, two types of secretory cells. The ultrastructure of these cells is in keeping with their being

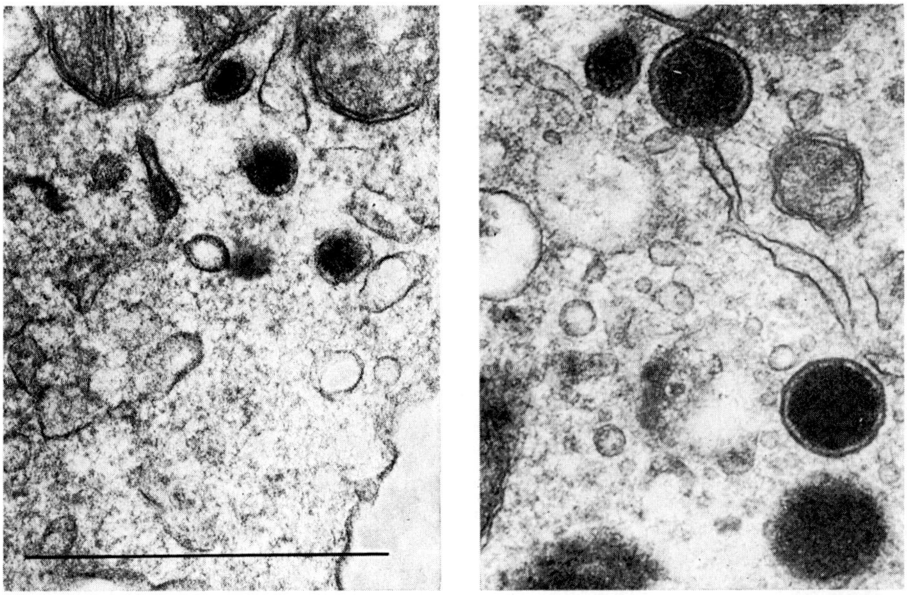

Fig. 1. Mouse embryo thymus 13 days gestation. A: prosecretory granules in type I epithelial cells from the compact peripheral zone; B: type 1 secretory granules. (The scale lines on all figs. represent 1 micron).

Department of Anatomy, The University of Newcastle-upon-Tyne, Newcastle-upon-Tyne. England

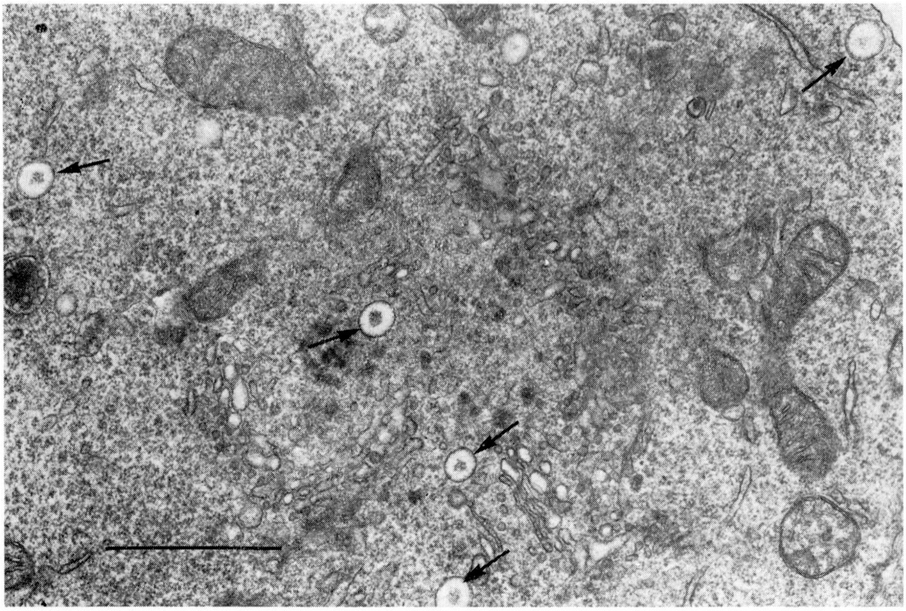

Fig. 2. Mouse embryo thymus 13 days gestation. Active Golgi area in type II secretory epithelial cell from central zone. Type II granules arrowed.

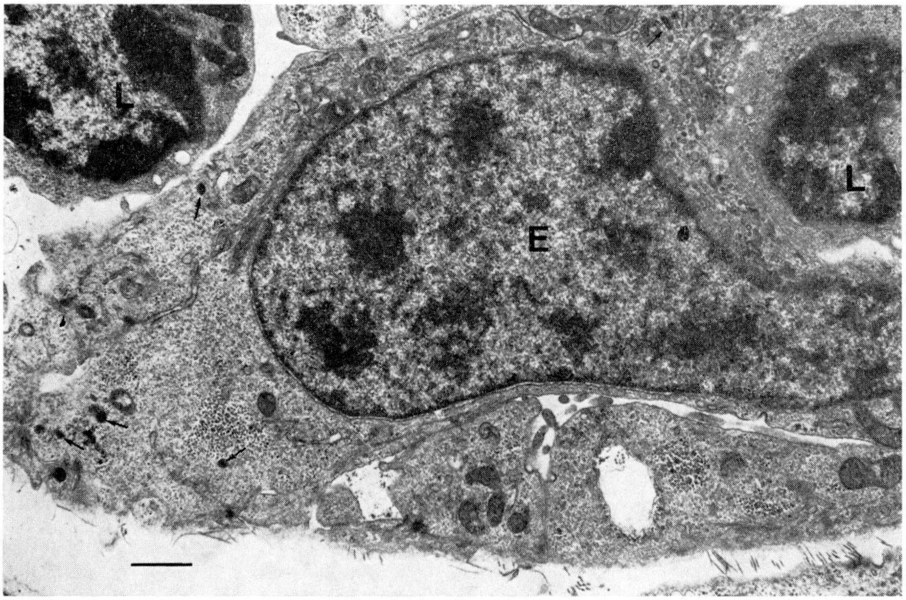

Fig. 3. Type I epithelial cell from 14-day mouse embryo thymus (E), in association with two developing lymphoid cells (L); granules in epithelial cell arrowed.

polypeptide producing cells. The epithelial thymus has a compact peripheral zone and a looser central area.

The first cell type (described as type I) is found in the peripheral zone of compact epithelium. These type I cells are characterized by the presence of single membrane bound secretory vesicles (230 nm in diameter) with a homogeneous dense core and a narrow clear halo. Smaller prosecretion vesicles (160 nm in diameter) are often present; these have been found to arise from the Golgi apparatus.

The second secretory cell (described as type II) is found more towards the central area and never in the compact periphery. The type II cell has prominent junctional complexes which include desmosomes and contain specific vesicles (250 nm in diameter) with a central electron dense core of varying density and a wide halo (reminiscent of insulin secretion in β cell of pancreatic islets).

In mouse embryo thymus (BALB/c) a similar morphological stage of histogenesis is found at 13/14 days of gestation. Large basophilic cells are regularly found in the epithelial thymus at 14 days of gestation and both secretory cell types are present. Type I in the periphery and type II in the central area.

The number of large basophilic cells rapidly increases and they are soon found in the peripheral zone of the thymic epithelium where they are often in close association with the type I secretory cells.

In the 14-day "nude" mouse embryo thymus (nude embryos of nude parents which have *not* been supplemented with thymus grafts) no large basophilic cells are found; indeed we have found *no* lymphoid cells in the thymus from

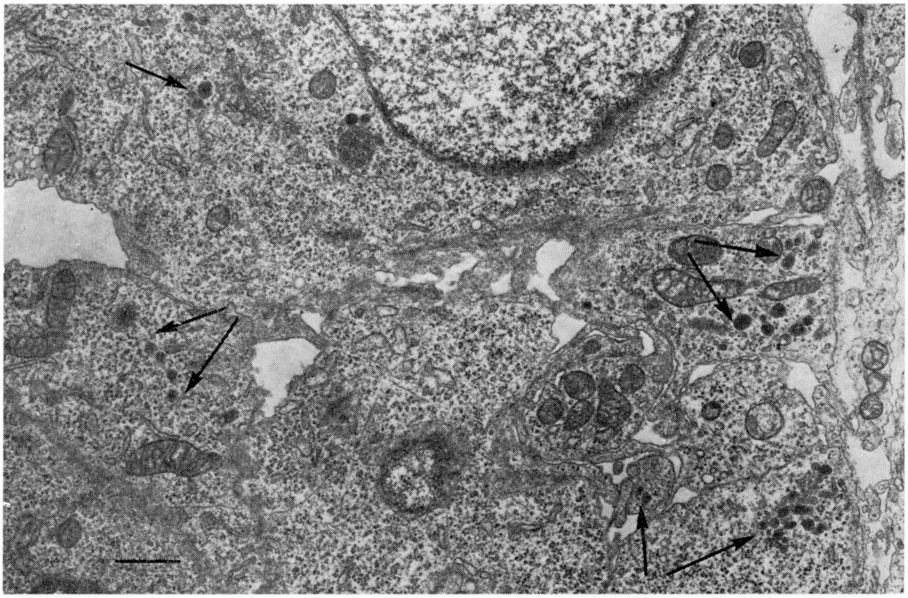

Fig. 4. Type I epithelial cell in peripheral zone of nude mouse embryo thymus of 14 days. Note increased numbers of secretory granules present (arrowed).

such mice at any time during foetal life. No type II cells have been found in the nude mouse embryo thymus (n.b. these observations are based on a limited number of specimens). However, type I cells are found at the periphery. The cells are normal, excepting for a high state of functional activity, typified by the large number of secretion and prosecretion granules (approx. 10× the normal). Furthermore, there are more granule-containing cells present in the periphery of 13-day "nude" mouse embryo thymus than in normal mouse thymus at the same time of gestation.

In conclusion, it is known that theta-positive cells are present in increasing numbers in mouse thymus from 14 days onwards and the appearance of these is dependent upon the initial presence of the large basophilic "blast" cells (Owen & Ritter 1969). Therefore a study of cell interactions at this stage of development should be of value in elucidating the nature of the intrathymic environment and its role(s) in thymocyte maturation.

REFERENCE

Owen, J. J. T. & Ritter, M. A. (1969) *J. exp. Med.* **129**, 431.

Biological Activity of Thymic Hormones

DISCUSSION

ZUCKER-FRANKLIN, New York

I would like to ask Dr. Jordan how he can be certain that the granules he has been discussing are secretory? After all, polymorphonuclear, leukocytes and platelets also have granules that are not secretory.

JORDAN, Newcastle-upon-Tyne

The evidence is indirect; we do see morphological signs of secretion, if you subscribe to the ideas of Lacy (Endocrinology, London, 1971) regarding insulin secretion and the roles of microtubules in release of insulin granules from β cells. Furthermore, the secretory granules are in the same size range as secretion products of other known peptide hormones such as calcitonin, gastrin, parathyroid hormone, insulin, and the like. I stress that all of our results at the moment are morphological and, until we know something about the stimulus which triggers secretion, it would be very difficult to examine this experimentally. I should say further that, if you regard the relationship between the initial lymphoid cells and the epithelial cells in the periphery as significant, the absence of this relationship in the nude mouse may suggest, taken together with the increase in numbers of granules seen, that the target system is absent and therefore the epithelial cells are trying to compensate for this by increasing their amounts of secretion. In other words, trying to reach a sort of an infinite functional demand and these observations could be interpreted in this way.

WARREN-JOHNSON, Copenhagen

My question is directed to Dr. de Sousa. The supernatant material, was this ultracentrifuged?

DE SOUSA, Glasgow

No. The supernatant from the human thymocytes was obtained from the washes of the cells (three times) which were done at 1,500 rpm. In the mouse experiments on T and B cell adhesiveness, the cells were maintained in Hank's or medium 199 for 2 h at room temperature or 3 h at 4 °C. The cells were then removed by centrifugation at ca. 300 g. The supernatants were sterile-filtered through membrane filters and usually concentrated using Amicon UM2 pressure dialysis membranes.

SNYDER, Nutley, N.J., USA

To Dr. de Sousa. The human data that you presented, was it from volunteers or patients and, if so, how many?

DE SOUSA, Glasgow

Normal blood donors!

CANTOR, Boston

Dr. de Sousa suggests that there is a feedback mechanism which regulates the intrathymic production of mature thymocytes. First, there is evidence consistent with this idea coming from work done by Dr. Richard Asofsky and myself (Nature, 1972). We were struck by the unexpected observation that, following depletion of peripheral T cells with ATS, the GvH-reactive cells in the thymus increase about 10-fold, suggesting as one possibility that feedback control of thymocyte production may be provided by ATS-sensitive peripheral lymphocytes. Therefore, I would like to ask Dr. de Sousa whether or not she has looked at the morphology of the thymus after ATS administration, something that we did not do after depleting peripheral T cells with ATS.

DE SOUSA, Glasgow

Not in a way that would satisfactorily answer your question. I have done the straight morphology of ALS treated mice, but what one should do is the autoradiography of the thymus of ATS-treated animals after ^{3}H-thymidine incorporation. Your observation is, however, very interesting and perhaps is a further example of what happens functionally in the absence or a decrease of the "regulatory" thymus cortical lymphocyte. Maroni and I observed in the thymus of pregnant mice at a time when Jean-Francois Bach finds high levels of serum TF that the decrease in the numbers of cortical lymphocytes is accompanied by a concomitant increase in the medullary lymphocyte population.

GOLDSTEIN, Galveston

I would like to direct my two comments to Dr. de Sousa's and Dr. Cantor's presentations. Several years ago, Dr. A. White and I found that, if thymosin fraction 3 was prepared from thymus glands obtained from older cows and steers (6-7 years old) instead of from young calves (6-8 weeks old), it was our general impression that per pound we would isolate more fraction 3. These results would be in agreement with your observation. My second comment is directed to Dr. Cantor. We have found that very high doses of thymosin (500-1000 mg/kg per day for 14 days) resulted in extreme atrophy of the thymus gland. We do not know if this involution is due to the stress of the megadoses or whether there is a specific feedback mechanism which turns off thymic epithelial cells.

RYGAARD, Copenhagen

Talking about morphology; I know that a lot of antisera have been made to thymic humoral factors and I would expect that a lot of people have tried to apply these in immunofluorescent assays to demonstrate the origin of the various factors. I know of one paper published in Nature a year and a half ago (a Hungarian one); who else did it?

WHITE, Palo Alto

In the October 4 issue of Nature (vol 251, page 421, 1974) Pyke & Gelfand described the culturing of human thymic epithelial cells. After 5 to 7 days of epithelial outgrowth, the medium was assessed for its ability to convert Isopaque-Ficoll gradient separated human bone marrow cells into cells that formed E rosettes with sheep erythrocytes. The results suggested that the medium from confluent human thymic epithelial monolayers was capable of increasing the capacity of human marrow cells to form rosettes. The data indicate that the human thymic epithelium may be a source of a factor or factors with biological activity similar to that of thymosin.

Biological Activity of Thymic Hormones

CHARACTERIZATION OF SUBCLASSES OF T LYMPHOCYTES AT DIFFERENT STAGES OF THYMUS-DEPENDENT DIFFERENTIATION

H. CANTOR & E. A. BOYSE

Stem cells migrate from yolk sac and liver in embrionic life (1) and from bone marrow in adult life (2) into the thymus, where they differentiate to thymocytes (3). Export of these "thymus-processed" cells to peripheral lymphoid tissues is necessary for the development and maintenance of the peripheral T cell pool. It is not clear, however, whether a) some emigrants leave the thymus at relatively early stages of maturation and continue to differentiate in the periphery, and b) whether this differentiation results in functionally different subclasses of T cells.

Do "Immature" Thymocytes Migrate to Peripheral Tissues?

The idea that some classes of immature thymocytes may migrate to peripheral tissues is supported, albeit indirectly, by several observations. First, in cows, cells in the thymic vein and thymic effluent lymph bear a cell surface marker (BTA) expressed on immature thymocytes and on less than 1 per cent of peripheral lymphocytes (4). Secondly, the degree of peripheral emigration of *in situ* labelled thymocytes in a cortisone-treated mouse is 100 times less than that seen in normal mice (5). This observation, of course, may reflect a direct effect of cortisone upon emigration mechanisms rather than simply the effects of lysing "immature" thymocytes. The third line of evidence comes from the demonstration by Komuro *et al.* that a) TL-negative mice produce anti TL antibody following injection of spleen cells from congenic TL positive mice, and b) injection of spleen cells into adult thymectomized (but immunocompetent) TL negative hosts did *not* result in the production of anti TL antibody (6). This observation indicates that maturation of thymic progenitors from TL positive donors was required for expression of the TL phenotype. Since intra-thymic expression of TL antigens is unlikely to lead to significant antibody formation, it is reasonable to suspect that sufficient numbers of TL positive cells migrated to the periphery to stimulate an antibody response. These observations, taken together, suggest that relatively immature thymocytes may migrate to the peripheral tissues.

Sidney Farber Cancer Center and Department of Medicine, Harvard Medical School, Boston, Mass. 02115, U.S.A. and Memorial Sloan-Kettering Cancer Center, 1275 York Avenue, New York, N.Y. 10021, U-S.A.

Evidence for Peripheral T Cells at Different Stages of Maturation - The Effects of Adult Thymectomy on Peripheral T Cells.

There is little or no effect on the recirculating population of T lymphocytes found mainly in thoracic duct within 6 months after adult thymectomy (ATx) (7). This finding, along with observations documenting the profound effects of neonatal thymectomy on the levels of recirculating cells, suggested that recirculating T lymphocytes were, in the main, long-lived and that once seeded to peripheral tissues would function in the absence of thymus. In order to examine the short term effects of ATx upon a population of T lymphocytes that did not rapidly recirculate, a group of 50 male CBA mice were thymectomized or sham-thymectomized at 6 weeks of age (8, 8a). At intervals thereafter, spleen, lymph node and thoracic duct cell suspensions prepared from mice in each group were incubated with anti Thy-1.2 and guinea pig complement. Within one month after thymectomy, the proportion of Thy-1.2^{+} cells in spleen had fallen to about 55 per cent of sham operated controls. Although the degree of reduced sensitivity to anti Thy-1.2 in spleen was quite variable during the first two weeks following thymectomy, by the fourth post-operative week a substantial and consistent depletion was noted. On the other hand, the concentration of Thy-1.2^{+} cells in peripheral lymph nodes and thoracic duct was not significantly altered during the first month following thymectomy. By the end of the second post-operative month, however, a 30 per cent reduction was noted in lymph node Thy-1.2^{+} cells. This observation is consistent with the idea that a portion of Thy-1.2^{+} cells in the spleen depended upon an intact thymus in adult life because they are short-lived and require continuous replenishment and/or because they depend upon a humoral factor elaborated by the thymus.

Studies of T lymphocytes which form rosettes with sheep erythrocytes (TRFC) have also suggested that antigen-binding T cells have different degrees of thymus-dependence, which may be correlated with circulating properties and anatomic locale (9, 10). These studies show that one population of TRFC, found mainly in thymus and spleen, appears to be easily inhibited with anti Thy-1.2 and decreases in the spleen shortly after adult thymectomy; this T cell subpopulation is relatively resistant to *in vivo* treatment with small doses of ALS. A second subpopulation of TRFC was found primarily in the lymph nodes and blood. These cells were 1) depleted following small doses of ALS *in vivo*, 2) relatively resistant to the inhibitory effects of anti Thy-1.2 *in vitro* and 3) did not decrease shortly after adult thymectomy. Since both kinds of RFC disappeared after neonatal thymectomy, Bach and Dardenne suggest that they represent two subpopulations of antigen binding T cells. The idea that ATx-sensitive TRFC found in spleen might be stimulated by antigen to become recirculating T cells no longer affected by ATx receives some support from the observation that ATx resistant, ALS-sensitive TRFC increased markedly after immunization. In this system, the subpopulation of TRFC sensitive to ATx is apparently not lost from the T cell pool, since cells with these properties reappear after *in vivo* or *in vitro* treatment with thymus extract or sera from normal mice. These findings suggest that a portion of TRFC are dependent upon the thymus in adult life for maintenance of cell surface characteristics.

Use of Ly Antisera to Define Peripheral Subsets of T Cells.

One direct approach to defining subsets of peripheral T cells at different stages of maturation is based upon the development of a panel of antisera by Boyse and colleagues that define cell surface antigens present on thymocytes and a portion of peripheral lymphocytes. Each antigen, termed Ly, is determined by a single genetic locus having 2 alleles (11, 12). Ly-1 has been located on chromosome 19, while Ly-2 and Ly-3 are closely linked but separately mutable sites on chromosome 6 (13).

Studies of the complement (C) mediated lytic effects of these antisera on C57BL/6 lymphoid cells (Ly phenotype 1.2, 2.2, 3.2) have revealed that approximately 85-90 per cent of thymocytes express all 3 Ly determinants. By contrast, a substantial portion of cortisone resistant thymocytes and peripheral cells do not express all 3 Ly determinants. In order to estimate the proportions of peripheral cells expressing different combinations of Ly determinants, the effects of sequential C-mediated lysis with different Ly antisera were examined. This approach is based upon the observation that maximum lysis with each Ly antiserum +C is achieved in a single incubation, as judged by the absence of further lysis above background upon a second incubation of the cells with the same antiserum +C. These studies indicated that a) virtually all peripheral Ly^+ cells also expressed Thy-1, b) 1/3 of Thy-1^+ cells expressed only Ly-1, c) approximately 1/2 expressed all 3 Ly antigens (Ly-123^+) and d) about 1/10 expressed Ly-23 (Table I). Within the limits of sensitivity of this assay, we

TABLE I

LY SURFACE ANTIGENS ON SPLEEN AND LN LYMPHOCYTES

	% of LN and Spleen
1. Association of Ly and Thy-1 determinants	
Thy 1^- Ly^+ cells	0–1
Thy 1^+ Ly^- cells	3–5
2. Expression of different Ly antigens on Thy 1^+ cells	
Ly Phenotype	*% of Thy 1^+ Cells (Spleen+LN)*
Ly-$1^+2^+3^+$	53
Ly-1^+	31
Ly-2^+3^+	7
Ly-2^+	0
Ly-3^+	1

were unable to detect significant numbers of cells expressing either Ly-2 or Ly-3. This finding is not unexpected in view of previous studies indicating that Ly-2 and Ly-3 determinants are very closely related on the cell surface, perhaps representing different antigens on the same macromolecule (11, 12, 14).

Studies of the ontogeny of Ly^+ cells in periphery showed that virtually all Thy-1^+ spleen cells in the first week of life were Ly-123^+. As the animal matured, the proportions of Ly-123^+ T cells declined in favor of Ly-1^+ and Ly-$2/3^+$ cells (Table II). The finding that Ly-123^+ cells were in highest concentration in the cortisone sensitive, TL positive fraction of thymus, and appeared early in ontogeny suggested that this subset represented relatively "young" thymus migrants. This view was supported by the finding that 4 weeks after adult thymectomy the concentration of this subset in spleen was reduced by 50 per cent. By contrast, the proportions of Ly-1^+ and Ly-23^+ cells are slightly increased 4 weeks after thymic ablation (Table II).

TABLE II

ONTOGENY OF LY^+ SUBSETS

Weeks after birth	*% in Spleen* 1	2	5	10	*ATx*	13
Ly Phenotype						
Ly-123^+	28	19	20	21		9
Ly-1^+	0	6	11	14		16
Ly-23^+	0	2	4	5		8

These data suggested that lymphocytes undergoing thymus-dependent differentiation can be divided into subclasses on the basis of expression of particular Ly differentiation determinants. Moreover, these subsets appeared to possess different biologic properties, perhaps representing cell types at different stages of thymus-dependent differentiation. In order to characterize these subsets with respect to immune function, the effects of depleting different Ly^+ subsets upon 1) the ability to generate helper activity and 2) the ability to generate a cytotoxic response were determined.

Depletion of Ly-1^+ cells from LN cells abolished subsequent helper activity to SRBC in adoptive, syngeneic irradiated hosts. Removal of Ly-23^+ or Ly-123^+ cells did not significantly alter the adoptive primary helper response (Table III). By contrast, depletion of Ly-23^+ cells but not Ly-1^+ cells or Ly-123^+ cells eliminated the ability of Thy-1^+ cells to generate killer activity both *in vivo* (in irradiated F_1 hosts) (Table III) and *in vitro* during a 5 day mixed lymphocyte culture. The idea that pre-killer T cells expressed Ly-23 determinants was also supported by the demonstration that the killer activity generated in MLC by normal T cells was sensitive to anti Ly-2 +C or anti Ly-3 +C but completely resistant to anti Ly-1 +C (data not shown).

These findings indicated that a) loss of different Ly surface components may

TABLE III

EFFECT OF LY ANTISERA UPON THE IMMUNOLOGIC ACTIVITY OF T CELLS*

Antiserum	*(Helper function Anti-SRBC PFC) Direct/Total (b)*	*% Lysis (a)*
NMS+C	1950/2410	51
anti Ly-1.2+C	140/100	56
anti Ly-2.2+C	2250/2605	4
anti Thy-1.2+C	40/0	3

* B6 LN cells were treated with Ly antisera+C, or NMS and then (a) injected into F_1 (BALB × B6) irradiated hosts and assessed for anti-H-2^d killer activity after 5 days or (b) injected into syngeneic irradiated hosts along with anti-theta+C-treated spleen cells, and 5×10^6 SRBC; PFC assays were done 6 days later.

accompany functional maturation of T cells and b) the capacity of T cell subclasses to express helper or killer activity is determined by differentiation events occuring *before* immunization with antigen. (15)

We have not directly established the relationship of Ly-123$^+$ cells to Ly-1$^+$ pre-helpers and Ly-23$^+$ pre-killers. It is most likely that Ly-123$^+$ cells are less mature and give rise to both Ly-1$^+$ cells and Ly-23$^+$ progeny, and that this maturation occurs both in the thymus and in peripheral lymphoid tissues (Fig. 1). Isolation of Ly-123$^+$ cells should allow this maturation scheme to be directly tested, and permit analysis of the contribution of this T cell subset to the regulation of the immune response.

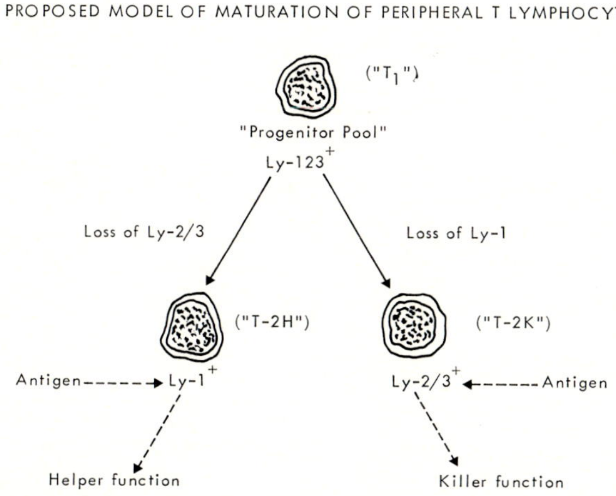

Fig. 1. Proposed Model of maturation of peripheral T lymphocytes

REFERENCES

1. Owen, J. J. T. & Reiter, M. A. (1969) *J. Exp. Med.* **129**, 431.
2. Ford, C. E., Micklem, H. S., Evans, E. P., Cray, J. G. & Ogden, D. A. (1966) *Ann. NY Acad. Sci.* **129**, 283.
3. Owen, J. J. T. & Roff, M. C. (1970) *J. Exp. Med.* **132**, 1216.
4. Williams, R. M., Chanana, A. D., Cronkite, E. P. & Waksman, B. H. (1971) *J. Immunol.* **106**, 1143.
5. Weissman, I. Personal communication.
6. Komuro, K., Boyse, E. A. & Old, L. J. (1973) *J. Exp. Med.* **137**, 533.
7. Miller, J. F. A. P. & Mitchell, G. F. (1969) *Transplant. Rev.* **1**, 3.
8. Simpson, E. & Cantor, H. (1975) *Eur. J. Imm.*, in press.

8a. Cantor, H. (1972) *2nd Lepetit Colloquium on Cell Interactions*, North Holland Press, Amsterdam.

9. Bach, J. F. & Dardenne, M. (1972) *Immunology* **6**, 394.
10. Greaves, M. F. & Hogg, N. (1971) In *Progr. in Immunol.* Ed. by B. Amos, Academic Press, New York.
11. Boyse, E. A., Miyazawa, M., Aoki, T. & Old, L. J. (1968) *Proc. Roy. Soc. B.* **170**, 175.
12. Boyse, E. A., Itakura, K., Stockert, E., Iritani, C. & Miura, M. (1971) *Transpl.* **11**, 351.
13. Itakura, K., Hutton, J. J., Boyse, E. A. & Old, L. J. (1972) *Transpl.* **13**, 239.
14. Boyse, E. A., Old, L. J. & Stockert, E. (1968) *Proc. Nat. Acad. Sci. US* **60**, 886.
15. Cantor, H. & Boyse, E. A. (1975) *J. Exp. Med.*, in the press.

Biological Activity of Thymic Hormones

DISCUSSION

DE SOUSA, New York

Harvey, from your data on the PFC, did you discover the identity of the suppressor cell? Because when you treated the spleen cells with the anti-Ly-2.2 +C the indication from your results was that you have in fact abolished some suppression.

CANTOR, Boston

I think that it is too early to tell. This result might be due to the fact that we were simply enriching for helper cells and depleting irrelevant cells. On the other hand, we have preliminary evidence in other systems that the "immature" Ly-1 2 3^+ cell may in certain cases exert regulatory effects.

TOURAINE, Lyon

Does the Ly-1 2 3^+ cell have a relatively high concentration of Thy-1 antigen?

CANTOR, Boston

I have not looked at that correlation; Ly-1 2 3^+ cells obviously have properties that in the past have been attributed to T cells having relatively high concentrations of the Thy-1 antigen.

GISLER, Basel

Do you know whether there is a difference in radiosensitivity between the Ly-1 and the Ly-2 3?

CANTOR, Boston

No, we don't.

BACH, Paris

I would like to report a recent finding by S. Andersson, P. Hayry, my wife, and me, as will appear soon in Nature, about the effect of adult thymectomy on the CML test which may be relevant to what Harvey Cantor has just told us. The finding is that CML is very much depressed (70 per cent depression) four weeks after adult thymectomy (much more than MLC, which is also depressed but to a much less extent). One can give two interpretations: either "pre-killer" T cells (Ly-2 3^+) are very thymus-dependent (much more than the classical long-lived T cell) or the cell which is altered by adult thymectomy is the Ly-1^+ amplifier cell, as Harvey Cantor's work might suggest, and the effect of adult thymectomy is due to the loss of these amplifier cells. Maybe Harvey would like to comment on that particular aspect?

CANTOR, Boston

I think that those questions as well as many other questions concerning a direct demonstration of this kind of maturation await techniques capable of separating out the adult thymectomy-sensitive Ly-1 2 3^+ cell, the putative precursor of both pre-killers and amplifier cells. Currently, we separate by a negative selection technique using the complement-mediated lytic effects of Ly-antisera. Thus, it is impossible for us to obtain Ly-1 2 3^+ cells following these procedures. We will approach this problem using the Cell Sorter, which is capable of positively selecting Ly-1 2 3^+ cells.

EIJSVOGEL, Amsterdam

If you put your Ly-1^+ cells alone in the mixed lymphocyte reaction, do you get DNA synthesis without generation of cytotoxic cells?

CANTOR, Boston

Yes.

WILLIAMS, Cambridge

I would like to ask whether there has been a correlation between degree of theta-ness and Ly-antigenicity.

CANTOR, Boston

We do not have any studies bearing on that question.

GOLDSTEIN, Galveston

Did you say whether Ly-1 2 3^+ cells are also found in the bone marrow?

CANTOR, Boston

We have not looked in bone marrow; I really cannot say. I believe that Dr. Boyse has looked at the ability of various tissues to absorb subsequent cytolytic activity of the Ly-antisera. I do not believe he found that bone marrow cells were capable of significant absorption, but you will have to ask him.

LUCKEY, Columbia

Have you checked Bursa and thymus for these three types of cell?

CANTOR, Boston

These alloantigens were produced over the last seven years in Dr. Boyse's laboratory using inbred strains of mice. It is possible that analogues may be found in other species, most significantly in man. I might point out that these are potentially very useful markers for studies of thymus-dependent differentiation. Unlike Thy-1, which is a differentiation antigen expressed on various tissues, Ly-antigens have been found so far only on thymocytes and peripheral Thy-1^+ cells. Thus, they are apparently only at the point where stem cells begin thymus-dependent differentiation.

WHITE, Palo Alto

Harvey, you spoke of the rapid disappearance of Ly-1 2 3^+ cells after adult thymectomy. Have you looked after neonatal thymectomy?

CANTOR, Boston

No.

WHITE, Palo Alto

Because after neonatal thymectomy there apparently are cells present which can function as helper cells.

CANTOR, Boston

I think that the critical question is how long after neonatal thymectomy one looks. If, for example, one looks 3 months after neonatal thymectomy, I doubt whether any helper activity would be detected.

EIJSVOOGEL, Amsterdam

When you have a cell which only carries Ly-23, are you sure that that cell never can regain Ly-1?

CANTOR, Boston

Whether or not cells can dedifferentiate is a question that people have been asking for many years, well before we knew about T and B cells. The only clear-cut example of dedifferentiation, to my knowledge, involves oncogenesis.

Biological Activity of Thymic Hormones

THE POSTTHYMIC PRECURSOR CELL

OSIAS STUTMAN

The observation that the restoration obtained with thymus grafts in neonatally thymectomized mice was mainly mediated by host cells (1) was interpreted as indicating that either the thymus produced some humoral factor (acting on the host) (2) or that the host cells were modified by migration through the thymus (3). Support for both of these views came with the description of several thymic extracts with apparent functional activity (see this volume) and by the direct demonstration that hemopoietic precursor cells could become competent T lymphocytes after passage through the thymus (4). In the present discussion, we will show evidence that, whatever the nature of the intrathymic event, a population of postthymic precursors is generated through thymus traffic and that such population in the peripheral tissues may be one of the prime targets for the action of the thymic humoral factor(s). The fact that indeed there is a thymic humoral factor detectable in the serum of man and mice (see J. F. Bach in the present volume) supports this view. Furthermore, it is apparent that both the thymic humoral factor detected in serum and a thymic factor extracted from the thymus (THF) act primarily on cells that have received some sort of thymic influence (i.e., postthymic cells) (5, 6).

During our analysis of the restoration of immune functions in neonatally thymectomized mice (7, 8), especially using thymus enclosed in diffusion chambers (DC), we observed that the animals became refractory when such treatment was delayed for 40 to 60 days after neonatal thymectomy (8) or when the animals were suffering postthymectomy wasting disease (7, 8). When we studied the effects of various cell supplements in augmenting the capacity of thymus grafts or thymus in DC to restore immune competence in 50-day-old neonatally thymectomized mice we observed: a) that lymphoid and hemopoietic cells from adult or newborn animals acted synergistically with thymus in DC in restoration of immune functions (9); b) that the actual content of immunologically competent cells in the different cell types used was not a factor, since tissues with low or no immunocompetent T lymphocytes (i.e., newborn liver, spleen, or adult marrow) were as effective as adult spleen in

Cellular Immunobiology Section, Memorial Sloan-Kettering Cancer Center, New York, N.Y. 10021 U-S.A.
The present work was supported by U.S. Public Health Service grants CA-08748 and CA-16899. I would like to thank M. Cuttito, W. Harrison, L. Tang, L. Stevenson, and J. Solomon for their able assistance.

such cooperative restoration (9, 10); and c) that embryonic hemopoietic cells (i.e., yolk sac, blood, liver), especially before day 14-16 of embryonation, cooperated in restoring immune functions only with free thymus grafts and not with thymus in DC (10). It should be stressed that all those embryonic cell types contain precursors that can generate competent T cells via thymus traffic (4). The results were interpreted then as indicative of a sub-population of cells, termed postthymic, present in the lymphoid and hemopoietic tissues of adult and newborn mice which were capable of cooperation with thymus in DC for the restoration of immune functions and generation of competent T cells (i.e., were sensitive to the humoral activity of the thymus). On the other hand, the early embryonic tissues contained mainly a population of cells, termed prethymic, that required contact with the thymic stroma through traffic for its further differentiation (i.e., was "insensitive" to humoral activity of the thymus). It is obvious that the intrathymic differentiation step may be, and probably is, mediated by humoral factors, thus the quotation marks. It also became apparent from these and other studies (11-13) that the postthymic population was incapable of self-renewal in the absence of thymic tissue and that such cells were generated as a consequence of traffic of prethymic cells to the thymus and subsequent emmigration to the peripheral lymphoid tissues (10-14). Thus, the unique traffic patterns of hemopoietic cells described by Ford *et al.* (15, 16) actually represent a process by which competent T lymphocytes are generated (4, 11-13). It is difficult at the present writing to define the magnitude of these differentiation steps under physiological conditions, especially if there are any quantitative or qualitative differences in early ontogeny versus adult life. Our own work indicates that, by temporary exposure to thymus, neonatally thymectomized animals can generate immunologically competent cells, but that this pool of cells is depleted with time in the absence of the thymus, i.e., are incapable of self-renewal (13).

Point (b) mentioned above suggested that the postthymic pool could be composed of both nonimmunocompetent (precursor or early postthymic cells) and competent postthymic T cells. These two subpopulations have contrasting differences as indicated in Table I (based on data from references 8, 9, 17, and 18) and are represented in different proportions in lymphoid and hemopoietic tissues of adult and newborn mice.

Before describing in detail the characteristics of the postthymic precursor cell presented in Table I, a brief presentation of our basic experimental model. In the experiments, 50-60-day-old neonatally thymectomized C3Hf, CBA/H, or A/J mice (see reference 7 for details about mouse strains and animal care) were injected intraperitoneally (IP) with cells derived from syngeneic mice of different ages (newborn mice in the majority of the present experiments). In many instances, the cells were derived from animals that had received some form of treatment *in vivo* (adult thymectomy, treatment with antilymphocyte serum), or were manipulated *in vitro* (treatment with different alloantisera, different cell separation procedures). Some of these animals were subsequently grafted IP with an empty DC or a DC containing a thymic lobe or a spleen

TABLE I

CHARACTERIZATION OF TWO SUBPOPULATIONS OF POSTTHYMIC CELLS IN MOUSE TISSUES

*Biological Characteristics**	*Early Postthymic Precursor Cell*	*Postthymic T Cell*
Tissue distribution (adult)	Spleen, marrow	Lymphoid tissues
(newborn)	Spleen, liver	–
Traffic patterns	Spleen-seeking	Lymph-node seeking
Recirculation (presence in TD)	No	Yes
Immunological competence	No	Yes
Capacity of adoptive restoration of thymectomized animals	No	Yes
Effect of adult thymectomy	Depletion (30-60 days)	None (within 60 days)
Effect of short term ALS treatment	None	Depletion
3H-Thymidine suicide	Yes	No, usually
BSA gradients	A-B layers	C-D layers
Sedimentation rate (adult spleen)	5.9 mm/hr	3.7 mm/hr
(adult marrow)	5.4 mm/hr	3.6 mm/hr
(newborn spleen)	5.8 mm/hr	?
Adherence to plastic	Yes, partial	No
Adherence to nylon wool	Yes	No
Surface antigens: Thy. 1	Yes	Yes
TL	No?	No
Ig	No	No

* See text and references 17 and 18 for details. TD: thoracic duct. BSA gradients: A-B layers (10 to 26 per cent) C-D layers (26-35 per cent BSA).

fragment (for details of preparation of DC and controls, see references 19 and 20). At different times after treatment, starting at 7 days (although the majority of the animals were tested at 30 days after treatment), the immune responses were measured in spleen, lymph nodes, and thoracic duct as the capacity to generate graft-versus-host reactions *in vivo* (GVH), response *in vitro* to phytohemagglutinin (PHA), or in mixed lymphocyte reactions (MLR). For details on these techniques, see references 7 to 12.

Ecology of postthymic cells.

In a recent review (21), the term "ecology" was borrowed from other sources and applied to the characterization of thymus-dependency. It was meant to suggest the "acting" of the thymus-derived cells in their different "stages" or "territories" (i.e. the thymus-dependent areas). Table I shows some of these territorial features, comparing the early postthymic cell (or postthymic precursor) with the "mature" postthymic T cell. The postthymic precursor is found mainly in the marrow and spleen in the adult and in the spleen, marrow, and liver of the newborn. Post-thymic precursor cells are present in the liver even for 3-5 days after birth (10). In the embryonic liver, post-thymic precursors are detected with ease in the 17-day-old embryo (10), i.e., approximately 5 days after the appearance of the thymus, while liver or blood from embryos at earlier ages show a predominance of prethymic precursor cells, i.e., require a free thymus graft for restoration of immune functions (10). When unfractioned newborn spleen or the purified fractions containing mainly postthymic precursors are labeled with ^{51}Cr and injected intravenously into adult syngeneic mice, the main component is detected in the spleen 4 h after injection. Thus, the precursor cells are mainly "spleen seeking" while the competent T cells are mainly "lymph node seeking", using accepted terminology (22). The early postthymic precursor cells are not recirculating and are not detected in the thoracic duct lymph; however, they can be detected in blood, especially in late embryos and newborn mice (17). Concerning their functional capacity as measured as immunological competence, the post-thymic precursor is incompetent (17, 18). Purified preparations of such cells from newborn spleen were incapable of generating GVH reactions *in vivo* or of helping bone marrow cells to generate responses to sheep red cells in irradiated hosts, even in cell doses 100-fold larger than those required for competent T cells. Similarly, such postthymic precursors are incapable of generating responses *in vitro* to PHA, Concanavalin A, or in the MLR. In accordance with this, postthymic precursors are incapable of producing adoptive restoration of neonatally thymectomized mice (17). Adoptive restoration is observed in neonatally thymectomized mice injected with immunologically competent syngeneic cells and is mediated exclusively by the donor cells (1, 23). In contrast with the results of thymus grafts or thymus in DC, adoptive restoration is easily achieved late after neonatal thymectomy and can even produce reversal of the postthymectomy wasting syndrome (23). When the cell donors were thymectomized as adults and their spleen or marrow cells were used in the model experiments, it was apparent that the postthymic precursor was depleted after adult thymectomy (17). Within 20-30 days after such treatment, there was a complete disappearance of the postthymic precursor from marrow (17). Conversely, short term treatment with ALS (0.5 ml IP and withdrawal of cells 48 h later) had no detectable effect on the postthymic precursors in adult spleen or marrow, while it had marked effects on the postthymic competent T cell (17). Due to the complexity of the experimental design, it is difficult to determine the half-life of the postthymic precursor cell (although their disappearance rate after adult thymectomy would indicate a rapid turnover). However, Table I indicates that indeed it must be a rapidly dividing population, since it can be eliminated by short pulses (24 h) with ^{3}H-thymidine of high specific activity, i.e., can commit "thymidine suicide" (17). The relative short life and rapid turnover is in accordance with our observation of the time-dependent refractoriness of neonatally thymectomized mice to treatment with thymus in DC (8).

Physical and surface characteristics.

Different separation procedures showed some clear differences between the postthymic precursor and the competent postthymic T lymphocyte, as Table I indicates. Using bovine serum albumin (BSA) gradients, the precursor cells are detected mainly in the A-B layers (10 to 26 per cent BSA) while the competent T cells are detected mainly in the dense C-D layers (26-35 per cent BSA) (17). The less dense bands are those also containing the cells that can be induced to express T cell surface antigens by thymic extracts (24). Similarly, using velocity sedimentation at unit gravity, it was apparent that the postthymic precursor is a cell larger than the competent T cell, which migrates much faster (5.9 mm/hr versus 3.7 mm/hr). For technical details on both separative procedures, see references 17 and 18. It is apparent from these studies that the postthymic precursor cell is less dense and larger than the immunologically competent postthymic T cell. Morphologically, the postthymic precursor cell looks like a middle-sized basophilic lymphocyte. In scanning electron-microscopy, the purified populations of postthymic precursor cells proved to be enriched for cells with a smooth surface (done in collaboration with Dr. C. M. Fenoglio). An interesting feature of the postthymic precursor cell is that it is adherent to nylon wool (in columns with low fetal calf serum, 5 per cent or less in the medium) while competent postthymic cells pass through such columns which are known to retain mainly non-T and B lymphocytes. As regards surface antigens, the postthymic precursor cell purified from newborn spleen has enough Thy. 1 (theta) antigen to be eliminated by *in vitro* treatment with anti-Thy. 1 and C (Table II). This is an important feature because it is the only direct evidence that the postthymic cell has indeed received thymic influence, i.e., is truly postthymic (experiments using chromosome markers are presently in progress to prove this point). The postthymic precursor cells may also have TL antigen (25), although this point requires

TABLE II

EFFECT OF ANTI-THY. 1.2 AND C ON THE CAPACITY OF NEWBORN C3Hf CELLS AND FRACTIONS SEPARATED IN VELOCITY SEDIMENTATION AT UNIT GRAVITY TO COOPERATE WITH THYMUS IN DC FOR RESTORATION OF GVH CAPACITY IN 50-DAY OLD NEONATALLY THYMECTOMIZED C3Hf MICE

*Cells**	*Pretreatment***	*Thymus in DC*	*Restoration of GVH****
Whole	None	No	0/13
Whole	Control	Yes	7/10 (70%)
Whole	Anti Thy. 1.2	Yes	0/11
5.0-7.0 mm/hr	None	No	0/12
5.0-7.0 mm/hr	Control	Yes	6/10 (60%)
5.0-7.0 mm/hr	Anti Thy. 1.2	Yes	1/10 (10%)

* Whole newborn spleen cells or the fractions that migrated 5.0-7.0 mm/hr in velocity sedimentation at unit gravity (see reference 17). All animals injected with 20×10^6 viable whole spleen cells or with 10×10^6 viable spleen fractions, IP.
** Cells preincubated with anti-Thy. 1.2 (theta C3H) or anti-Thy. 1.1 (theta AKR) as controls with rabbit C. Dead cells were removed by centrifugation in whole fetal calf serum (see reference 17). The actual percent of lysed cells was 6 per cent (4-14 per cent) in unfractioned spleen and 9 per cent (6-17 per cent) in the velocity fraction.
*** Measured 20 days after treatment using (C3Hf × C57BL/6) F1 hybrids as test mice (see references 8–9).

further study. Using CBA/H mice, we could not detect any effect by pretreatment with anti-TL and C (17). However, using A/J mice, which are TL+ (25), we could show a reduction in functional capacity when the purified newborn spleen cells were pretreated *in vitro* with anti-TL and C and subsequently used in the model system.

When purified postthymic precursor cells obtained from the spleen of newborn CBA/HT6T6 mice were injected into 60-day old neonatally thymectomized CBA/H mice which also had a thymus in DC, we could show that the precursor cells indeed differentiated into competent cells in the peripheral tissues of the CBA/H mice (17, 18). When tested 30 days after treatment, a high proportion of cells in lymph nodes and thoracic duct which were responding *in vitro* to PHA or MLR had the chromosome type of the postthymic precursor (17, 18). These experiments indicate that, as a consequence of a "maturation" event which is probably regulated by thymic humoral factors (i.e., thymus in DC) and which is time-dependent (the earliest restoration was observed at 6 to 8 days after treatment), cells with the chromosome type of the postthymic precursor showed: a) recirculating capacities (i.e., were detected in thoracic duct lymph); and b) could respond to PHA and generate MLR, suggesting immunological competence (17, 18). The fact that the target for thymic function (even with free thymus grafts) may be the postthymic precursor population in the periphery is suggested when the timing for restoration is compared with the present model versus neonatally thymectomized animals or nude athymic mice. As was mentioned above, when cells are supplemented, detectable restoration is observed within 7 days after treatment. When thymus grafts are implanted into neonatally thymectomized mice at 30 days of age, restoration is also obtained at a relatively rapid pace, within 7-15 days after treatment (14). However, when nude mice are treated with a thymus graft, restoration is detected only after 20 days or more of treatment (26). It should also be stressed that nude mice are totally refractory to restoration with thymus in DC (26). Studies on the effects of cell supplementation in nude mice in association with thymic function are presently in progress. The refractoriness of nude mice to immunological restoration with thymus in DC or with some thymic extracts (26) supports our view that the prime target for the thymic humoral factors may be a postthymic precursor cell in the periphery, which is absent or diminished to nonfunctional levels in the nude mouse.

Table III shows our attempts to demonstrate that the postthymic precursor cell, or a subpopulation within those cells, can be driven into differentiation by exposure to antigens. Fifty-day-old neonatally thymectomized C3Hf mice were injected with precursor cells only (whole newborn spleen, the 5.0-7.0 mm/hr fraction from velocity sedimentation, or the 3.0-4.0 mm/hr fraction which is enriched for Thy. 1 positive cells and competent T cells). It is apparent that repeated immunization (3 weekly injections) with allogeneic or xenogeneic embryonic fibroblasts generated cytotoxic cells capable of destroying specific target cells *in vitro* (target cell loss of 10 per cent or more is considered positive) in lymph nodes (and spleen; not shown in Table). Treatment *in vitro* with

TABLE III

POSTTHYMIC PRECURSOR CELLS IN NEWBORN SPLEEN: EFFECT OF ANTIGENIC STIMULATION ON GENERATION OF COMPETENT T CELLS IN THE ABSENCE OF THYMUS FUNCTION

*Cells**	*Immunization***	*Percent target cell loss*			
		Rat	*C57BL/6*	*CBA/H*	*C3Hf*
Whole	No	4	4	3	4
Whole	Yes (Rat × 1)	7	4	5	5
Whole	Yes (Rat × 3)	39	13	11	6
Whole	Yes (SRBC × 3)	5	5	5	7
5.0-7.0 mm/hr fr.	No	4	4	4	5
5.0-7.0 mm/hr fr.	Yes (Rat × 1)	5	5	ND	4
5.0-7.0 mm/hr fr.	Yes (Rat × 3)	48	16	7	5
5.0-7.0 mm/hr fr.	Yes (C57BL/6 × 3)	9	44	12	6
5.0-7.0 mm/hr fr.	Yes (SRBC × 3)	6	4	ND	5
3.0-4.0 mm/hr fr.	No	6	6	ND	ND
3.0-4.0 mm/hr fr.	Yes (Rat × 1)	34	6	ND	5
3.0-4.0 mm/hr fr.	Yes (Rat × 3)	67	11	ND	7

* 50-day-old neonatally thymectomized C3Hf mice were injected IP with 20×10^6 whole spleen or velocity sedimentation fractions. Immunization started 1 week after injection.
** Immunization SC by injection of 1×10^6 Lewis rat or C57BL/6 embryonic fibroblasts or by 10^8 sheep red blood cells (SRBC) either one single dose or 3 weekly doses. Lymph node cells tested 8-10 days after last immunization, using 3H-proline prelabeled target cells as described in refer ence 27.

anti-Thy. 1 and C completely eliminated the cytotoxic capacity of such cells (not shown in Table III). When the same experiments were done using the 3.0-4.0 mm/hr fraction (which in adult spleen contains the competent Thy. 1 positive T cells), results were comparable, although these cells could generate cytotoxic lymphocytes even after a single immunization. This fraction contains the small numbers of competent T cells in newborn spleen. It is apparent that further characterization of these subsets of cells is mandatory, since small contamination of the precursor fraction with competent T cells plus specific expansion of such population by hyperimmunization may explain the present results.

The characterization of possible "target" cells for the thymic humoral factors seems a necessary step for understanding the interactions that lead to T cell differentiation. It may help to design rational assays for the extracts, to define specific (i.e. extract-dependent) versus nonspecific steps of differentiation (20, 24), and it may help to clarify the discrepancies existing between the functional activity of different extracts or between *in vivo* versus *in vitro* assays using such extracts (20). Dogmatic presentations of results usually act more as barriers than as helpers in clarifying controversial issues. The proliferation of reviews sometimes crystalize as fact pieces of information which may be termed preliminary or handled more cautiously when included in an experimental paper. By simple repetition of statements, some of these incomplete data become "established" and the danger of the rule-of-three, "What I tell you three times is true" (Lewis Carroll in *The Hunting of the Snark*), becomes apparent. However, it is through collaborative work as well as workshops such as this that discrepancies will be eliminated.

REFERENCES

1. Dalmasso, A. P., Martinez, C., Sjodin, K. & Good, R. A. (1963) *J. Exptl. Med.* **118**, 1089.
2. Osoba, D. & Miller, J. F. A. P. (1963) *Nature* **199**, 653.
3. Harris, J. E. & Ford, C. E. (1963) *Lancet* **I**, 389.
4. Stutman, O. & Good, R. A. (1971) *Transplant. Proc.* **3**, 923.
5. Bach, J. F. & Dardenne, M. (1973) *Immunology* **25**, 353.
6. Lonai, P., Mogilner, B., Rotter, V. & Trainin, N. (1973) *Eur. J. Immunol.* **3**, 26.
7. Stutman, O., Yunis, E. J., Martinez, C. & Good, R. A. (1967) *J. Immunol.* **98**, 79.
8. Stutman, O., Yunis, E. J. & Good, R. A. (1969) *J. Exptl. Med.* **130**, 809.
9. Stutman, O., Yunis, E. J. & Good, R. A. (1970) *J. Exptl. Med.* **132**, 583.
10. Stutman, O., Yunis, E. J. & Good, R. A. (1970) **132**, 601.
11. Stutman, O. (1970) in *Proceedings of 5th Leukocyte Culture Conference*, Ed. J. Harris, Academic Press, New York, p. 671.
12. Stutman, O. & Good, R. A. (1971) in *Morphological and Functional Aspects of Immunity*, Eds. K. Lindhal-Kiessling, G. Halm & M. G. Hanna, Plenum Press, New York, p. 129.
13. Stutman, O. (1972) in *Membranes and Viruses in Immunopathology*, Eds. S. B. Day & R. A. Good, Academic Press, New York, p. 437.
14. Stutman, O., Yunis, E. J. & Good, R. A. (1972) *J. Exptl. Med.* **135**, 339.
15. Harris, J. E. & Ford, C. E. (1964) *Nature* **201**, 884.
16. Ford, C. E. (1966) in *The Thymus*, Eds. G. E. W. Wolstenholme & R. Porter, Churchill, London, p. 131.
17. Stutman, O. (In press) *Ann. N.Y. Acad. Sci.*
18. Stutman, O. (In press) *Transplant. Proc.*
19. Stutman, O., Yunis, E. J. & Good, R. A. (1969) *J. Natl. Cancer Inst.* **41**, 499.
20. Stutman, O. & Good, R. A. (1973) in *Contemporary Topics in Immunobiology, Vol. 2*, Eds. A. J. S. Davies & R. L. Carter, Plenum Press, New York, p. 299.
21. de Sousa, M. A. B. (1973) in *Contemporary Topics in Immunobiology, Vol. 2*, Eds. A. J. S. Davies & R. L. Carter, Plenum Press, New York, p. 119.
22. Zatz, M. M. & Lance, E. M. (1970) *Cell. Immunol.* **1**, 3.
23. Stutman, O., Yunis, E. J. & Good, R. A. (1969) *J. Immunol.* **102**, 87.
24. Scheid, M. P., Hoffman, M. K., Komuro, K., Hammerling, U., Abbot, J., Boyse, E. A., Cohen, G. H., Hooper, J. A., Schulof, R. S. & Goldstein, A. L. (1973) *J. Exptl. Med.* **138**, 1027.
25. Boyse, E. A., Old, L. J. & Stockert, E. (1966) in *IVth International Symp. Immunopathol.*, Eds. P. Grabar & P. Miescher, Schwabe, Basel, p. 23.
26. Stutman, O. (1974) *Fed. Proc.* **33**, 736.
27. Bean, M. A., Pees, H., Rosen, G. & Oettgen, H. F. (1973) *Natl. Cancer Inst. Monogr.* **37**, 41.

Biological Activity of Thymic Hormones

DISCUSSION

CANTOR, Boston

A question on the last two slides which were intended to show antigenic stimulation responsible for maturation of postthymic cells. How do you exclude the possibility that you have a contaminant population of mature T cells which have been cloned up by antigen, especially after hyperimmunization?

STUTMAN, New York

Yes, we cannot exclude that. Within the limits of whatever we test, that is, ability to generate GvH *in vivo*, ability to respond to PHA, Con A, LPS, or to generate MLC or CML reactions *in vitro*, this purified fraction of newborn spleen is "incompetent". However, I agree that hyperimmunization may enrich contaminating competent subpopulations. We cannot exclude that. It would be interesting to look at Ly-types.

GOLDSTEIN, Galveston

Did you say that both the T_0 and T_1 are your postthymic cell?

STUTMAN, New York

Postthymic, you see, is everything outside the thymus and actually it is a very bad word, because it obviously includes the competent T cell which we know, although thymus-derived, is thymus-independent for its function. So, it is a terrible word; but I will keep this terminology.

GOLDSTEIN, Galveston

Will both the T_0 and the T_1 cells, if they are two separate populations, be driven by antigen?

STUTMAN, New York

I would assume that one, the T_0, is not and the other, T_1, is.

GOLDSTEIN, Galveston

Now, the obvious question is, and I guess you asked it, have you checked with Dr. Cantor to see whether his precursor cell is a T_0 or a T_1 cell, or are we talking about the same (postthymic) cell population?

CANTOR, Boston

Well, I think something very useful may be gained if someone discusses the terminology problems based on Dr. Stutman's, Dr. Bach's, and my own nomenclature which are a bit different, but perhaps refer to similar cells.

BACH, Paris

I will show you now a slide (Fig. 1) on the comparison of the terminologies used to define T cell subsets. There is some agreement in terms of prethymic (the name is the same), but there is a difference in the evaluation of theta-positivety, Roelants and myself finding a small but significant amount of theta on prethymic cells, whereas Stutman and Cantor do not find any theta antigen in these cells. This may just simply be due, however, to differences in tech-

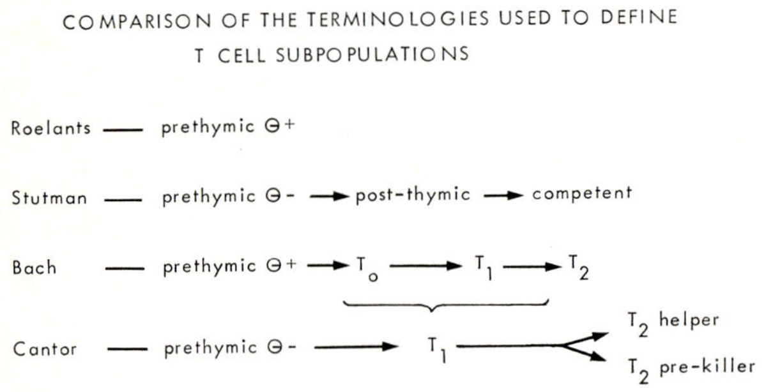

niques, since Roelants uses immunofluorescence and we use antigen-binding inhibition which are much more sensitive techniques than cytotoxicity assays or even function inhibition as used by Stutman and Cantor. The other maturation stages are still confused, since we have postthymic cells for Stutman, T_0 and T_1 in our mind, and T_1 in Cantor's view. The way it is indicated in the slide shows an overlapping between these different subsets and there is probably a cell population which, in our interpretation, may have two different metabolic states, possibly related to the presence of the thymic humoral function. Finally, it may very well be that Stutman's postthymic cells and our T_0 cell, are equivalent and not very much different from Cantor's T_1 cell The Stutman's competent, our T_2 and Cantor's T_2 helper and killer on the right hand side of the fig. are probably the same cells.

STUTMAN, New York

One of the questions that came out of this discussion is that we have a super stem cell that can give rise to everything and we have clear evidence, or at least very suggestive evidence, that we have commitment stages in which certain stem cells become committed stem cells that would mainly differentiate along a single pathway. So question one was whether the prethymic commitment, if there is such a commitment, is an intrathymic or extrathymic event. I think that is a good open question. As for target cells for hormone activity, I think that the fact that you have "contamination" with postthymic cells in practically every adult tissue, and in every newborn tissue that you treat, is an important factor to consider that these are cells that are already primed to be sensitive to hormonal stimulation. And, to my mind, some of the data presented concerning effects of cells other than postthymic cells are not too strong, although some of the *in vitro* antigenic conversions by Boyse have shown that they induce intrathymic markers such as TL on those cells, suggesting that perhaps one can reproduce the type of intrathymic event *in vitro*.

Biological Activity of Thymic Hormones

THE HELPER CELL ACTIVITY OF T CELLS FROM DIFFERENT SOURCES

W. B. VAN MUISWINKEL*, O. B. ZAALBERG°, G. MAJOOR°, F. H. LUBBE°, P. L. VAN SOEST* & J. J. VAN BEEK*.

The helper cell activity of different T cells was studied both *in vivo* and *in vitro*. Three types of T cells were used:

a. Normal thymocytes (NT) derived from 5-6 weeks old (DBA/2×C57BL/Rij) F_1 mice.

b. Corticosteroid-resistant thymocytes (CRT) derived from mice 48 h after i.p. injection of 30 mg/kg dexamethasone-21-phosphate (Merck and Co., Inc., Rahway, N.J., U.S.A.).

c. Educated T cells (EdT) obtained from spleens of mice 6 or 7 days after irradiation and i.v. injection of 5×10^7 NT and 4×10^8 sheep red blood cells (SRBC) (1).

d. Spleen cells enriched for T cells (Spleen T) were obtained by incubation of normal spleen cells in nylon wool columns for 45 minutes at 37 °C (2).

The helper cell activity of the different T cells was studied *in vivo* by means of cell transfer experiments. Irradiated recipients were i.v. injected with 4×10^8 SRBC, 3×10^7 spleen cells from adult thymectomized, irradiated and bone marrow-reconstituted mice (B cells) and various numbers of T cells. The spleen of the recipients was removed on day 7 and the number of IgM-, IgG- and IgA-plaque forming cells (PFC) was determined with the plaque assay (3, 4). The number of PFC was considered as a measure of the helper cell activity of the T cells.

It was observed that optimal PFC responses could be obtained when 10^7 CRT or 3×10^6 EdT were transferred (Table I). However, suboptimal IgG-PFC responses were observed when the usual number of NT (5×10^7) was injected. Even 10^8 NT did not show the same helper activity as 10^7 CRT. Due to the occurrence of embolism higher numbers of NT could not be injected into the recipients. These observations indicate that the use of CRT or EdT as helper cells should be preferred to obtain optimal PFC-responses in an *in vivo* transfer system.

The helper cell activity of the different T cells was studied *in vitro* by using the culture system of Mishell and Dutton (5). Normal mouse spleen cells were incubated *in vitro* with SRBC (10^7) in the presence of NT, CRT, EdT or spleen T cells. The response in control cultures containing only normal spleen

* Dept. of Cell Biology and Genetics, Erasmus University, Rotterdam, and
° Medical Biological Laboratory TNO, Rijswijk Z.H., The Netherlands.

TABLE I

THE HELPER CELL ACTIVITY OF DIFFERENT T CELLS *in vivo*

Cells transferred		*PFC/recipient spleen*		
T cells ($\times 10^6$)	*B cells* ($\times 10^6$)	*IgM*	*IgG*	*IgA*
–	30	1.540	3.450	950
100 NT	30	16.460	49.160	11.630
10 CRT	30	18.900	130.400	21.350
–	30	220	600	220 (n.s.)
50 NT	30	5.140	13.910	950 (n.s.)
3 EdT	30	13.000	201.000	10.000

n.s.=The number of indirect plaques (IgM-PFC+IgA-PFC) did not differ significantly from the number of direct plaques (IgM-PFC).

cells and SRBC was 1000 to 2000 IgM-PFC/dish on day 5. It is known that the T cell is the limiting cell type in mouse spleen cell cultures (6). Therefore an enhanced response could be expected when T helper cells are added to the cultures. However, the number of IgM-PFC decreased when 1 to 5 $\times$ 10^6 NT 2 $\times$ 10^6 CRT or 1 to 10$\times$$10^6$ spleen T cells were added. A clear increase in the PFC response was observed when 0.5 to 2$\times$$10^6$ EdT were added as helper cells. This stimulating effect of the addition of EdT was reduced when 4$\times$$10^6$ NT, EdT were used (Table II).

It is obvious that NT and high numbers of CRT affect a suppressive influence on the humoral response *in vitro* and a stimulating influence on the response *in vivo*. Possibly the NT and CRT population contains only relatively undif-

TABLE II

THE EFFECT OF T CELLS ON THE IMMUNE RESPONSE OF NORMAL SPLEEN CELLS CULTURED *in vitro*

T cells ($\times 10^6$)	*Normal spleen cells* ($\times 10^6$)	*IgM-PFC/dish* (*Fraction of control*)
1 NT	19	0.86
2 NT	18	0.50
5 NT	15	0.39
0.2 CRT	20	1.02
0.5 CRT	20	0.91
2 CRT	18	0.54
0.5 EdT	20	2.82
2 EdT	18	3.23
4 EdT	16	1.29
1 Spleen T	10	0.90
5 Spleen T	10	0.87
10 Spleen T	10	0.75

ferentiated T cells (T_1) which have to differentiate to more active T cells (T_2) before they can act as helper cells. The lymphoid organs in the animal probably provide a more suitable micro-environment for the differentiation from T_1 to T_2 than the culture dish. Factors which play a role in the differentiation from T_1 to T_2 could be antigens and thymic hormones.

REFERENCES

1. Mitchell, G. F. & Miller, J. F. A. P. (1968) *Proc. Natl. Acad. Sci. (Wash.)* **59**, 296.
2. Julius, M. H., Simpson, E. & Herzenberg, L. A. (1973) *Eur. J. Immunol.* **3**, 645.
3. Zaalberg, O. B., van der Meul, V. A. & van Twisk, M. J. (1968) *J. Immunol.* **100**, 451.
4. Benner, R., Meima, F., van der Meulen, G. M. & van Muiswinkel, W. B. (1974) *Immunology* **26**, 247.
5. Mishell, R. I. & Dutton, R. W. (1967) *J. Exp. Med.* **126**, 423.
6. Vann, D. C. & Dotson, C. R. (1974) *J. Immunol.* **112**, 1149.

Biological Activity of Thymic Hormones
© Kooyker Scientific Publications, Rotterdam, The Netherlands

THE IMMUNOCONVERSION OF PRECURSOR CELLS BY THE PERFUSED THYMIC GLAND

Studies in the acquisition of functional cell-mediated immunological characteristics in vitro

RAPHAEL H. LEVEY & RICHARD BURLESON

In the past ten years, a wide variety of thymic extracts of varying biological activity have been described. These substances are polypeptides and have been classified as thymic hormones. However, there has been no clear demonstration of the site of action of these materials and no general agreement as to the cell upon which they act. The classic definition of a hormone requires that it is a product of living cells that circulates in body fluids and produces a specific effect on the activities of cells *remote* from its point of origin. This definition does not preclude the possibility that the substance acts at a very short distance, and it is possible that the thymus naturally exercises its action within the gland itself rather than at a great distance. This hypothesis does not negate the internal validity of those experiments in which active compounds have been isolated from calf thymuses or from the sera, but only suggests that in the intact animal the primary sequence of events that leads to the acquisition of immunocompetence are intrathymic in nature and do not occur at the periphery. An extension of this theory is that further steps in differentiation and/or modulation could indeed occur in the lymph nodes, spleen, etc., but such alterations would not be possible without the initial intrathymic events.

In an attempt to mimic *in vitro* the steps that lead to *in vivo* acquisition of immunological competence, we have taken advantage of the blood supply to the thymus to establish the gland in whole organ culture by retrograde perfusion of the aorta. Each lobe of the thymus is fed by vessels arising from the subclavian artery, internal carotid artery, and internal mammary artery. Six days of organ culture lead to selective depletion of medullary lymphocytes. However, the epithelial reticular elements remain intact. Transplantation of the gland after 5 days of perfusion into neonatally thymectomized hosts leads to a reconstitution of the test animals. The kinetics of cell release from the thymus and the behavior of cells added to the perfusion circuit have shown that it is possible to clearly recognize those cells that are added exogenously

Department of Surgery, Harvard Medical School, Children's Hospital Medical Center, Boston, Massachusetts, U.S.A.
Supported by American Cancer Society Grant No. IM-36A, United States Public Health Service Grant No. AM16392-02, and the Charles E. Merrill Trust Fund

to the circuit, and those cells that are recovered, and to attribute any observed effects to passage of the cells through the gland itself.

In order to demonstrate acquisition of immunocompetence by incompetent precursor cells, two sources of such cells were chosen: 1) spleen cells from neonatally thymectomized mice, and 2) a subpopulation of bone marrow cells recovered by discontinuous albumin gradient centrifugation of whole marrow, using only those cells which have no biological attributes of thymus-derived lymphocytes. Of course, neither of these two cell groups excludes the possible inclusion of "postthymic cells".

Spleen cells from neonatally thymectomized mice passaged through the *in vitro* perfusing rat thymus gland acquired the ability to mount graft versus host reactions in appropriate recipients. Incubation of these cells in a perfusate which had previously percolated through the gland for up to 48 h failed to confer this reactivity. Furthermore, passage through a syngeneic spleen was also ineffective in bestowing competence.

Using an entirely syngeneic circuit in which C57Bl/6 marrow stem cells (*vide supra*) were perfused through a C57Bl/6 thymus, similar results were obtained in two test systems. The first involved the ability to mount a graft versus host reaction in F_1 recipients and the second measured the capacity of such passaged cells to adoptively break neonatal transplantation tolerance in adult-thymectomized recipients. Only passage through the gland itself led to acquisition of these abilities and incubation in the perfusate failed to do so.

Newborn mice had been rendered tolerant by the intravenous injection of hybrid cells within 24 h of birth, grafted at 5 weeks of age with second parental skin, and thymectomized 5 weeks later. Only those animals bearing healthy skin grafts 50 days after grafting were considered highly tolerant. The acquisition of immunocompetence in this regard was striking, and the inoculation of perfused cells led to prompt graft breakdown.

We had previously demonstrated that the thymus gland could be repopulated with cells active in delayed hypersensitivity responses by chronic treatment of the host animal with heterologous antilymphocyte serum. Furthermore, the depleted population could be promptly restored by the intravenous injection of appropriate marrow precursor cells. This substantiated the concept that the marrow is the source of stem cells upon which the thymus exerts its effect. The other salient feature of this system was the reappearance of immunocompetent cells in the animal chronically treated with antilymphocyte serum, first in the thymus and only after a significant lag in peripheral lymphoid organs, suggesting export of competent cells rather than conversion of precursors at the periphery.

Taken together, these data indicate that the thymus produces immunocompetence in stem cells within the thymus itself and that physical traffic through the gland is a crucial event in the life history of the thymus-derived cell. Also, on a cell-to-cell basis, passage through the gland *in vitro* restores a level of competence equal to that seen in a subpopulation of cells recovered from the thymus by discontinuous albumin gradient centrifugation.

We have no evidence that the thymus is secreting active substances into the perfusate and have been unable to demonstrate immunoconversion by perfusion of the cells through a syngeneic spleen.

The results show that cell-to-cell contact within the thymus is the means by which the thymus exercises its guiding role in the immunological processes in the intact animal. We cannot exclude the possibility that other means of differentiation and modulation play a role in the development of the thymus-derived cell. Further analysis of the secretory activity of the epithelial reticular elements *in situ* will be necessary to shed light on these questions.

REFERENCES

Burleson, R. & Levey, R. H. (1971) *Transplant. Proc.* **3**, 918.
Levey, R. H. & Burleson, R. (1972) *Cellular Immunology* **4**, 305.
Levey, R. H. & Burleson, R. (1972) *Cellular Immunology* **4**, 316.
Burleson, R. & Levey, R. H. (1972) *Cellular Immunology* **4**, 333.
Levey, R. H. & Burleson, R. (1974) Submitted to *Cellular Immunology*.
Levey, R. H. & Burleson, R. (1974) Submitted to *Cellular Immunology*.

Biological Activity of Thymic Hormones

DISCUSSION

STUTMAN, New York

The fraction 3 is the BSA gradient fraction, right?

LEVEY, Boston

Yes.

CANTOR, Boston

The question of ALS being unphysiologic is certainly a real one and we did note that the increased activity seen in the thymus after ALS was not accompanied by a reduction in the cellularity of the tissues, thus the kind of steroid mediated stress effects that one might anticipate after injection of foreign serum were not present. As to the multiple transplant experiments, I agree with Dr. Levey that with all those thymuses, the lack of any increased T dependent activity must be telling us something about feedback regulatory mechanisms controlling the production of immunocompetent T cells.

VAN BEKKUM, Rijswijk

In connection with the remark of Dr. Levey, I would like to recall the experiments of Mark Dabrowski (*Transplantation 14* (1972) pp. 321-324), who noticed that neonatally thymectomized rats do not show any T cell function for the first 3 months after birth, but when they grow, keeping them under protective conditions, their T cell functions such as PHA responsiveness, gradually reappear after about 1 year.

ROELANTS, Basel

Those cells seem to have specific receptors for antigen already.

Biological Activity of Thymic Hormones

DEPENDENCY OF THYMUS LYMPHOCYTE KINETICS ON AGE AND PERIPHERAL ANTIGENIC STIMULATION

M. W. HESS, B. J. BRYANT* & H. COTTIER

The thymus is considered to be largely autonomous in its relation to other lymphoid organs and to the animal's experience with peripheral antigen exposure. Intrathymic lymphocyte production and differentiation – under intrinsic and humoral control – yield immunocompetent cells whose configurations of antigen receptors are determined by genetic rather than environmental factors. As Dr. White would put it, there is an alternative hypothesis, and I should like to point to some data that suggest an additional subtle, but significant, role of the antigenic environment in thymic activities, as assessed by kinetic studies.

The general notion that most newly-produced thymocytes appear to die in the thymus lingers on. However, the incidence of thymic pyknotic nuclei or fragments in SPF Swiss mice during their first days of life is in the order of 5 per 10,000 cells, while in conventional animals this figure is from 40 to 50 times higher. This difference is apparent shortly after birth, i.e., before adrenocortical steroids are secreted. It suggests that environmental factors may promote thymocyte death. Is this due to penetration of antigenic material into the thymus? There are no real hard data to support the notion of an impenetrable thymic barrier. And there is some evidence to indicate that with advancing age this incomplete barrier function may become increasingly compromised. Primary stimulation of 15-month-old Swiss mice with tetanus toxoid via footpads is followed by an early lymphoproliferative response in the thymus, preceeding by 24 h proliferative changes in regional lymph nodes. Peripheral administration of PHA, properly absorbed and filtered, to young adult mice caused a massive efflux of small lymphocytes from the thymus to the periphery within a day (1, 2).

These observations suggest that the thymus may respond to changes in peripheral demand for new thymus-derived cells. Environmental antigens encountered in the first postnatal days, especially the enormous antigenic challenge from a developing intestinal flora, may underlie the greatest such demand during the life-span of the animal. Accordingly, massive emigration of thymus lymphocytes to gut-associated lymphoid organs has been demonstrated to correlate with an early peak of thymic lymphocytes which exhibit initial labeling

Institute of Pathology, University of Bern, CH-3010 Bern, Switzerland and *Department of Pathology, Wayne State University, Detroit, Mich. 48201, U.S.A.

with tritiated thymidine. The fraction of the emigrant population that survives as long-lived cells in the periphery decreases to 1 per cent or less in adult mice. This decreased survival correlates not only with decreased demand but also with a lengthening of intrathymic transit of small lymphocytes from 54 to 72 h and a fall in the initial labeling index from 19 to 13 per cent. The survival of thymus-derived cells thus seems to be tuned to demand while demand – in developing animals – also appears to influence thymocytokinetics (3). This mutual dependence – even if it is unknown at present how it is brought about – should be kept in mind when speculating on thymic functions.

REFERENCES

1. Bryant, B. J. (1972) *Europ. J. Immunol.* **2**, 38.
2. Bryant, B. J., Hess, M. W. & Cottier, H. (1975) *Immunology* (in press).
3. Bryant, B. J., Hess, M. W. & Cottier, H. (in press) *Proc. Hanford Symposium*, Richland, Wash. 1974.

Biological Activity of Thymic Hormones

DISCUSSION

WHITE, Palo Alto

Would you consider at some future date trying to answer the question of whether the word "demand" lies on the level of the hypothesis.

HESS, Bern

What do you mean?

WHITE, Palo Alto

Whether the response to a stimulus is the basis of the hypothesis.

HESS, Bern

O.K., I agree.

CANTOR, Boston

It might be useful to note that the type of thymocyte that migrates to the periphery is not clear. For example, the work of Elliott suggests that medullary cells never seem to migrate, at least in the 60 days he studies. The experiments using calf thymuses suggest that cells having antigens comparable to TL in the mouse are found in high concentrations in thymic effluent, lymphatics, and veins. So, I think it might be appropriate to ask what kind of cells emigrate from the thymus and are they in fact limited to the so-called mature subset.

HESS, Bern

I have never said that medullary thymocytes emigrate. To my mind, the medulla of the thymus is at least partly hooked on to the recirculating lymphocyte pool. If you study the kinetics of lymphocyte production in the thymus, you find that newly produced cells from the outer cortex migrate towards the corticomedullary junction from where they leave. They are small lymphocytes and they are certainly Thy-1 cells.

DE SOUSA, New York

We labelled the thymus of rats *in situ* to see whether we could detect reasonable numbers of cells eventually in the thoracic duct lymph and in fact we failed to find this. The question, I would like to put to all of you, that is, to Max Hess, Stutman, Jean-Francois Bach, Harvey Cantor: if one is going to discriminate between the lymphocyte in the thymus cortex and in the periphery whether anybody has done experiments with local irradiation of the thymus and looked at the change of Ly-1 lymphocyte in the blood.

CANTOR, Boston

I have not done, but Dr. I. Weismann from Stanford has done the following experiment: he has administered cortisone to mice and asked what effect the cortisone has on the rate of migration of cells from the thymus to the peripheral lymphoid tissues. He found that after cortisone the rate of migration was reduced about 90 per cent, suggesting that either cortisone-sensitive cells are the main emigrants from the thymus or that cortisone has some direct effect on the migratory capacity of thymocytes.

HESS, Bern

For how long was this effect observed?

CANTOR, Boston

I think between 2 and 3 days after cortisone.

BACH, Paris

To complicate the problem further; when looking at the serum level of circulating thymic factors after cortisone treatment or irradiation we show a decrease in the serum level of the factor and thus probably a depression of the epithelial thymic function, although not dramatic and readily reversible.

Biological Activity of Thymic Hormones

A CANDIDATE FOR A T COMMITTED PRETHYMIC LYMPHOCYTE

G. E. ROELANTS, K. S. MAYOR, L-B. HÄGG & F. LOOR

Results obtained in congenitally athymic nude mice and in surgically T deprived mice define a new type of lymphocyte characterized by:

a) a low membrane density of the θ antigen as well as TL in TL^+ strains

b) the absence of surface Ig detectable by immunofluorescence

c) a slow electrophoretic mobility similar to that of thymocytes and not of peripheral T cells

d) its presence in all lymphoid organs of nude or T deprived mice, especially spleen where it may represent 20 per cent of all lymphocytes

e) it is not recirculating through the thoracic duct but is present in peripheral blood

f) it has a very rapid turn over with a half life of 1-2 days

g) it bears specific receptors for antigen but does not appear to be functioning as a mature T lymphocyte

This cell is present in nude mice born from homozygous nude mothers.

The possibility that it represents a prethymic T cell precursor is supported by the fact that it appears rapidly after thymic deprivation and disappears rapidly after thymus grafting. Moreover, the absence of these cells only one or two days after thymus insertion in a millipore diffusion chamber suggests an hormonal regulation of its production.

REFERENCES

Loor, F. & Roelants, G. E. (1974) *Nature* **251**, 229.

Roelants, G. E., Loor, F., von Boehmer, H., Sprent, J., Hägg, L-B., Mayor, K. S. & Rydén, A. (In press) *Eur. J. Immunol.*

Basel Institute for Immunology, CH-4058, Basel, Switzerland.

Biological Activity of Thymic Hormones

DISCUSSION

LEVEY, Boston

I like to make two points, partly bearing on this and partly on a point that was brought up earlier. If one looks at patients with the Di-George syndrome, that is, with no demonstrable thymic function, and thymus tissue (as proven by detailed exploration of the mediastinum) and one follows those patients long enough, then 50 per cent of those patients will spontaneously turn themselves on, slowly regaining different parameters of T cell function. The second point I would like to make is one that Dr. Cantor raised, namely, the matter of feedback. If one takes an adult mouse and grafts it with up to 20 syngeneic thymuses, these thymuses will all take and look perfectly healthy as well, but the recipients are not superthymic. They will still reject a skin graft in a normal time. We have repeated this work in the course of some other experiments, but it was originally described by Metcalf. One has to be very careful about the manipulations to which one subjects a mouse with injections of substances which may be unphysiological.

DICKE, Rijswijk

So you want to say that these cells do not have the Ly-1 2 3^+ antigens on their cell surface.

ROELANTS, Basel

We did not look at that.

DICKE, Rijswijk

This would be extremely important, because then you would not have described a new cell, but it would fit in completely with the theory of Dr. Cantor that you have detected a precursor T_1 cell.

ROELANTS, Basel

Yes sir, we don't know that. Maybe it is still before his T_1 that this cell really expresses a little bit of theta and a little bit of TL as a kind of a passport to enter the thymus, but I doubt the maturation will start maybe in the Ly-antigen, only when it enters the thymus. We don't know that.

Biological Activity of Thymic Hormones

CHARACTERISTICS OF THF, A THYMIC HORMONE

NATHAN TRAININ, MYRA SMALL, DOV ZIPORI, TEHILA UMIEL,
ABRAHAM I. KOOK & VARDA ROTTER

1. INTRODUCTORY REMARKS

It has been demonstrated in different laboratories, including ours, that the impaired capacity of neonatally thymectomized (NTx) animals to reject skin grafts and to induce a graft-versus-host (GvH) response is partially restored either by implantation of cell-impermeable diffusion chambers containing thymus tissue (1-6), or by injection of cell-free thymic extracts (7-11). Moreover, it has been recently shown in our laboratory that THF increases the cytotoxic reactivity of lymphoid cells against syngeneic tumors *in vitro* and *in vivo* (12, 13).

THF was also shown to restore cellular GvH reactivity and the ability of spleen cells from NTx mice to produce a primary immune response to sheep red blood cells (14-17). It was found that a brief *in vitro* contact between syngeneic or xenogeneic thymic preparations and incompetent lymphoid cells confers immune maturation upon young immature thymus and thymus derived cells, and that this induction of immunocompetence by THF occurs prior to antigenic stimulation (14-17).

With this background information, several related questions have been raised recently in our laboratory. What is the chemical nature of the active humoral factor of the thymus? What are the biochemical mechanisms involved in the induction of immune maturation of lymphoid cells? How does THF modify the behaviour of cells of the lymphoid system or of the hemopoietic compartment in additional biological models?

The following is a brief account of work done to elucidate these points.

2. CHEMICAL NATURE OF THF

The bioassay routinely used to evaluate the activity of THF is the *in vitro* GvH model adopted from Auerbach & Globerson (18). It was shown in our laboratory that spleen cells from NTx mice are incompetent to react in this assay (14). Therefore, the biological activity of THF is expressed by its ability to induce competence in these cells to react in the *in vitro* GvH test. In the following isolation procedure, cultures of spleen cells of NTx parental C57BL/

Department of Cell Biology, The Weizmann Institute of Science, Rehovot, Israel.

6 mice and of control syngeneic (C57BL/6×C3H/eb) F_1 mice were simultaneously exposed to THF preparations from calf thymus.

The standard procedure used in our laboratory for preparation of THF was as follows: Fresh thymus was homogenized in 2 volumes of 0.005 Na phosphate buffer, pH 7.4. The homogenate was centrifuged at 2500 rpm for 20 min and the supernatant was further centrifuged at 105.000×g for 5 h. This supernatant was then dialyzed against 20 times larger volume of water for 60 h. The THF passed through Union Carbide dialysis sacs No. 27/32 or 23/32, suggesting that the M.W. of the active material is roughly 6000 or less (15). The dialyzate was lyophylized and diluted to standard protein concentration for biological tests. Further purification was achieved along the following steps. The lyophylized dialyzate is fractionated by gel filtration through G-10 Sephadex column, where the activity is recovered in the void volume (Fig. 1, A). This activity is further fractionated by gel filtration on G-25 Sephadex column and the peak containing the active material is chromatographed on DEAE Sepha-

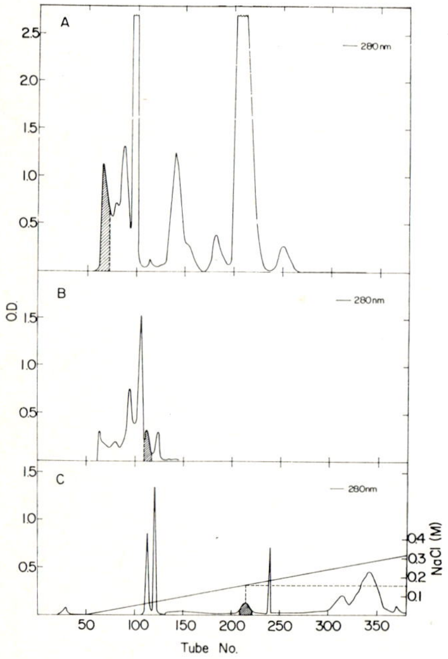

Fig. 1. A. The elution pattern of the dialyzate obtained from supernatant of homogenized calf thymus on Sephadex G-10 columns (2.75×135 cm). 5 ml were collected per tube at a rate of 0.5 ml/min. Outer volume 330 ml. Shaded area represents activity eluted from the column. B. The elution pattern of the active peak obtained from A on a Sephadex G-25 fine column (2.75×135 cm). 5 ml were collected per tube at a rate of 0.5 ml/min. Shaded area represents activity eluted from the column. C. The elution pattern of the active peak obtained from B on DEAE Sephadex A-25 column (2.42×55 cm). The column was equilibrated with 0.1 M Tris-HCl pH 8.0 buffer and the material eluted with a linear gradient of NaCl. 3 ml were collected per tube at a rate of 0.5 ml/min. Shaded area represents activity eluted from the column.

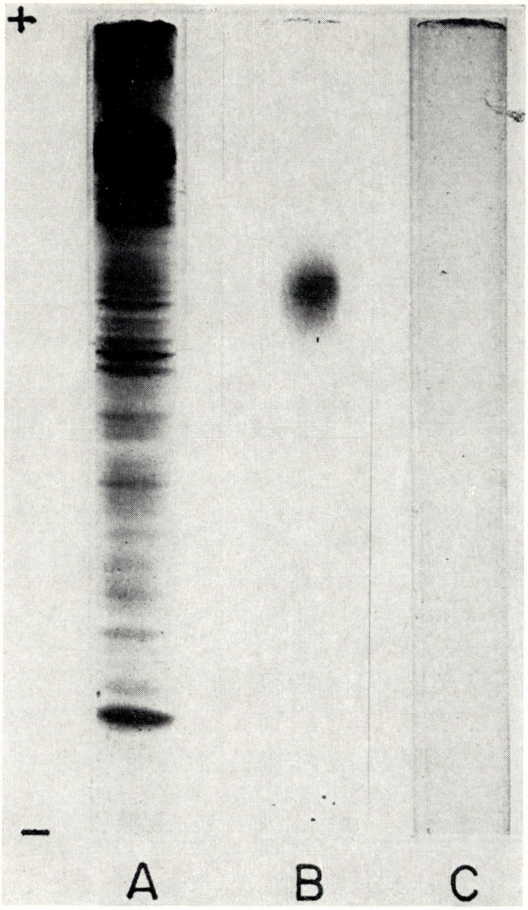

Fig. 2. Isoelectric focusing on 7.5 per cent polyacrylamide gels of *A*. 80 μg protein of the dialysate of calf thymus extract fixed with trichloroacetic acid and stained for protein with Coomassie blue. *B*. 80 μg protein of the active peak eluted from the anion exchange chromatography column fixed with trichloroacetic acid and stained for protein with Coomassie blue. *C*. 80 μg protein of the active peak eluted from the anion exchange chromatography column fixed with trichloacetic acid, oxidized in periodic acid, washed with potassium metabisulfite and stained for glycopeptides with Alcian blue. The measured pH gradient ranged from 3.5 at the anode to 8.4 at the catode poles.

dex A-25 anion exchanger developed with a linear concentration gradient of NaCl (Fig. 1, B and C). The activity which is concentrated in one peak eluted at 0.15 M NaCl, is represented by one active protein species having a pI of 5.7-5.9 as analyzed by isoelectric focusing on polyacrylamide gels (Fig. 2). Calibration of the G-25 Sephadex column with insulin (M.W. 5700), glucagon (M.W. 3460) and bacitracin (M.W. 1400), revealed the THF to be a polypeptide of M.W. of approximately 3000. The activity of the preparation is abolished by pronase treatment but not with DNase or RNase. No glycopeptide was

TABLE I

ANALYSIS OF AMINO ACID COMPOSITION OF THF*

Amino acid residue	*nmol*	*No. of residues (Leucine = 1)*
Asp:	160.98	4
Thr:	45.02	1
Ser:	186.07	5
Glu:	280.20	8
Pro:	72.50	2
Gly:	170.60	5
Ala:	66.30	2
Leu:	36.44	1
Lys:	49.64	1
Arg:	57.65	2
		Sum: 31

* The amino-acid analysis (320 μg protein of THF) shows no unusual amino acids. Based on Leucine as unit, the minimal molecular weight is 3220.

detected on the gels. Analysis of the amino acid composition of THF revealed the presence of 31 residues of 10 amino acids. The M.W. based on the amino acid composition is 3220 (Table I). The acidic nature of the peptide is expressed by the relatively high proportion of acidic amino acids. Thus, out of 31 residues glutamic acid, serine and aspartic acid constitute 8, 5 and 4 residues respectively.

3. INTRACELLULAR EVENTS OF BIOCHEMICAL NATURE INVOLVED IN INDUCTION OF MATURATION OF TARGET CELLS BY THF

These experiments were aimed at the understanding of the mechanism by which THF induces immune competence in immature lymphoid cells, the *in vitro*

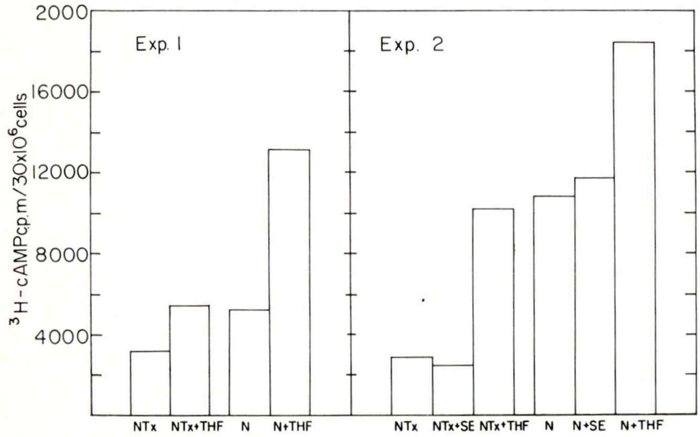

Fig. 3. The effect of THF on adenyl cyclase activity in spleen cells from NTx and normal (N) C57BL/6 mice. Spleen extract (Spl. Ex.) was used as control. Cells were incubated in the presence of 20 μg protein per ml of THF or Spl. Ex. for 1 h at 37 °C in E.M.

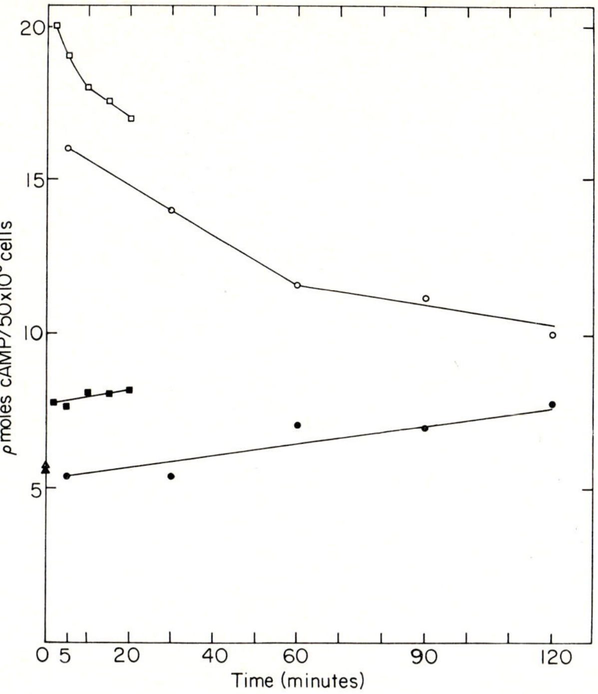

Fig. 4. The effect of THF on intracellular levels of cAMP in thymocytes of C57BL/6 mice. 50×10^6 cells were incubated in 2 ml of E.M. at 37 °C. Incubation started by addition of 50 μg protein per ml of THF. (○——○), (□——□), THF present; (●——●), (■——■) THF absent; (△), (▲) normal levels of cAMP.

GvH model being used for this purpose. It was found that THF induces a rapid activation of membranal adenyl cyclase (Fig. 3), in spleen cells from NTx and normal mice, and an increase in cellular levels of cAMP in thymocytes (Fig. 4). The induction of adenyl cyclase activity is probably due to structural

TABLE II

EFFECT OF VARIOUS CONCENTRATIONS OF DIBUTYRYL CAMP (D-B CAMP) ON THE INDUCTION OF IN VITRO GVH RESPONSE BY SPLEEN CELLS OF NTX C57BL/6 MICE

Substance tested	*Concentration (μg/ml medium)*	*Incidence of reactive cultures*	*Culture response* (%)
–	–	0/5 1/8 0/5	6
THF	20+	4/5 6/8	77
D-B cAMP	0.0005*	0/5 0/8	0
D-B cAMP	0.001*	3/5 6/8 3/5	67
D-B cAMP	0.005*	1/5 1/8	15

+ μg of protein per 1 ml culture medium added at the start of cultures.
* μg of D-B cAMP per 1 ml culture medium added at the start of cultures.

TABLE III

THE EFFECT OF THEOPHYLLINE ON THE INDUCTION OF IN VITRO GvH RESPONSE BY SPLEEN CELLS OF NTx C57BL/6 MICE

Substance tested	*Concentration (μg/ml medium)*	*Incidence of reactive cultures*		*Culture response* (%)
–	–	1/5	0/5	10
THF	20 μg protein	3/5	4/5	70
Theophylline	0.001 μg	4/5	5/5	90

changes induced in the cell membrane by THF (19). (The THF preparation itself does not contain any detectable amounts of cAMP). The level of adenyl cyclase activity was found to be low in spleen cells from NTx mice and was restored to that of spleen cell population from intact mice, following exposure of the cells to THF (Fig. 3). The activation of adenyl cyclase and the increase in cellular levels of cAMP were found to be directly related to the process of induction of immune competence in spleen cells of NTx mice by THF. Thus, substances which were found to increase intracellular levels of cAMP such as DBcAMP, theophylline (an inhibitor of cyclic nucleotide phosphodiesterase known to increase cellular levels of cAMP (20)), or prostaglandin E_2 (PGE_2), were found to mimic the effect of THF and confer reactivity to spleen cells from NTx mice in the *in vitro* GvH assay (Tables II, III and IV). These substances exhibited a dose response curve, typical to effects mediated via cAMP. Moreover, it was found that the increase in cellular cAMP levels is an obligatory event in the process of induction of immune competence by THF. Thus, the ability of spleen cells from NTx mice to respond to allogeneic stimulation was abolished when the increase of cellular cAMP was prevented, while the immune competence of spleen cells from intact mice was not impaired under this condition (21) (Table IV).

TABLE IV

THE INDUCTION OF GvH RESPONSE IN SPLEEN CELLS OF NTx C57BL/6 MICE BY INCUBATION WITH PGE_2 AND INHIBITION OF THE EFFECT BY FLUFENAMIC ACID

Substance (concentration)	*Source spleen cells**	*Incidence of reactive cultures*			*Culture response* (%)
–	NTx	0/5	0/5		0
THF (50 μg protein/ml)	NTx	4/5	3/5		70
PGE_2 (5 μg/ml)	NTx	5/5	4/5	4/5	87
PGE_2 (5 μg/ml) + flufenamic acid (75 μg/ml)	NTx	1/5	0/5	1/5	13
Flufenamic acid (75 μg/ml)	NTx	1/5	0/5		10
–	Intact	4/5	5/5	5/5	93
Flufenamic acid (75 μg/ml)	Intact	4/5	5/5	5/5	93

* 25×10^6 spleen cells obtained from either NTx or intact mice were incubated with or without the substances tested in 1 ml E.M. for 30 min at 37 °C. Following incubation the cells were washed and tested in the GvH assay.

TABLE V

In vitro GVH RESPONSE OF SPLEEN CELLS OBTAINED FROM NTx C57BL MICE AFTER PREINCUBATION WITH THF OR THEOPHYLLINE*

Substance tested	*Concn. (μg/ml of medium)*	*Incidence of reactive cultures*	*Culture response (%)*
–	–	0/5 0/5 1/5	7
THF	20+	3/5 3/5 4/5	67
Theophylline	0.001	4/5 5/5 4/5	87

* Cells were incubated for 30 min at 37 °C in E.M. or E.M. with THF, or with theophylline. After incubation, the cells were washed in organ culture medium (O.C.M.) and 1×10^6 live cells tested in the GVH assay.
\+ μg protein per 1 ml culture.

These results are consistent with the postulates established by Sutherland to define hormonal action mediated by cAMP (22), and permit the classification of THF as a thymus hormone.

Results of experiments performed in our laboratory (14), demonstrate that THF itself does not provide antigenic stimulation to immature spleen cells from NTx mice. Moreover, it was possible to show that exposure of immature spleen cells to THF, or theophylline for 1 h before their stimulation by alloantigens restored the ability of the cells to react in the *in vitro* GvH assay (Table V) (21). Thus, the induction of immune competence by THF occurs prior to antigenic stimulation, and is unrelated to antigenic challenge. Our working hypothesis was, therefore, that THF exerts its effect on nonimmunocompetent thymus and thymus derived cells by inducing them to differentiate into mature immunoreactive cells, and that the differentiation and/or matura

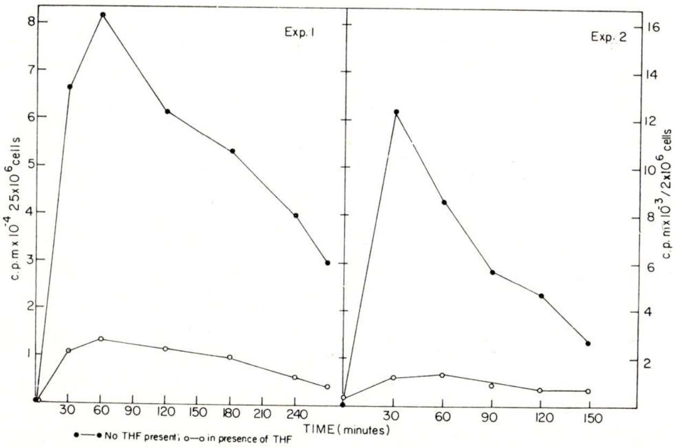

Fig. 5. The effect of THF on the incorporation of ^{3}H-thymidine into DNA of thymocytes (Exp. 1) and of spleen cells from NTx C57BL/6 mice (Exp. 2). Cells were incubated in 1 ml E.M. in presence of 20 μg protein per ml of THF. A 30 min pulse of 2 μCi ^{3}H-thymidine was given before each time point determination.
●—● no THF present; ○——○ in presence of THF.

TABLE VI

THE EFFECT OF CYCLOHEXIMIDE ON PROTEIN SYNTHESIS IN MUSCLE AND LYMPHOID CELLS*

					Cycloheximide (20 μg/ml)				
								Inhibition (%)	
Exp.	*Cell type*	^{14}*C-C.P.M.*	*Protein (mg)*	^{14}*C-C.P.M./mg protein*	^{14}*C-C.P.M.*	*Protein (mg)*	^{14}*C-C.P.M./mg protein*	^{14}*C-C.P.M.*	^{14}*C.P.M./mg protein*
I	muscle	39952	0.79	50587	3262	0.76	4303	92	92
II	spleen cells of intact mice	12732	2.90	4390	10822	2.85	3797	15	14
III	spleen cells of intact mice	15895	–	–	13352	–	–	16	–
IV	spleen cells of NTx mice	10563	–	–	6138	–	–	42	–
V	spleen cells of NTx mice	12339	–	–	7359	–	–	40	–
VI	spleen cells of NTx mice	15667	4.34	3615	9260	4.15	2234	41	38

* Each experiment was done in triplicates. 20×10^6 spleen cells from normal or NTx C57BL/6 mice and 2×10^6 muscle cells from normal rat were incubated for 1 hr at 37 °C in 1 ml E.M. with 2 μCi 1-^{M}C-Leucine in presence or absence of 20 μg cycloheximide. The results shown are averages.

TABLE VII

THE INDUCTION OF GVH RESPONSE IN SPLEEN CELLS OBTAINED FROM INTACT OR NTX C57BL/6 MICE FOLLOWING PREINCUBATION IN PRESENCE OF THF AND CYCLOHEXIMIDE

Substance tested (concentration)	*Source of spleen cells*	*Time of cycloheximide addition following start of incubation (min)*	*Incidence of reactive cultures*			*Culture response (%)*
–	Intact	–	4/5	4/5	4/5	80
cycloheximide (20 μg/ml)	Intact	0	5/5	5/5	4/5	93
–	NTx	–	0/5	0/5	0/5	0
THF (20 μg protein/ml)	NTx	–	4/5	3/5	4/5	73
cycloheximide (20 μg/ml)	NTx	0	0/5	0/5	0/5	0
THF (20 μg protein/ml) + cycloheximide (20 μg/ml)	NTx	−15	0/5	1/5	0/5	6
THF (20 μg protein/ml) + cycloheximide (20 μg/ml)	NTx	0	0/5	0/5	0/5	0
THF (20 μg protein/ml) + cycloheximide (20 μg/ml)	NTx	+15	0/5	0/5	0/5	0

20×10^6 cells per ml were incubated for 1 h at 37 °C in E.M. in presence or absence of THF. Cycloheximide was added 15 min prior to addition of THF, with THF or 15 min after addition of THF. Following incubation the cells were washed twice in O.C.M. and 1×10^6 live cells tested in the GvH assay.

TABLE VIII

THE EFFECT OF THF AND OF SPLEEN EXTRACT (SPL. EX.) ON THE INCORPORATION OF ^{3}H-THYMIDINE INTO DNA OF LYMPHOID CELLS FROM C57BL/6 MICE

Cell type	*Substance tested**	*^{3}H-C.P.M./10×10^6 cells*
Thymocytes	–	25958
	Spl. Ex.	23915
	THF	2069
Spleen cells from NTx mice	–	9672
	Spl. Ex.	9995
	THF	2176
Spleen cells from intact mice	–	5579
	Spl. Ex.	5544
	THF	1675

* Cells were incubated in 1 ml E.M. for 1 h at 37 °C in presence of 20 μg protein of spleen extract (Spl. Ex.) or 20 μg protein of THF. A 30 min pulse of 2 μCi ^{3}H-thymidine was given before incubation was ended. The results shown are averages of two such experiments showing a close pattern.

tion is initiated by a rise in cellular cAMP levels. The observation that immune maturation takes place in the absence of antigenic stimulation allowed the investigation of biochemical events which lead to the acquisition of immunocompetence and which follow the rise in cellular levels of cAMP induced by THF. Indeed, it was possible to demonstrate, using cycloheximide as a reversible inhibitor of protein synthesis (19), that a protein synthesis step is initiated following the rise in cellular cAMP which is a prerequisit for spleen cells from NTx mice to acquire immune maturation (Tables VI and VII). It was thus concluded that, in agreement with established modes of differentiation, a protein synthesis step is involved in the chain of biochemical events induced by THF via cellular cAMP, which lead to maturation of lymphoid cells and acquisition of cell-mediated immune capacity.

Since the effect of intracellular levels of cAMP on cell cycle is well documented (23-25), it was of interest to investigate the effect of THF on DNA synthesis in lymphoid cells. It was found that both thymocytes and spleen cells from NTx mice exposed to THF exhibited increased levels of cAMP and adenyl cyclase activity which persisted for the duration of the preincubation period and were accompanied by a marked reduction in DNA synthesis (Fig. 5 and Table VIII) and the proliferative activity of these cells. Mitomycin-C is a well known inhibitor of DNA synthesis and cell division. However, in contrast to THF, the presence of mitomycin-C during the preincubation period, did not induce spleen cells from NTx mice to respond in the *in vitro* GvH reaction and abolished the reactivity of spleen cells from intact mice in this assay (19).

These results suggest that the inhibitory effect of THF on DNA synthesis in lymphoid cells is a physiological step resulting from a rise in intracellular cAMP levels. Moreover, by preventing cell proliferation, THF via elevated levels of cAMP stimulates protein synthesis and induces the cells to acquire immunocompetence allowing the otherwise immature spleen cells from NTx mice to respond the *in vitro* GvH assay.

It can then be hypothesized that differentiation processes take place during the G_1 or G_2 phases of the cell cycle and/or that the capacity to respond to allogeneic challenge depends on the existence of the cells in one or both phases of their cycle. This implies that cellular levels of cAMP in a lymphoid cell population could determine the ability of the cells to respond to antigenic stimulation.

4. BIOLOGICAL PROPERTIES OF THF

a. *Effect on lymphoid cell reactivity in MLC.*

The observation that DNA synthesis in lymphoid cells is inhibited in the presence of THF led us to assume that immunological reactions which involve intensive and repeated cell divisions should be inhibited by the presence of THF during the assay. Indeed it has been demonstrated that agents that activate adenyl cyclase strongly inhibited the response of lymphoid cells in im-

TABLE IX

MIXED LYMPHOCYTE CULTURE (MLC) BY SPLEEN CELLS PREINCUBATED OR IN THE PRESENCE OF THF

Exp.	*Cell mixture**	*THF§*	*cpm ±S.E.*	*Stimulation index*
Incubation**	ab→abm	—	4,099 ± 1,558	
	ab→abm	+	7,317 ± 889	
	a→abm	—	68,075 ± 8,212	16.6
	a→abm	+	30,172 ± 5,176	4.12
	ab→abm	—	2,865 ± 542	
	ab→abm	+	4,068 ± 248	
	a→abm	—	18,465 ± 3,083	6.4
	a→abm	+	12,984 ± 2,690	3.1
Preincubation***	ab→abm	—	1,530 ± 60	
	ab→abm	+	1,742 ± 64	
	a→abm	—	17,707 ± 462	11.5
	a→abm	+	27,609 ± 684	15.8
	ab→abm	—	3,583 ± 1,223	
	ab→abm	+	3,847 ± 713	
	b→abm	—	11,183 ± 1,125	3.1
	b→abm	+	26,730 ± 1,935	7.0

* a = 10^6 C57BL/6 spleen cells ab = 10^6 (C3H/eb × C57BL/6) F_1 spleen cells b = 10^6 C3H/eb spleen cells. m = mitomycin—C 25 μg/ml cell suspension.
§ 20 μg protein/ml.
** THF present in the culture medium during the MLC assay.
*** Preincubation for 1 h at 37 °C before exposure to MLC.

munological reactions (26, 27, 28, 29). Our hypothesis on the mechanism of THF activity was therefore tested in a one way MCL assay (30). This model was preferred since by pretreatment of the stimulator cells by mitomycin-C the effect measured refers mainly to the degree of immunological competence of the responding cells. Table IX summarizes the results of one way MLC assay in which responding spleen cells from intact mice were exposed to THF duiing the MLC reaction or by 1 h preincubation with THF. It was found that the presence of THF during the MLC reaction significantly decreased the response of the effector cells in the assay. On the contrary preincubation with THF raised the response of these cells over and above that seen in the controls. These results are in line with the concepts previously stated on the mechanism of cellular activation by THF. The results presented point to the fact that preincubation with THF markedly increased the reactivity of spleen cells from intact mice in the MLC assay. This suggests that the spleen of normal mice contains cells which could still be activated by THF. This effect of THF on spleen cells from intact mice could not be measured in the *in vitro* GvH response which by nature is an all or non type of response. Since the MLC response is a cellular immunological event mediated by T lymphocytes, the above experiments suggested that THF increases the activity and/or the number of responding T cells. As the lymphoid cell population of spleens of NTx and intact mice contain a mixture of thymus derived and bone marrow derived cells, two alternative hypotheses could explain THF activity in the above experiments. THF could either influence the differentiation of bone marrow derived cells towards T reactive cells able to respond in MLC reactions, or alternatively THF could induce functional maturation and/or proliferation of cells already possessing T cells properties. To distinguish between these two possibilities, 10^6 bone marrow derived spleen cells obtained from thymectomized irradiated bone marrow reconstituted mice (B cells) were incubated

TABLE X

EFFECT OF THF ON MLC REACTION BY BONE MARROW DERIVED SPLEEN CELLS FROM C57BL/6 MICE

Exp. #	*Cell mixture*[a]	*THF*[b]	*CPM ± SE*	*Stimulation index*
1	a→a_m	—	10804 ± 1360	
	a→ab_m	+	14959 ± 1715	1.3
	a→ab_m	—	14332 ± 3954	1.32
2	a→a_m	—	2557 ± 3894	
	a→a_m	+	3189 ± 2686	
	a→ab_m	—	4437 ± 9684	1.7
	a→ab_m	+	5320 ± 209	1.6
3[c]	a→a_m	—	7853 ± 1021	
	a→a_m	+	7212 ± 350	
	a→ab_m	—	9546 ± 601	1.2
	a→ab_m	+	13625 ± 503	1.8

[a]) a=C57BL/6 ab=(C3H/eb × C57BL/6) F_1 m=mitomycin-C
[b]) preincubation of responding cells in THF for 1 h
[c]) 2×10^6 of each stimulating and responding cells.

with THF and then tested in the MLC response. As seen in Table X, B cells failed to respond in the MLC reaction and further treatment of these cells with THF did not modify this incompetence. Activation was neither observed when the number of B cells participating in the MLC reaction was raised up to 2×10^6 cells (Table X, exp. #3).

The cell population of the thymus is heterogeneous and contain elements at different levels of maturity. Still, they are composed in their majority by immature elements of the lymphoid line with a low competence to participate in immune responses (31, 32, 33). We tested then whether THF could raise the competence of thymocytes to respond in MLC reactions. Two concentrations (1×10^6 and 2×10^6) of thymocytes were tested. While no apparent increase of competence was observed with 10^6 thymic cells after incubation with THF, a striking elevation in the response was obtained when 2×10^6 cells were

TABLE XI

EFFECT OF THF ON MLC REACTION BY THYMOCYTES FROM C57BL/6 AND C3H/eb MICE

Exp. #	*Cell mixture*[a]	*Extract*[b]	*CPM* ± *SE*	*Stimulation index*
1	ab→ab_m	–	3508 ± 164	
	ab→ab_m	THF	3380 ± 143	
	a→ab_m	–	3907 ± 55	1.1
	a→ab_m	THF	3568 ± 353	1.0
2	ab→ab_m	–	3668 ± 54	
	ab→ab_m	THF	3271 ± 1268	
	a→ab_m	–	6300 ± 1620	1.7
	a→ab_m	THF	6352 ± 1256	1.9
3[c]	ab→ab_m	–	1647 ± 197	
	ab→ab_m	THF	1558 ± 117	
	a→ab_m	–	3516 ± 367	2.1
	a→ab_m	THF	12836 ± 1325	8.2
4[c]	ab→ab_m	–	7002 ± 671	
	ab→ab_m	THF	2133 ± 571	
	b→ab_m	–	10060 ± 813	1.43
	b→ab_m	THF	17594 ± 1370	8.2
5[c]	ab→ab_m	–	2044 ± 126	
	ab→ab_m	S.E.	2779 ± 325	
	a→ab_m	–	6639 ± 1340	3.2
	a→ab_m	S.E.	6796 ± 210	2.4

a) a=C57BL/6 b=C3H/eb ab=(C3H/eb × C57BL/6) F_1
m=mitomycin-C

b) preincubation of responding cells in THF or in SE for 1 h.

c) 2×10^6 of each stimulating and responding cells.

used (Table XI). These results suggested therefore that the thymus contain a population of cells which are targets for THF activity. In a further step to check the identity of the cells which within the thymus are the targets for THF activity, we tested the effect of THF on cortisone resistant thymocytes which have already the characteristics of peripheral T cells (34). Table XII shows that while the MLC responding capacity of cortisone resistant thymocytes was about 9 times higher than that of the average thymus cell population, there was no increase in their MLC stimulation index following treatment with THF. These results indicate that the target cells for THF activity are not in the cortisone resistant compartment of the thymus population, but rather among the cortisone sensitive thymocytes which represent about 95 per cent of the thymus cell population. Finally the effect of THF was tested on peripheral lymph node cell population composed in their majority by mature lymphocytes. Lymph node cells were treated with THF as in the previous experiments. The results shown in Table XIII indicate that no augmentation in the MLC response of these cells could be detected following treatment with THF, thus further

TABLE XII

EFFECT OF THF ON MLC REACTION BY CORTISONE RESISTANT THYMOCYTES FROM C57BL/6 MICE

Cell mixture[a]	*THF*[b]	*CPM ± SE*	*Stimulation index*
a→a_m	−	6916 ± 760	
a→a_m	+	7657 ± 642	
a→b_m	−	63670 ± 4892	9.2
a→b_m	+	70122 ± 2526	9.1

[a]) a = C57BL/6 thymocytes b = C3H/eb
m = mitomycin-C
[b]) incubation of responding cells in THF for 1 h.

supporting the concept that the target cells for THF activity are among the less mature lymphoid cell population.

b. *Increased mitogenic reactivity of normal spleen cells to T lectins by THF*

It has been shown that lymphocytes at various stages of maturation react differently to PHA and Con A (35, 36). This prompted us to study the effect of THF on cell reactivity to T-mitogens such as phytohemagglutinin (PHA) and Concanavalin A (Con A) (37), since this may serve as a direct way for evaluating cell maturation. Spleen cells of normal F_1 (C3H/eb × C57BL/6) F_1 mice were suspended in culture medium containing 20 μg THF/ml and exposed to mitogens. As shown in Table XIV, when THF was present in culture medium, a reduction was observed in the reactivity to Con A and PHA as compared to control cultures without THF. However, the response to LPS, a B-mitogen was not changed at all, thus suggesting that the reduced reactivity of spleen cells to T-lectins in the presence of THF was not the result of a toxic effect but rather an expression of antagonism between THF and T-lectins in the activation of the T-cell population. This inhibitory effect was also observed

TABLE XIII

EFFECT OF THF ON MLC REACTION BY LYMPH NODE CELLS FROM C57BL/6 MICE

*Cell mixture**	*THF***	*CPM ± S.E.*	*Stimulation index*
ab→ab_m	−	1204 ± 141	
ab→ab_m	+	1262 ± 258	
a→ab_m	−	52477 ± 834	43.5
a→ab_m	+	40364 ± 1077	32.0

* a = C57BL/6; ab = (C3H/eb × C57BL/6) F_1;
m = mitomycin-C.
** preincubation of responding cells in THF for 1 h.

TABLE XIV

REDUCED REACTIVITY OF SPLEEN CELLS TO T-MITOGENS IN THE PRESENCE OF THF[a]

Mitogens	*Control*		*THF*	
	CPM ±SE	*Ratio of transformation*	*CPM ±SE*	*Ratio of transformation*
–	7811 ± 461	–	9458 ± 312	–
PHA	240208 ± 1145	30.7 ± 2.7	157851 ± 4005	16.6 ± 0.9[b]
Con A	293985 ± 3449	37.6 ± 2.2	147269 ± 11516	15.5 ± 1.6[b]
LPS	53354 ± 3507	6.8 ± 0.7	57101 ± 521	6.0 ± 0.2[c]

a) 20 μg THF/ml in the culture medium
b) $P < 0.001$
c) P = Not significant

when different concentrations of THF were tested in the presence of a constant amount of T-lectins. As seen in Fig. 6, the reduction in the mitogenic reactivity of the treated spleen cells was already observed when a low concentration such as 0.01 μg THF/culture was used. Moreover, the reduction in the activity to the mitogens was found to be proportional to the THF concentration tested. These results suggest that simultaneous administration of both THF and T-lectins exerts an inhibitory effect on the mitogenic reactivity of spleen cells at any concentration of THF used.

As stated before, one hour preincubation of parental cells in THF provoked an increased mixed lymphocyte culture (MLC) reaction. It was, therefore, of interest to investigate whether in the present experimental system 1 h pre-

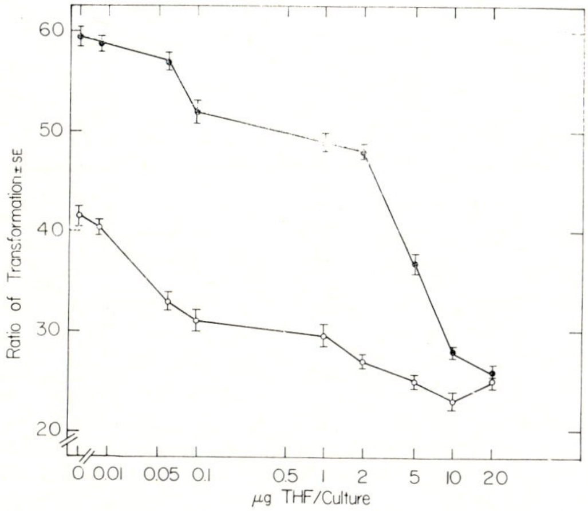

Fig. 6. Reduced mitogenic response of spleen cells in the presence of various concentrations of THF.
● Con A ○ PHA

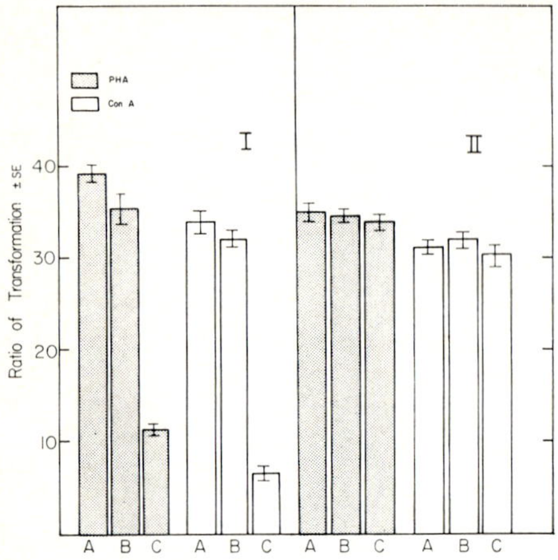

Fig. 7. Mitogenic response of spleen cells treated with THF.
I: THF present in culture medium. II. 1 h preincubation in THF.
A: Control B: Spleen extract C: THF.

incubation in THF will also increase the reactivity of spleen cells to T-lectins. Spleen cells were incubated for 1 h in medium containing THF, then transferred into regular culture medium and the cells were finally submitted to PHA and Con A stimulation. In contrast to the increased response observed in the MLC system, 1 h preincubation in THF did not induce any increase in mitogenic reactivity (Fig. 7). Moreover, no suppressive effect was observed under these conditions, thus suggesting that the inhibitory activity of THF on the response of spleen cells to T-lectins occurs only in the presence of THF.

As previously shown, lymphocyte activation by THF is mediated by an increase in cyclic AMP level in T lymphocytes. On the other hand, lymphocyte activation by T-lectins such as PHA or Con A was shown to result in an increased level of cyclic GMP (38, 39). Therefore, the suppressed activity to T-mitogens observed by simultaneous exposure of cells to THF and T-lectins could be the expression of an antagonism (40, 41) between cyclic AMP induced by THF on one hand and cyclic GMP induced by the mitogen on the other hand. Since both of the above phenomena were shown to occur in the cell immediately after exposure to these substances (21, 38), such an antagonism may exist. It was necessary to test the action of THF on target cells under conditions which could permit the completion of THF effect before the rise in cyclic GMP induced by the mitogens. Spleen cells were therefore incubated for 24 h in culture medium containing 20 μg/ml THF assuming that during this time interval the chain of events induced by THF leading to cell maturation could be completed. After this, the medium was changed and PHA, Con A or LPS were added. Control cell cultures were incubated in regular medium or in medium containing 20 μg/ml spleen extract.

As shown in Table XV, 24 h preincubation in THF caused a marked increased reactivity of spleen cells both to PHA and Con A, as compared to

TABLE XV

INCREASED REACTIVITY OF SPLEEN CELLS TO T-MITOGENS FOLLOWING 24 H PREINCUBATION WITH THF[a]

Mitogens	*Control CPM ±SE*	*Ratio of transformation*	*THF CPM ±SE*	*Ratio of transformation*	*Spleen extract CPM ±SE*	*Ratio of transformation*
–	4480 ± 939	–	5893 ± 1006	–	4690 ± 876	–
PHA	69400 ± 5134	15.5 ± 4.1	179743 ± 9526	30.5 ± 6.7[b]	59925 ± 18010	12.7 ± 6.0
Con A	149039 ± 1443	33.2 ± 7.2	290638 ± 1505	49.3 ± 8.6[c]	134402 ± 1343	28.6 ± 5.1
LPS	58387 ± 2965	13.0 ± 3.2	70203 ± 1583	11.9 ± 2.2[d]	47963 ± 5895	10.2 ± 3.0

a) Culture medium containing THF and controls was changed after 24 h and mitogens were added.
b) $P \leq 0.001$
c) $P = 0.005$
d) P = not significant

TABLE XVI

INFLUENCE OF VARIOUS PERIODS OF PREINCUBATION OF SPLEEN CELLS IN THF ON THEIR RESPONSE TO T-MITOGENS

	CPM ±SE	*PHA CM ±SE*	*Ratio of transformation*	*Con A CPM ±SE*	*Ratio af transformation*
Group A					
–	4466 ± 281	250188 ± 1431	56.0 ± 3.6	338203 ± 25531	75.7 ± 10.2
THF	4549 ± 648	250208 ± 16959	55.0 ± 11.4[a]	313050 ± 22568	68.8 ± 14.7[a]
Spleen extract	5523 ± 211	252458 ± 11079	45.7 ± 3.3	311320 ± 19271	56.3 ± 5.0
Group B					
–	6147 ± 891	74050 ± 5295	12.0 ± 2.1	122440 ± 8100	19.6 ± 3.4
THF	7502 ± 1124	65350 ± 4135	8.7 ± 1.8[a]	123258 ± 11328	16.4 ± 3.7[a]
Spleen extract	7019 ± 411	58952 ± 1281	8.3 ± 0.7	114840 ± 3236	16.3 ± 1.4
Group C					
–	4701 ± 710	299780 ± 1001	63.7 ± 9.7	431518 ± 7999	91.7 ± 15.4
THF	8941 ± 950	230371 ± 2466	25.7 ± 2.8[b]	233739 ± 8066	26.1 ± 3.6[b]
Spleen extract	5829 ± 158	309768 ± 364	53.1 ± 1.5	474273 ± 35911	81.3 ± 7.8
Group D					
–	5700 ± 1373	60813 ± 2470	10.6 ± 2.9	107912 ± 4398	18.9 ± 1.8
THF	6000 ± 130	108696 ± 4021	18.1 ± 1.0[b]	156606 ± 2530	26.1 ± 0.9[b]
Spleen extract	5821 ± 996	67248 ± 201	11.5 ± 1.9	100319 ± 1408	17.2 ± 3.1

Group A: THF and spleen extract were present in culture medium for 1 h, medium was changed and mitogens added.
Group B: Like group A but mitogens were added after 23 h.
Group C: THF and spleen extract were present in culture medium throughout the experiment.
Group D: THF & spleen extract were present in the culture medium for 24 h, then medium was changed & mitogens added.
a) P = not significant b) $P < 0.005$.

cells preincubated in regular medium or in medium containing spleen extract. This increased reactivity was more pronounced vis-a-vis PHA than to Con A. Moreover, as seen in same Table XV, the increased mitogenic reactivity was limited to T-mitogens only, since under the same experimental conditions no change was observed in the response of THF treated cells to LPS a well established B-mitogen. It was then important to elucidate whether 24 h preincubation of cells in THF is essential for the expression of reactivity, or 1 h preincubation is enough provided that the mitogens are added after a further 23 h interval. Therefore, one group of cultures was incubated for 1 h in the presence of THF, the medium was then replaced by normal medium and mitogens were added immediately to half of the cultures (group A), while to the rest mitogens were added 23 h later (group B). THF and mitogens were added together to cultures in group C and in group D, medium containing THF was changed after 24 h and mitogens were then added. As shown in Table XVI, THF increased the reactivity to mitogens only when present for 24 h prior to mitogen stimulation (group D). No increased mitogenic response was observed after 1 h preincubation either when mitogens were added immediately after the incubation period (group A) or when added 23 h later (group B). These results suggest that increased mitogenic response of lymphoid cells to PHA and Con A requires a longer period of THF preincubation than that required by MLC.

c. *Control of autoreactivity by THF*

Early suggestions that self-reactive clones are eliminated during ontogeny must be questioned following the demonstration that potentially autoreactive lymphocytes do exist in adult rodents and that these cells manifest reactivity when removed from normal control mechanisms (42, 43). What then prevents such cells from reacting against self under normal conditions? One mechanism was suggested by previous work in our laboratory which pointed to a role for THF in preventing sensitization against self antigens (44). It was found that spleen cells of normal mice sensitized *in vitro* on syngeneic fibroblast monolayers manifested cytotoxicity against syngeneic tumor cells while addition of thymic extract to the sensitization cultures resulted in a striking inhibition of cytotoxic activity. The interest of this finding in increasing our understanding of the process of autoreactivity as well as the therapeutic implications involved prompted further investigation of the role of THF in controlling antiself reactivity.

The first experiments were performed to evaluate autoreactivity of lymphocytes sensitized against self components by testing their ability to induce a GvH reaction against syngeneic tissue, and to determine the effect of THF on this process. For this purpose, we modified the *in vitro* GvH response usually used to measure allogeneic reactivity, in order to measure the response induced against syngeneic tissue by autosensitized lymphocytes. Thus, the relative enlargement of a newborn C57BL spleen explant challenged by autosensitized

C57BL spleen cells as compared with a paired reference explant exposed to nonsensitized syngeneic spleen cells reflected the response to challenge by autoreactive cells. Spleen cells of C57BL mice were sensitized on fibroblast monolayers of either C57BL or Balb/c origin and these cells were tested against newborn C57BL spleen explants. Sensitized lymphocytes were tested after four days or after 24 hours of sensitization. In both cases, as can be seen in Table XVII, C57BL lymphocytes sensitized on C57BL monolayers induced a GVH reaction against syngeneic tissue, while C57BL cells sensitized on Balb/c monolayers did not show autoreactivity. When THF in the form of thymic extract was introduced into the autosensitization cultures, the response of autosensitized lymphocytes against syngeneic tissue was clearly inhibited in all cases (Table XVII). Thus, lymphocytes sensitized on syngeneic monolayers were found to induce splenomegaly against syngeneic spleen explants while the presence of THF during sensitization prevented this reaction.

TABLE XVII

IN VITRO GVH RESPONSE AGAINST SYNGENEIC TISSUE BY SPLEEN CELLS SENSITIZED ON SYNGENEIC FIBROBLASTS WITH AND WITHOUT THF

Donor of graft cells	*Sensitizing monolayer*	*THF during sensitization*	*Host spleen explants*	*Incidence of reactive cultures**	
	C57BL	—	C57BL	5/6	7/8
Intact C57BL+	C57BL	+	C57BL	1/6	1/8
	Balb/c	—	C57BL	1/6	
	C57BL	—	C57BL	5/6	4/6
Intact C57BL†	C57BL	+	C57BL	1/6	1/5
	Balb/c	—	C57BL		1/6

* Number of cultures with a spleen index ≥ 1.2 per total number of cultures tested.

\+ THF at a concentration of 20 μg/ml was added to the medium for the duration of the sensitization. Cells were harvested after 4 days of sensitization and 1×10^6 sensitized lymphocytes were assayed in comparison to 1×10^6 nonsensitized syngeneic spleen lymphocytes.

† Lymphocyte suspensions were supplemented with THF at a concentration of 50 μg/ml for 1 hour prior to sensitization. The cell suspensions+THF were added to the monolayer without washing. Cells adhering to the monolayer were harvested after 24 hours of sensitization by removal of medium with nonadherent cells and vigorous pipetting of adherent cells. $.5 \times 10^6$ sensitized lymphocytes were assayed in comparison to $.5 \times 10^6$ nonsensitized syngeneic spleen lymphocytes.

In the next experiments the spleen cells submitted to sensitization were obtained from neonatally thymectomized mice. This enabled simultaneous comparison of the effect of THF on lymphoid cells participating in autoreactivity or alloreactivity. C57BL cells were harvested after 24 h of autosensitization and aliquots of each sample were tested in parallel against syngeneic or allogeneic spleen explants. Autosensitized C57BL cells exhibited the capacity to induce a GVH response against syngeneic tissue in nearly all of the assay

TABLE XVIII

IN VITRO GVH RESPONSES OF SPLEEN CELLS FROM NEONATALLY THYMECTOMIZED MICE SENSITIZED ON SYNGENEIC FIBROBLASTS WITH AND WITHOUT THF*

Donor of graft cells	*THF during sensitization*	*Host spleen explants*	*Incidence of reactive cultures***		
			Exp. I†	Exp. II§	
	− (π)	C57BL	6/6	5/6	(92%)
Neonatally	+ (II)	C57BL	3/6	2/6	(42%)
Tx C57BL	− (π)	Balb/c	0/5	1/6	(9%)
	+ (II)	Balb/c	5/6	4/7	(69%)

* Cells adhering to the monolayer were harvested after 24 h of sensitization by removal of medium with nonadherent cells and vigorous pipetting of adherent cells.

** Number of cultures with a spleen index ≥ 1.2 per total number of cultures tested.

† THF at a concentration of 20 μg/ml was added to the medium for the duration of the sensitization. 1×10^6 sensitized lymphocytes were assayed in comparison to 1×10^6 nonsensitized spleen lymphocytes syngeniec with the host spleen explants.

§ Lymphocyte suspensions were supplemented with THF at a concentration of 50 μg/ml for 1 hour prior to sensitization. The cell suspensions ±THF were added to the monolayer without washing. $.5 \times 10^6$ sensitized lymphocytes were assayed in comparison to $.5 \times 10^6$ nonsensitized spleen lymphocytes syngeneic with the host spleen explants.

π, II: Aliquots of respective lymphocyte suspension were tested either against syngeneic or allogeneic spleen explants.

replicates, but not against the allogeneic Balb/c tissue (Table XVIII). Addition of THF to the autosensitization cultures reduced the autoreactivity by 50 per cent. It can also be seen in Table XVIII that under the influence of THF these cells from neonatally thymectomized C57BL source acquired allogeneic

TABLE XIX

IN VITRO GVH RESPONSE AGAINST SYNGENEIC TISSUE BY THYMOCYTES SENSITIZED ON SYNGENEIC FIBROBLASTS WITH AND WITHOUT THF*

Graft cells	*Extract during sensitization*	*Host spleen explants*	*Incidence of reactive cultures***	
			Exp. I+	Exp. II§
Sensitized C57BL	none	C57BL	3/5	5/6
thymocytes	THF	C57BL	0/4	1/5

* Suspensions of thymocytes were supplemented with THF at a concentration of 50 μg/ml for 1 h prior to sensitization. The cell suspensions with or without THF were added to the monolayers without washing. Cells adhering to the monolayer were harvested after 24 h of sensitization by removal of medium with nonadherent cells and vigorous pipetting of adherent cells.

** Number of cultures with a spleen index ≥ 1.2 per total number of cultures tested.

\+ 3×10^6 sensitized thymocytes were assayed in comparison to 3×10^6 nonsensitized syngeneic thymocytes.

§ 1×10^6 sensitized thymocytes were assayed in comparison to 1×10^6 nonsensitized syngeneic thymocytes.

reactivity which was manifested against Balb/c spleen explants. The next two experiments were performed with autosensitized thymocytes. In Table XIX it can be seen that when the total thymocyte population was sensitized on syngeneic monolayers, these autosensitized cells also induced a GvH reaction against syngeneic tissue. This anti-self reactivity of the thymocytes was prevented by addition of THF to the sensitization cultures. On the other hand, autosensitization of cortisone-resistant thymocytes, which are known to be enriched in more differentiated T-cells (45, 46) did not result in anti-self reactivity in the GvH assay (Table XX).

TABLE XX

IN VITRO GVH RESPONSE AGAINST SYNGENEIC TISSUE BY SENSITIZED THYMOCYTES COMPARED TO SENSITIZED CORTISONE-RESISTANT THYMOCYTES

*Graft cells**	*Sensitizing monolayer*	*Host spleen explants*	*Incidence of reactive cultures***	
Sensitized thymocytes C57BL	C57BL	C57BL	5/6	3/5
Sensitized cortisone-resistant thymocytes C57BL†	C57BL	C57BL	1/4	0/4

* Cells adhering to the monolayer were harvested after 24 h of sensitization by removal of medium with nonadherent cells and vigorous pipetting of adherent cells. 1×10^6 sensitized lymphocytes were assayed in comparison to 1×10^6 nonsensitized syngeneic thymocytes.

** Number of cultures with a spleen index ≥ 1.2 per total number of cultures tested.

† Thymocytes remaining 48 h after i.m. injection of 5 mg hydrocortisone acetate.

Assuming that autoreactivity is an attribute of immature cells which is lost during differentiation of lymphocytes to a more mature state, exposure of cells to THF prior to sensitization should suffice to inhibit self reactivity. In Table XXI, it can be seen that incubation of spleen cells in THF prior to 24 h autosensitization decreased the subsequent autoreactivity of these cells.

At this point, we wished to confirm these results by examining directly the proliferative reaction of autosensitized lymphocytes in an MLC response. This was done to complement the estimation of autoreactivity measured by the GvH counter-reaction (that benefits from the advantage of detecting cumulative activity and of eliminating differences in physiologic properties of the populations tested). Spleen cells from intact donors sensitized with or without THF on syngeneic fibroblasts under the same conditions as described above were tested in a one-way mixed lymphocyte culture against syngeneic spleen cells. As is shown in Fig. 8, autosensitized cells showed an uptake of ^{3}H-thymidine which was 4 fold that of control nonsensitized syngeneic cells, and the reaction was significantly reduced though not abolished under the conditions tested when the cells were autosensitized with the addition of THF.

These results suggested that the presence or absence of THF might deter-

TABLE XXI

EFFECT OF THF PRIOR TO SENSITIZATION ON THE IN VITRO GVH RESPONSE OF SENSITIZED SPLEEN CELLS AGAINST SYNGENEIC TISSUE

Graft cells	*Treatment with THF*	*Host spleen explants*	*Incidence of reactive cultures**	
Sensitized spleen cells from intact C57BL mice	none	C57BL	5/6	4/6
	prior to sensitization**	C57BL	1/7	2/6
	prior to and during sensitizations§	C57BL	1/6	1/5

* Number of cultures with a spleen index ≥ 1.2 per total number of cultures tested.

** Lymphocyte suspensions were supplemented with THF at a concentration of 50 μg/ml for 1 h prior to sensitization. Cells were washed and sensitized without added THF. Cells adhering to the monolayer were harvested after 24 h of sensitization by removal of medium with nonadherent cells and vigorous pipetting of adhering cells. $.5 \times 10^6$ sensitized lymphocytes were assayed in comparison to $.5 \times 10^6$ nonsensitized syngeneic lymphocytes.

§ Lymphocyte suspensions were supplemented with THF at a concentration of 50 μg/ml for 1 h prior to sensitization. The cell suspensions + THF were added to the monolayer without washing. Cells adhering to the monolayer were harvested after 24 h of sensitization by removal of medium with nonadherent cells and vigorous pipetting of adherent cells. $.5 \times 10^6$ sensitized lymphocytes were assayed in comparison to $.5 \times 10^6$ nonsensitized syngeneic lymphocytes.

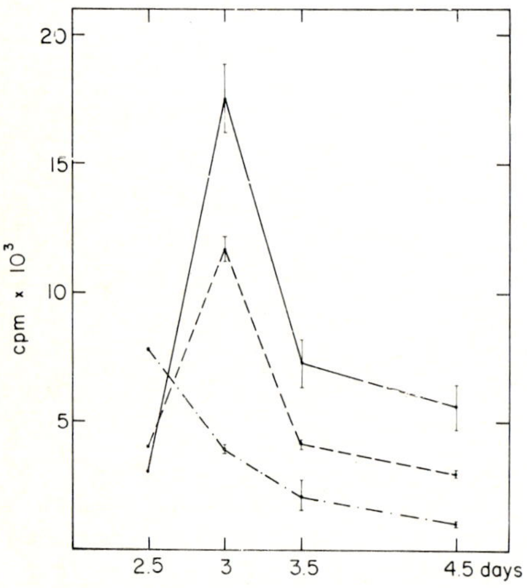

Fig. 8. Incorporation of ^{3}H-thymidine in MLC response against syngeneic spleen cells. Responding C57BL spleen cells were nonsensitized (. — . —), sensitized on syngeneic monolayers for 36 h (———) or sensitized on syngeneic monolayers with addition of THF (– – – –). The lymphocyte suspension supplemented with THF at a concentration of 50 μg/ml for 1 h prior to sensitization, was added to the monolayer without washing.

mine whether or not autoreactivity develops. Since it was shown in the present work that spleen cells from neonatally thymectomized mice are potentially autoreactive, and shown previously that serum of thymectomized animals failed to prevent such reactivity (44), we reasoned that spleen cells of thymusless mice might undergo a spontaneous autosensitization process *in vivo* and be able to induce a response against syngeneic tissue without further sensitization. This idea was submitted to test in the following experiments. Suspensions of spleen cells from individual neonatally thymectomized C57BL mice were incubated for 1 h in Eagle's medium with or without the addition of THF. These cells were washed and tested in the *in vitro* GvH assay against syngeneic

TABLE XXII

EFFECT OF THF ON THE IN VITRO GVH RESPONSE AGAINST SYNGENEIC TISSUE BY SPLEEN CELLS FROM NEONATALLY THYMECTOMIZED MICE

Donor of graft cells	*Sensitizing monolayer*	*Extract during incubation**	*Incidence of reactive cultures***			
Neonatally Tx C57BL	none	none	6/6	3/5		3/6
	none	THF	2/6	0/5	0/5	0/5
	none	SE		4/5	4/5	

* Suspensions of spleen cells from each neonatally thymectomized mouse were incubated for 1 h at 37° in EM with or without THF or spleen extract (SE) at a concentration of 50 μg/ml. After washing, 1×10^6 lymphocytes were assayed in comparison to 1×10^6 spleen cells from an intact syngeneic mouse also incubated in EM for 1 h.

** Number of cultures with a spleen index ≥ 1.2 per total number of cultures tested. Each column represents one experiment in which spleen cells from the same donor mouse were tested against newborn C57BL spleen explants.

tissue, in comparison to syngeneic spleen cells from intact mice. As can be seen in Table XXII, spleen cells from mice deprived of the thymus had indeed developed reactivity against components of self, and this autoreactivity was prevented by exposure of the cells to the thymic humoral factor. The results shown in Table XXII also indicate that this action of THF could be exerted after the sensitization process had taken place.

d. *Stimulation of B.M. stem cell cycling by THF*

It was found in our laboratory that neonatal thymectomy causes a reduction in the number of colony-forming cells (CFU-S) present in the bone marrow of mice (47, 48). We suggested that this change may be due to a reduced proliferative capacity of bone marrow cells from thymectomized mice, since the radioprotective effect and the rate of DNA synthesis of the progeny of these cells were found to be impaired (49). We tested here the sensitivity of bone marrow CFU-S from thymectomized mice to *in vivo* administration of chlorambucil (a nitrogen mustard derivative) and to the *in vitro* killing effect of ^{3}H-thymidine.

TABLE XXIII

THE EFFECT OF CHLORAMBUCIL (CB) TREATMENT ON THE TOTAL NUMBER OF CFU-S* IN THE BONE MARROW OF THYMECTOMIZED MICE

Bone marrow donor	*Total number of CFU-S in the bone marrow** *Before CB*	*8 days after CB*	*15 days after CB*
Thymectomized	4,620 ± 250	4,348 ± 679	5,733 ± 730
Normal	7,800 ± 600	2,967 ± 700	5,960 ± 413

* Calculated as follows: average number of colonies in spleens of recipients was multiplied by total number of nucleated cells counted in the marrow of the donor and divided by 2×10^4, i.e., number of bone marrow cells injected to the recipient.

The colony-forming capacity of bone marrow cells was determined by the spleen colony assay of Till & McCulloch (50). Two month old female C3H/eb mice, thymectomized 3 days after birth, and intact controls were injected with a single dose of chlorambucil. Mice at 8 and 15 days post treatment with chlorambucil, and untreated controls, were killed, and bone marrow of these mice injected into groups of lethally irradiated recipients. Eight days later, the spleens were removed, fixed, and macroscopic spleen colonies were counted.

As seen in Table XXIII, thymectomized mice had a reduced average number of CFU-S in their bone marrow, as compared to that in normal mice. Moreover, while a significant decrease was observed in the number of CFU-S of normal bone marrow 8 days after chlorambucil treatment, no change was observed in the bone marrow of similarly treated thymectomized mice. In the same experiment, nucleated bone marrow cells were counted in chlorambucil-

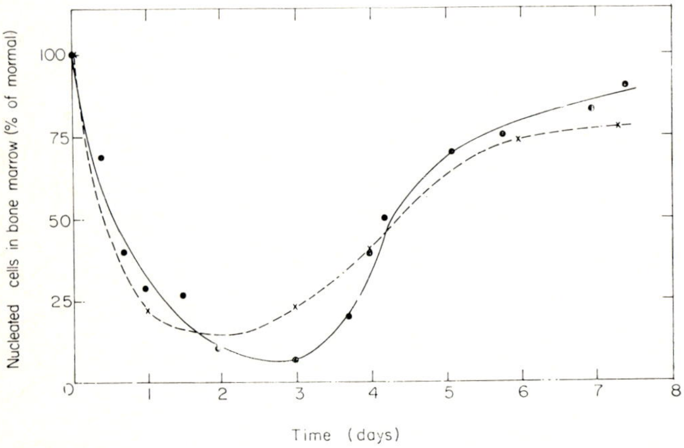

Fig. 9. Effect of chlorambucil treatment on the cellularity of the bone marrow of thymectomized mice.
Each point on the curves represents the average cell counts from 2-4 animals. The cellularity of the marrow at each time point is represented as percentage from the total marrow cellularity before treatment with chlorambucil. ●—normal; ×—thymectomized.

treated thymectomized and normal mice at different intervals, as indicated in Fig. 9. As seen in the Fig. 9, 3 days after injection of chlorambucil, the cellularity of the marrow of normal mice dropped to less than 10 per cent of the initial level, and was restored at about 8 days post-treatment. Almost the same curve was obtained when thymectomized mice were similarly treated with chlorambucil. Considered together, these experiments indicate that though the total bone marrow cell populations of normal and thymectomized mice react similarly to chlorambucil treatment, the stem cell population of thymectomized mice is less sensitive than that of normals to the cytotoxic action of the drug. Since the effect of chlorambucil is exerted on dividing stem cells (51), its lack of influence on stem cells from thymectomized mice suggests that these cells are in a resting phase.

We studied then the sensitivity of bone marrow CFU-S to the *in vitro* killing effect of ^{3}H-thymidine (52). Bone marrow cells from thymectomized or normal mice were pooled separately, and incubated with or without 200 μCi/ml of ^{3}H-thymidine (12-13 Ci/mmole) for 30 min at 37 °C, injected into irradiated recipients. Eight days later, the number of CFU-S was estimated. The proportion of stem cells in S phase was obtained from the percent loss of CFU-S in bone marrow suspensions after incubation with ^{3}H-thymidine (53). As seen in Table XXIV, only 6.7 per cent of the CFU-S in bone marrow of neonatally thymec-

TABLE XXIV

INFLUENCE OF THYMECTOMY AND OF *in vitro* ADDITION OF THF ON SENSITIVITY OF BONE MARROW CFU-S TO THE *in vitro* KILLING EFFECT OF ^{3}H-THYMIDINE

*Source of BM cells**	*Extract*	*^{3}H-thymidine (200 μCi/ml)*	*Average No. of colonies ± SE***	*% Reduction of CFU-S caused by ^{3}H-thymidine*	*p****
Normal	—	—	10.7 ± 0.4	25.7	< 0.005
		+	7.9 ± 0.3		
	THF†	—	11.4 ± 0.7	19.9	< 0.05
		+	9.1 ± 0.6		
	Spleen† extract	—	11.8 ± 0.7	14.7	< 0.05
		+	10.0 ± 0.6		
Thymectomized	—	—	8.7 ± 0.3	6.7	N.S.
		+	8.0 ± 0.4		
	THF†	—	9.8 ± 0.7	33.2	< 0.005
		+	6.6 ± 0.4		
	Spleen† extract	—	7.8 ± 0.5	11.2	N.S.
		+	6.9 ± 0.4		

* In each of 13 experiments performed, bone marrow from 5 normal or 5 thymectomized mice were pooled.

** Averaged from 13 experiments.

*** Significance of the reduction in number of colonies after *in vitro* treatment with ^{3}H-thymidine was determined by Student's t test (N.S. = non significant).

† 25 μg protein/ml.

tomized mice were in S phase as compared to 25 per cent in normal bone marrow. This is in agreement with the results obtained by *in vivo* administration of chlorambucil, thus indicating that CFU-S of thymectomized mice are in a resting phase. Since thymus reimplantation restores the colony-forming capacity of bone marrow from thymectomized mice (49), it was of importance to study the effect of THF, on the cycling of CFU-S from thymectomized mice. Bone marrow samples from normal and thymectomized mice were preincubated *in vitro* 30 min in the presence of THF, and then they were exposed to the killing effect of ^{3}H-thymidine. In the bone marrow of thymectomized mice THF elevated the percentage of cells sensitive to the killing effect of ^{3}H-thymidine from 6.7 per cent to 33 per cent, while it had no effect on CFU-S of normal mice (Table XXIV).

Induction of cycling of CFU-S by THF is a fast process which occurs within the 30 min incubation period, therefore, resembling from the kinetic point of view, the effects of some hormones, drugs (54) and prostaglandin E_2 (55) on the cycling of CFU-S. Despite this similarity, the effect of THF on CFU-S is restricted to bone marrow from thymectomized mice while normal CFU-S are not affected.

5. CONCLUSIONS

Our present knowledge suggests that THF exerts its influence on immature lymphocytes and regulates a step in the process of differentiation leading to mature T cells. As a result of the THF-dependent step, biochemical changes occur in target lymphocytes which acquire the properties necessary for response to allogeneic antigens in GvH and MLC reactions, for reaction to T-cell mitogens, for helper function in the response to sheep erythrocytes, and for development of characteristics which facilitate antitumor activity. The results presented are compatible with the unifying hypothesis that loss of reactivity against "self" may also result from the maturation of lymphocytes under the influence of THF, as outlined in Fig. 10.

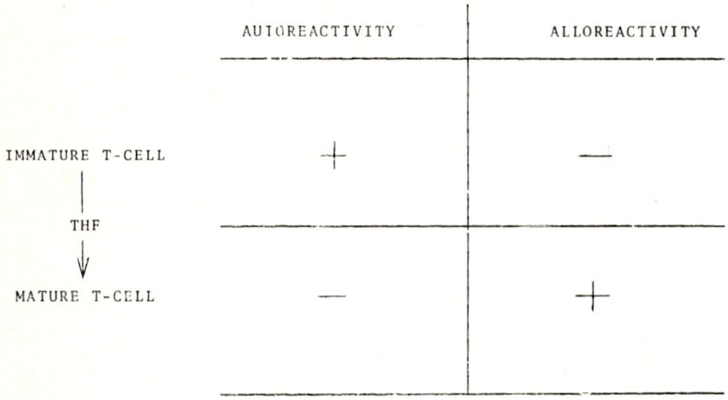

Fig. 10. Proposed scheme of development of immune characteristics under the control of THF.

In addition, THF seems to regulate the proliferation of some of the CFU-S present in the bone marrow.

REFERENCES

1. Levey, R. H., Trainin, N. & Law, L. W. (1963) *J. Natl. Cancer Inst.* **31**, 199.
2. Osoba, D. & Miller, J. F. A. P. (1963) *Nature* **199**, 653.
3. Law, L. W., Trainin, N., Levey, R. H. & Barth, W. F. (1964) *Science* **143**, 1049.
4. Aisenberg, A. C. & Wilkes, B. (1965) *Nature* **205**, 716.
5. Sherman, J. D. (1967) *Arch. Pathol.* **83**, 251.
6. Trench, C. A. H., Watson, J. W., Walker, F. C., Gardner, P. S. & Green, C. A. (1966) *Immunology* **10**, 187.
7. Trainin, N., Bejerano, A., Strahilevitch, M., Goldring, D. & Small, M. (1966) *Israel J. Med. Sci.* **2**, 549.
8. Trainin, N., Burger, M. & Kaye, A. (1967) *Biochem. Pharmacol.* **16**, 711.
9. Trainin, N. & Linker-Israeli, M. (1967) *Cancer Res.* **27**, 309.
10. De Somer, P., Denys, P. Jr. & Leyten, R. (1963) *Life Sci.* **2**, 810.
11. Goldstein, A. L., Slater, F. D. & White, A. (1966) *Proc. Natl. Acad. Sci.* **56**, 1010.
12. Carnaud, C., Ilfeld, D., Brook, I. & Trainin, N. (1973) *J. Exp. Med.* **138**, 1521.
13. Small, M. & Trainin, N. (Submitted for publication).
14. Trainin, N., Small, M. and Globerson, A. (1969) *J. Exp. Med.* **130**, 765.
15. Trainin, N. & Small, M. (1970) *J. Exp. Med.* **132**, 885.
16. Lonai, P., Mogilner, B., Rotter, V. & Trainin, N. (1973) *Eur. J. Immunol.* **3**, 21.
17. Rotter, V., Globerson, A., Nakamura, I. & Trainin, N. (1973) *J. Exp. Med.* **138**, 130.
18. Auerbach, R. & Globerson, A. (1966) *Exp. Cell. Res.* **42**, 31.
19. Kook, A. I. & Trainin, N. (In press) *J. Immunol.* **114**.
20. Sutherland, E. W. & Robinson, G. A. (1968) *Circulation* **37**, 279.
21. Kook, A. I. & Trainin, N. (1974) *J. Exp. Med.* **139**, 193.
22. Sutherland, E. W. (1972) *Science* **177**, 401.
23. Froehlich, J. E. & Rachmeler, M. J. (1974) *Cell Biol.* **60**, 249.
24. Millis, A. J. T., Forrest, G. & Pious, D. A. (1972) *Biochem. Biophys. Res. Commun.* **49**, 1645.
25. Millis, A. J. T., Forrest, G. A. & Pious, D. A. (1974) *Exp. Cell. Res.* **83**, 335.
26. Henny, C. S. & Lichtenstein, L. M. (1971) *J. Immunol.* **107**, 610.
27. Henny, C. S., Bourne, H. E. & Lichtenstein, L. M. (1972) *J. Immunol.* **108**, 1526.
28. Strom, T. B., Deisseroth, A., Morganroth, J., Carpenter, C. B. & Merrill, J. P. (1972) *Proc. Natl. Acad. Sci. U.S.A.* **69**, 2995.
29. Hadden, J. W., Hadden, E. M., Haddox, M. K. & Goldberg, N. D. (1972) *Proc. Natl. Acad. Sci. U.S.A.* **69**, 3024.
30. Bach, F.-H. & Voynow, K. (1966) *Science* **153**, 545.
31. Howe, M. L., Manziello, B., Goldstein, A. L. (1972) in *Proceeding of the Sixth Leucocyte Culture Conference*. ed. M. Roy Schwarz Academic Press, New York, p. 599.
32. Blomgren, H. & Andersson, B. (1969) *Exp. Cell. Res.* **57**, 185.
33. Cohen, J. J., Fischbach, M. & Claman, H. N. (1970) *J. Immunol.* **105**, 1146.
34. Raff, M. C. (1971) *Transplant. Rev.* **6**, 52.
35. Stobo, J. D. & Paul, W. E. (1972) *Cell. Immunol.* **4**, 367.
36. Stobo, J. D. & Paul, W. E. (1973) *J. Immunol.* **110**, 362.
37. Stobo, J. D., Rosenthal, A. S. & Paul, W. E. (1972) *J. Immunol.* **108**, 1.
38. Hadden, J. W., Hadden, E. M., Haddox, M. K. & Goldberg, N. D. (1972) *Proc. Natl. Acad. Sci. U.S.A.* **69**, 3024.
39. George, W. J., Polson, J. B., O'Toole, A. G. & Goldberg, N. D. (1970) *Proc. Natl. Acad. Sci. U.S.A.* **66**, 398.
40. May, D. C. (1969) *J. Allerg.* **43**, 163.
41. Hadden, J. W., Hadden, E. M. & Middleton, E. Jr. (1970) *Cell. Immunol.* **1**, 583.
42. Cohen, I. R., Globerson, A. & Feldman, M. (1971) *J. Exp. Med.* **133**, 834.
43. Cohen, I. R. & Wekerle, H. (1973) *J. Exp. Med.* **137**, 224.
44. Trainin, N., Carnaud, C. & Ilfeld, D. (1973) *Nature New Biol.* **245**, 253.
45. Blomgren, H. & Andersson, B. (1970) *Cell. Immunol.* **1**, 545.
46. Weissman, I. L. (1973) *J. Exp. Med.* **137**, 504.
47. Trainin, N. & Resnitzky, P. (1969) *Nature* **221**, 1154.

48. Resnitzky, P., Zipori, D. & Trainin, N. (1971) *Blood* **37**, 634.
49. Zipori, D. & Trainin, N. (In press) *Expl. Haematology.*
50. Till, J. E. & McCulloch, E. A. (1961) *Radiat. Res.* **14**, 213.
51. Dunn, C. D. R. & Elson, L. A. (1970) *Cell Tissue Kinet.* **3**, 131.
52. Becker, A. J., McCulloch, E. A., Siminovitch, L. & Till, J. E. (1965) *Blood* **26**, 296.
53. Byron, J. W. (1970) *Nature* **228**, 1204.
54. Byron, J. W. (1973) *Nature New Biol.* **241**, 152.
55. Feher, I. & Gidali, J. (1974) *Nature* **247**, 550.

Biological Activity of Thymic Hormones

THE CIRCULATING THYMIC FACTOR (TF). BIOCHEMISTRY, PHYSIOLOGY, BIOLOGICAL ACTIVITIES, AND CLINICAL APPLICATIONS. A SUMMARY.

JEAN-FRANÇOIS BACH, MARIE-ANNE BACH, JEANNINE CHARREIRE, MIREILLE DARDENNE, CATHERINE FOURNIER, MARTINE PAPIERNIK & JEAN-MARIE PLEAU

Normal serum of several species contains a polypeptidic factor secreted by the thymus, provisionally called "thymus factor" (TF) (1, 2, 3). We would like to present in this short review a summary of the present state of our TF knowledge. No detail or experimental data will be given, thus the reader will have to refer to original references. This review should be considered in the final analysis as an explicative listing of data obtained in our laboratory. We shall first present the basis of the rosette assay on which TF definition and isolation have been established.

I THE SHEEP CELL ASSAY FOR TF EVALUATION

A large percentage of Rosette Forming Cells (RFC) as found, for example, in the normal mouse spleen are T cells as indicated by their inhibition by anti-theta serum (AθS) (1, 2), their presence in the steroid-resistant thymocyte pool (3), the absence of θ-positive RFC in neonatally thymectomized or nude mice (1, 2), and the enrichment of θ-positive RFC after filtration on anti-immunoglobulin (Ig) antibody-coated columns (4). The absence of a major involvement of cytophilic antibodies in the phenomenon is suggested by the RFC antigen specificity (5) and the SRBC-induced rosette capping (6). Lastly, the involvement of a portion of RFC in antigen recognition is indicated by the specific unresponsiveness to SRBC induced in normal spleen cells by SRBC-RFC depletion using centrifugation on Ficoll after SRBC rosette formation (7). It has been shown that AθS sensitive RFC were also inhibited by low concentrations of azathioprine (AZ), a purine analogue (2, 8).

Unexpectedly, adult thymectomy proved to suppress AθS and AZ sensitivity of spleen RFC within a week (2, 9). This observation suggested that RFC sensitivity to AZ and AθS might depend on thymic hormonal influence. Evidence for this hypothesis was the correction of normal AZ and AθS sensitivity in spleen RFC from adult thymectomized mice by *in vitro* or *in vivo* treatment with thymic extracts kindly provided by A. L. Goldstein & A. White (10) and N. Trainin (11). Thymic extracts were active *in vitro* in less than 60 min. Spleen, liver, and muscle extracts and endotoxin were inactive (10). A correla-

INSERM U 25, Hôpital Necker, 161, rue de Sèvres, 75730 Paris Cedex 15

tion was found in various fractions between the thymic extract concentrations active on RFC and in a graft versus host reaction (GVH) assay (10). In spite of the controls mentioned above, some doubt still persisted about the specificity of the observation, since one can never ascertain the exclusive thymic origin of a thymic extract, even if, for example, spleen extracts are essentially inactive in the assay.

The evidence for such specificity was brought about by the demonstration of "thymic-like" activity in normal mouse serum (12, 13).

In brief, normal serum, previously ultrafiltered on Amicon membranes with molecular weight (Mol Wt) cut-off of 60,000, in order to remove large Mol Wt inhibitors, induced the appearance of sensitivity to AZ and AθS in spleen cells from adult thymectomized mice, whereas serum from thymectomized or nude mice was totally inactive (12, 13). Concentration of the serum on Amicon UM 2 membrane, which increased serum activity up to 100 times, did not reveal activity in thymectomized mouse serum (14).

The details of the assay used routinely to evaluate serum TF levels as well as to pick up active fractions in chemical procedures are described elsewhere in this volume (15). In brief, spleen cells from mice thymectomized as adults 2-6 weeks earlier are incubated with the test sample and AZ at a concentration intermediate between that providing RFC inhibition in normal and adult thymectomized mice (e.g. 10 μg/ml). Without TF activity, RFC are not inhibited by AZ, whereas RFC are inhibited by AZ in the presence of TF activity. The assay is very reproducible. It could be used successfully on several occasions without mistakes in blind studies (14, 15). Furthermore, it is highly sensitive; concentrations of purified TF as low as 2 pg/ml can be detected (16).

II BIOCHEMISTRY OF THE CIRCULATING TF

Biochemical characteristics · TF activity in normal mouse serum persists after diafiltration of the serum through CF 50, PM 30, and PM 10 Amicon membranes. Conversely, no significant activity is found after filtration through UM 2 and UM 0.5 membranes. This data, although only indicative, suggests that the TF Mol Wt might range between 500 and 5,000 daltons (13). TF is dialysable against distilled water or phosphate buffer (0.2 M-pH 7.3) (16).

Serum TF stability at various temperatures is very weak when using total serum (16). Thus, if TF is stable at −20 °C and at 4 °C for several days, it is not stable at higher temperatures, since most of the activity disappears after 5 h at room temperature, 2 h at 37 °C, and a few min at 80 °C (a difference with thymic extracts such as thymosin which are heat stable). However, when TF is purified as will be detailed later, its stability is much better; it is possible to maintain TF activity for more than 8 h at 37 °C. Interestingly, TF resists lyophilization which provides an easy method for storage and chemical procedures. TF is relatively resistant to extremes pH. We have shown that it is possible to keep most of the activity at pH ranging from 2 to 10.

TF was destroyed by trypsin-chymotrypsin and pronase after 60 min incubation at 37 °C at pH 7.3. Control experiments included non-TF-containing Hanks samples treated in the same way and TF incubated under identical conditions without enzymes. Ribonuclease used under similar conditions did not alter TF activity. Destruction of TF by proteolytic enzymes has been obtained for both mouse and pig TF and was obtained with crude serum preparations as well as with purified factor (16).

Mouse and pig TF-containing serum has been fractionated on various Sephadex columns. In all cases, the serum samples were first purified on Amicon membranes (consecutively PM 30 and PM 10) and then concentrated 10 to 40 times on UM 2 membranes. It was shown in both the mouse and the pig that TF was eluted with the void volume in G 10 and was separated from the bulk of proteins in other Sephadex beads (G 15, G 25, G 50). The best separation was obtained with Sephadex G 25 where TF was eluted after cytochrome and peroxidase and with angiotensin in phosphate buffer (0.2 M, pH 7.3). These Sephadex data which have been confirmed using Sephadex G 25 with 50 per cent acetic acid suggest that TF Mol Wt is between 700 and 2,000 (16, 17).

When applied to a carboxy methyl cellulose column, mouse or pig TF bound to CM cellulose and was eluted with sodium chloride at a molarity of 0.12 M in 0.01 M phosphate buffer, pH 6.0. TF was not retained on DEAE cellulose at pH 8.3. When electrophoresis was performed using the CM cellulose eluate, it was shown that TF had an isoelectric point (pHi) of 7.5 in pyridine acetate buffer.

In summary, serum TF appears to be a relatively neutral polypeptide (pHi 7.5) with a Mol Wt of about 1,000 daltons.

Isolation and purification (16, 17): Isolation of the polypeptide has been achieved by the successive operations: 1) defibrination; 2) dialysis; 3) concentration on UM 2 Amicon membrane; 4) G 25 Sephadex filtration; 5) CM cellulose chromatography; 6) thin-layer chromatography; and 7) electrophoresis. Each of these steps will be briefly described. The routine fractionation procedure utilizes a starting batch of 8 liters of pig blood, but it must be realized that, in order to obtain 20 μg of pure TF, 180 liters of blood must be used. Normal 3-4 month-old pigs are lethally bled at a local abattoir where blood is immediately *defibrinated* by mechanical agitation. It is then cooled at 4 °C and brought to the laboratory where it is centrifuged to obtain the serum. Biological activity of the serum, as determined by the rosette assay after defibrination, is 1/128.

Dialysis is the following step: 3.6 liters of serum are dialyzed in the cold room under ultrafiltration conditions. The membrane used is a polyacrylonitrile membrane (a product of Rhône-Poulenc). The serum is circulated with a pump and the ultrafiltrate is collected in the outside compartment of the dialyzer by a second pump equipped with an automatic outflow and pressure device (N. K. Man to be published). The biological activity of the ultrafiltrate is 1/128.

Four hundred ml of serum ultrafiltrate are placed in Amicon diafiltration chambers. After 8 h, when the membrane is dry, the chamber is filled with phosphate buffer and agitated to dissolve the product in the buffer. The activity is enriched to 1/25,000.

The pooled samples are then applied on a G 25 Sephadex column and eluted with phosphate buffer 0.2 M, pH 7.3 Fractions active in the rosette assay are found with an elution volume between 2 and 2.5 the void volume. Active fractions show activity up to the dilution of $1/2 \times 10^6$, suggesting removal of inhibitory molecules.

The active fractions obtained in the Sephadex chromatography are *desalted* using Amicon UM 2 membranes and the retentate is then applied on a CM cellulose column equilibrated with phosphate buffer (0.01 M, pH 6.3). TF is eluted with a step-wise NaCl gradient from 0.05 M to 0.4 M. Active fractions are eluted at NaCl molarity of 0.1 to 0.15 M and show activity diluted $1/10^6$.

CM cellulose eluates are then separated on 3 successive *thin layer chromatographies* including chromatographies in butanol-pyridine, methanol-chloroform-ammonia and rechromatography in the latter solvent (J. M. Pleau *et al.* in preparation).

The last stage of purification involves *high voltage electrophoresis* in diluted formic acid at pH 1.9.

The product thus obtained appears to be pure in TLC performed in 5 different solvents using fluorescamine staining. Studies are in progress to ascertain whether the product is indeed a pure entity (determination of amino acid terminals and amino acid composition). It should be emphasized that all of these fractionation procedures are made easy by the very high sensitivity of the rosette assay and that, at the end, the amount of material recovered from serum is low, which complicates direct TF characterization. The products used in biological studies (discussed below) have been fractionated to the 5th step, that is to say, the CM cellulose chromatography.

It should also be stressed that one single peak of biological activity has been detected in all fractionation procedures, indicating that TF activity is indeed associated with a single product.

Relationship to other thymic hormones: The relationship of the serum TF characterized on the basis of the rosette assay to other thymic hormones isolated and characterized by other authors is still a matter of speculation. It is interesting to note that all products considered have proved to be polypeptides but of different Mol Wt. A. Goldstein & A. White have reported the isolation of a polypeptide with a Mol Wt of 12,500 (18) which showed some activity in the rosette system but at a much higher molarity than the purified serum TF (100 ng/ml of the best fraction (10)). Similarly, G. Goldstein reported the isolation of three proteins with respective Mol Wt of 11,000 (prothymin) and 7,000 (thymin I and thymin II) (19). These products, isolated on the basis of their activity on neuromuscular transmission, did show some activity on lymphocytes (θ conversion of θ negative spleen cells). Lastly, one may mention the thymic humoral factor (THF) isolated by Trainin & Kook (20), on the basis of an *in vitro* GVH assay, which appears to be a polypeptide with a Mol Wt of 3,000. This latter product is certainly the closest to ours.

Several hypotheses can be put forward to explain the possible relationship between thymosin and thymins and serum TF. It may be that thymosin or thymin are polymers or aggregates of TF. It is also possible that thymin or thymosin are precursors of TF since they are obtained from the thymus gland itself, whereas we work with serum. The fact that thymosin is more active *in vivo* than could be expected from *in vitro* experiments is in favour of such an hypothesis. Lastly, it is possible that thymosin or thymin, and TF are different entities, either all active in the rosette assay (at least for thymosin) or that TF contaminates thymosin which could also be a TF carrier as, suggested by the fact that thymosin is an acidic protein, whereas TF is a basic peptide. It is difficult to chose at the present time among these various possibilities.

We have been engaged in the preparation of thymic extracts from the pig using Trainin's technique which includes dialysis as a first step. Results showed that some "TF-like" activity was recovered in the dialysate but that amounts of active products recovered for one whole thymus gland was not much more than that recovered from half a liter of serum. This might be due again to the predominant presence in the thymus of precursors which rapidly release the active product once split. It might also be due to the binding of active factors to other molecules from which they are not separated by fractionation procedures (16).

Serum TF inhibitor: Total mouse serum examined in the test described above does not possess the activity reported for serum ultrafiltrate. This activity only appears after elimination of molecules with Mol Wt between 100,000 and 300,000, as assessed by diafiltration on Amicon membranes (13). Therefore, there seems to exist a TF inhibitor with high Mol Wt in normal serum and separable from TF by simple dialysis or diafiltration. The molecule responsible for this inhibitory activity in normal serum is not known but it has been shown that it was active at very low concentrations, since total serum diluted 1/5,000 maintains its inhibitory activity (13). The thymic origin of the serum inhibitor has been investigated in the mouse. It was first thought that the inhibitor might be of thymic origin, since, when mixing directly retentate of thymectomized mouse serum on XM 100 Amicon membrane with normal serum ultrafiltrate, one did not find inhibitory activity in the retentate. The disappearance of inhibitory activity after thymectomy paralleled that of TF (13). However, when incubating "thymectomized" retentate and "normal" ultrafiltrate for 30 min at 37 °C before adding it to spleen cells from adult thymectomized mice for the rosette assay, the inhibitory activity was recovered (13). The extra-thymic origin of the TF inhibitor has been confirmed by the demonstration that nude mice injected with serum TF recovered serum activity within a few hours after the injection when tested after diafiltration, but that nondialyzed serum did not show activity (our unpublished results).

These data suggest that TF binds to the inhibitory molecule, as is the case for thyroxin, the *in vitro* function of which is inhibited by its specific binding protein. This hypothesis is supported by the data presented in the paragraph on TF metabolism.

III PHYSIOLOGY OF TF SECRETION

The availability of an *in vitro* assay for TF serum level evaluation proved to be a useful tool to study the physiology of TF secretion.

Demonstration of the thymic epithelial origin: The thymic origin of the circulating factor assessed by the rosette assay is demonstrated by its absence in nude mice, its rapid disappearance from the serum of normal mice after thymectomy, and its rapid reappearance after thymus grating (whether subcutaneous or intraperitoneal). A lag-time of 2 to 3 days is however observed before reappearance of normal serum factor level, probably due to the initial necrosis of the thymus graft. Grafting a neonatal thymus in a thymectomized mouse leads to a very long-lasting recovery of serum TF level.

It is also possible to induce the reappearance of TF level in the serum of thymectomized mice by injection of dissociated thymocytes, but high numbers of thymocytes must be injected (14), probably because thymus cell dissociation leads to the loss of a majority of epithelial cells which are not easily separated from the reticular epithelium. Lastly, injection of thymic extracts can also induce a restoration of TF level. The injection of thymic-cell-free extracts however gives only a temporary restoration of TF level (11).

The thymus contains two cell types: lymphocytes and epithelial cells. The epithelial origin of TF could be suspected in view of the secretory activity of normal thymic epithelial cells demonstrated in electron microscopy and in view of the absence of serum TF in young adult NZB mice, which exhibit an early atrophy of the thymus epithelium (21). This epithelial origin has been demonstrated by the significant reconstitution of serum TF level in adult thymectomized mice obtained by grafting a relatively small number of epithelial cells (14). These pure epithelial cells were obtained after *in vivo* incubation of two neonatal thymus lobes in a Millipore chamber in an intermediate host for 7 days. The absence of lymphocytes was verified histologically. Whether grafted directly into adult thymectomized mice or inside the Millipore chamber, the epithelial thymus restored by serum TF levels significant within 2 days. The restoration was even more clear-cut 5 days after grafting (14). Similarly, grafting thymectomized mice with 10^6 epithelial thymoma cells resulted in a highly significant recovery of serum TF. Grafting an identical number of normal thymocytes did not produce a detectable level of TF. In addition, only transient restoration was obtained with 2×10^6 thymocytes.

In a more direct approach to this problem, we have studied with M. Papiernik the changes undergone by spleen cells from adult thymectomized mice after incubation on thymic reticular epithelium cultures (22). Thymus fragments were explanted in plastic flasks in Eagle's medium. Rings of epithelial cells were visible at the explant periphery within 2-3 days. Electron microscopy studies, performed after 8 days of culture, confirmed the absence of lymphoid cells and the epithelial nature of the remaining cells in which tonofilaments were seen. Fibroblasts cultures were used as controls. The cultures were shown to induce the appearance of sensitivity to AθS in RFC from the spleen of adult thymectomized mice. Control fibroblast cultures did not induce significant changes in AθS sensitivity of spleen RFC. Similar results were obtained when the spleen cells were placed in a Millipore chamber on the culture, avoiding direct contact between epithelial cells and spleen cells.

Metabolism of serum TF: Serum TF level decreases rapidly after thymectomy and TF activity is no longer found in the serum after 6 days. However, this decrease is biphasic. During the first 6 h, serum TF varies from 1/64 to 1/8 with a half-life of 2 1/2 h. It remains at this level for 5 days. On the 6th day, a new fall is observed down to a dilution of 1/2-1/4. The second decrease on the 6th day is a significant one and occurs simultaneously with a drop in spleen RFC sensitivity to AZ and AθS. Similar results have been obtained in Swiss, CBA, C3H, and AKR mice; in all cases, sera collected 8-10 days after thymectomy showed TF levels lower or equal to 1/4 (13).

Whereas splenectomy alone has no effect on serum TF, when it is performed 2 days before thymectomy it modifies serum TF kinetics following thymectomy. Splenectomy suppresses the plateau observed between day 1 and day 6 after thymectomy alone. The significance of this effect is not known but may be eventually explained by binding and protection of TF in the spleen with slow and progressive release after thymectomy. It is interesting to note that the relatively slow decrease in TF level after thymectomy has also been observed in other species such as the pig and the human.

When normal mouse serum is injected i.p. into adult thymectomized mice, one can observe the reappearance of serum TF for a few hours. Similar data are obtained with serum filtered through XM 300 or XM 100 membranes, with respective Mol. Wt cut-off of 300,000 and 100,000. However, when serum is ultrafiltered through CF 50 (Mol. Wt cut-off: 50,000) PM 30, or PM 10 membranes (Mol. Wt: 30,000 and 10,000), activity is absent from the serum, except when one uses the i.v. route and looks at the serum within the first 5 min after the injection (13).

This rapid TF elimination represents a difficult problem when using purified TF completely separated from other serum proteins, since no *in vivo* effects of ultrafiltered TF are noted, a finding in keeping with the absence of serum activity. To avoid these difficulties in using *in vivo* purified TF, various vehicles have been tried in order to bind and protect TF from degradation. Among these, CM cellulose, Dextran, BSA, and serum from thymectomized mice proved to be the most efficient (our unpublished observation). The best prolongation of TF half-life was obtained with CM cellulose equilibrated at pH 6.3 in phosphate buffer 0.01 M, that is, the exact conditions of the CM cellulose chromatography used in the isolation procedure. CM cellulose-bound TF half-life is of 4-6 hours. Interestingly, when a sufficient half-life is obtained, the *in vivo* effects previously noted with thymic extracts or total serum are again obtained (correction of the normally low sensitivity to AθS of the spleen RFC). This method of injecting serum TF has been adopted in all *in vivo* biological studies further reported using purified TF (13).

Age dependence: The level of serum thymic hormone depends on age as does thymus weight. Thymic hormone level is stable in most strains of mice until the age of 6 months, after which it progressively declines. After 12 to 15 months, serum activity is no longer detectable. This decrease in thymic hormone level, which parallels the decrease in thymus weight, precedes by several months the decrease in cell-mediated immunity and eventually of humoral immunity observed with aging (12, 13).

Effect of pregnancy: The adult level of thymic hormone is already reached at birth. The fact that thymic hormone is secreted by the fetus, already suggested by the normal birth level, is further confirmed by the reappearance of the serum thymic hormone in the blood of pregnant thymectomized mice (26). In these mice, no activity is detected until the 14th or 15th day of gestation, after which there is a progressive increase in TF level with a peak immediately before parturition. In the hours following parturition, TF level becomes nil again. This data, which is very much in favour of TF secretion by the fetal thymus after the 15th day of gestation (that is the time when the thymic epithelium is already well formed and eventually colonized by a few lymphoid stem cells), would need, however, more direct demonstration, since one cannot exclude TF activity in the mother's serum due to various secretions related to pregnancy, including placental secretion.

Species specificity: The activity of thymic extracts and sera from various species has been tested on mouse RFC. A TF-like activity has been found in thymic extracts of mice, calves, pigs, and humans (10, 11) as well as in the sera of calves, sheep, pigs (23), rats, and men (24). For pig and human sera, the disappearance of TF-like activity after thymectomy allowed the ascertainment that biological activity detected was well due to thymic secretion (23, 24). Biochemical studies have so far shown no difference in TF characteristics in the mouse, the pig, and the human.

Serum TF has also been recently shown to be present in the serum of Urodeles. This data was obtained in 60 normal and thymectomized *Triturus alpestris*, *Pleurodeles waltlii*, and *Ambystoma mexicanum* (25). Sera of these Urodeles contain a factor with TF-like activity which disappears after thymectomy. This activity of amphibian TF in the mouse is reminiscent of the activity of certain mammalian hormones in amphibians.

Effects of ALS, irradiation, and steroids: Antithymocyte serum (ALS) decreases serum TF when given at large doses (our unpublished data). It is not known, however, whether this effect is due to direct ALS action on the thymic epithelium or to TF peripheral destruction. The long time needed for recovery (4-6 weeks) argues in favour of the former hypothesis. Irradiation (800 r) (our unpublished data) and steroids (1-10 mg of hydrocortisone succinate) (27) also decrease serum TF level, but only modestly (70 per cent decrease) and very transiently (3-10 days), indicating a relative radio- and steroid resistance of the thymic epithelium in comparison to thymus lymphocytes, as already known from other experiments. It should be noted, however, that these treatments do significantly alter thymic epithelium for some time.

IV BIOLOGICAL ACTIVITIES

The effects of pig TF have been studied in various *in vivo* and *in vitro* systems. It should be emphasized that all of the studies which will be mentioned have been performed with fairly purified preparations (up to the CMC step inclusive) which are active *in vivo* and *in vitro* at ng levels, at variance with experiments reported by other authors using rather unfractionated preparations (even when purified material had been made available for biochemical studies) at μg or even mg levels.

Theta conversion: Purified TF can induce the appearance of the θ antigen on previously θ-negative RFC. However, it may be shown with some very active AθS batches that there is in fact some inhibition of the TF-sensitive RFC, as seen in normal bone marrow or in spleen from adult thymectomized or nude spleen. In that case, TF increases θ antigen expression rather than provoking its appearance (2, 13, 28, 29).

Similar data have been obtained in normal spleen cells at ng levels using a cytotoxic assay after cell fractionation on a BSA gradient as described by Komuro & Boyse (30). These results (28, 29) must, however, be interpreted with caution, since θ conversion can be obtained by incubating the cells at 37 °C without any added material, suggesting a possible fragilization of cells containing small amounts of θ antigen, making them more sensitive to otherwise noncytotoxic concentrations (28, 31). This criticism does not apply to the sheep cell rosette assay which does not involve BSA fractionation and long-term incubation.

The mechanism of action of TF on RFC θ conversion has been investigated with regard to the cAMP system. In brief, TF effects are mimicked by low (and physiological) concentrations of cyclic AMP, theophylline, and prostaglandins (29, 32, 33). One can even show a synergy between cAMP and TF both used at subliminal levels (33). Lastly, indomethacin, a prostaglandin synthetase inhibitor, blocks TF effects (29, 34, 35) as well. When injected into normal mice, it transiently decreases the number of θ positive cells in the spleen (but interestingly not in lymph nodes (29, 34, 35). Finally, it appears that θ antigen expression has a rapid turnover and is probably regulated by agents altering cyclic AMP synthesis, TF possibly acting in this system through stimulation of cAMP synthesis, eventually through prostaglandin stimulation in view of indomethacin data.

Mitogen responses: TF has been shown to induce some responsiveness to Concanavalin A (Con A) and, to a lesser degree, to PHA in nude mouse spleen cells (16) and in low density normal spleen cells separated on a Ficoll gradient (P. Hayry & J. F. Bach, in preparation). However, one should emphasize that the increase although significant was not dramatic ($\times 2$-$\times 4$).

Similarly, a 2 week treatment with TF significantly increased Con A and PHA responses in the spleen of NZB mice at an age where they show decreased mitogen responses (35). Interestingly, a similar restoration was obtained by grafting a thymus in a Millipore chamber (37).

Autologous Rosettes: A small percentage of normal mouse lymphocytes form rosettes when mixed with autologous (or syngeneic) erythrocytes (38). These Autologous Rosette Forming Cells (ARFC) normally predominate in the thymus. Interestingly, their number increases with age and especially after adult thymectomy within a few days after the operation, ARFC level reaching its peak 30-45 days after the operation ($\times 20$ increase). TF normalizes the ARFC level in adult thymectomized mice when injected *in vivo* (39, 40, 41) or after *in vitro* (40) incubation. ARFC characteristics indicate that they belong to the pool of postthymic or T_0 cells (42). The significance of the ARFC phenomenon is still obscure but might have some relevance to autoantigen recognition. Anyhow, autologous rosette formation appears to be a marker of T_0 cells and the effects of TF on this marker can be utilized as a useful TF assay (41).

Suppressor T cells: NZB mice show an abnormally high antibody response to polyvinyl pyrrolidone which increases with age, probably due to the loss of suppressor T cells. *In vivo* TF treatment (500 ng) 3 times weekly for 3 weeks has been shown to normalize anti-PVP antibody responses in 6-9-month-old NZB mice (36). Interestingly, a one week treatment had no effect, suggesting that suppressor T cell maturation takes 2-3 weeks.

Tumour rejection: Thymectomized, irradiated, bone-marrow-reconstituted mice do not reject Moloney Virus sarcoma. *In vivo* TF treatment restored the ability of rejecting these tumours. However, when TF treatment was stopped, tumour recurrence was noted in the last mice which had clinically rejected their tumours (16).

Other TF effects: Purified TF has also been shown to reduce the density of steroid receptors on thymocytes (27, 43) and to enable spleen RFC from adult thymectomized mice to cap in the presence of SRBC (44). Moreover, TF has proven capable at ng levels to enable spleen cells from neonatally thymectomized mice to induce a GvH reaction *in vitro* (45).

Conclusions. TF target cell: Purified TF has been shown to possess several biological activities in addition to the sheep cell assay utilized for its purification. The *in vivo* data obtained at low doses (100-500 ng) indicate a possible physiological role in the periphery.

The TF target cell is not definitively known. However, one is struck by the relative ease with which biological activities are shown in T cell functions altered by adult thymectomy (autologous rosettes, suppressor T cells). Conversely, it appears to be much more difficult to obtain similar effects in nude mice, where 10-20 higher doses are needed (16). Moreover, data showing restoration of helper function, *in vivo* GvH or skin graft rejecting capacity, have not yet been obtained with TF. This may prove a fairly difficult task, since it takes several weeks (4-8) to obtain the immunological reconstitution of thymectomized mice with a fully functional thymus graft (46). In other words, it will probably be necessary to give chronic long term TF treatments over several weeks. This has not been easy to achieve so far. Finally, as discussed elsewhere in this volume (42), the TF target cell could be a T_0 cell as found in the thymus cortex or prethymic cells as found in nude mice needing a direct thymic traffic to find high concentrations of thymic factor (47).

V APPLICATIONS TO AUTOIMMUNITY

Experimental data: NZB mice and B/W (F1) hybrids have a normal level of serum TF at birth, but this level decreases prematurely between the 3rd and 6th week of life (21). At two months, NZB and B/W (F1) mice have no significant circulating TF. Six weeks after the decline of serum TF, NZB mice show a disappearance of θ-positive lymph node RFC and, two weeks later, a progressive decrease in spleen RFC sensitivity to AθS and AZ, as present in neonatally thymectomized mice. Interestingly, normal AZ and AθS sensitivity of spleen and lymph node RFC is reconstituted by *in vitro* and *in vivo* treatment with thymic extracts (21).

The etiology of the thymic lesions causing premature disappearance of serum hormonal activity is not known. The possible role of thymocytotoxic autoantibodies early in life in NZB mice is one among several possible hypotheses. Such antibodies, however, do not act, if they do play a role, by elimination of hormone produced in normal amounts, since injection of thymic extracts corrects both serum TF and sensitivity of spleen and lymph node RFC to AZ and AθS in NZB mice (21). Moreover, when grafting a neonatal NZB thymus into young or old NZB mice, one can rapidly reconstitute a normal level of serum TF (37). Interestingly, the duration of the reconstitution is between 2 to 4 weeks, which is identical to the spontaneous lifespan of thymus secretion in NZB mice. This short lifespan is in contrast with the long lifespan of thymus grafts in other strains.

Spontaneously autoimmune mice can also be obtained by genetic selection for spontaneous antibody production against nuclear antigens. Such mice have been obtained by Monier *et al.* by genetic selection bearing on an initial stock of outbred Swiss mice (48). Autoimmune mice thus obtained exhibit high titers of antinuclear antibodies at the age of 3 months and ultimately glomerulonephritis with immune complex deposits. Interestingly, the genetic selection also induces an early cessation of TF production, similar to that noted in NZB mice (49). As a control for these experiments, it has been shown that Swiss mice genetically selected as "high" and "low" responders for antisheep RBC haemagglutinin production did not differ from ordinary Swiss mice with regard to serum TF level (49).

Finally, these data indicate an early deficiency in TF secretion in NZB, B/W, and Swiss mice which precedes all other T cell abnormalities and the ultimate onset of autoimmunity. The possible role of this deficiency in the pathogenesis of autoimmunity is suggested by the correction of responsiveness to mitogen afforded by thymus grafting or TF *in vivo* treatment (36, 37) and the normalization of anti-PVP antibody response by *in vivo* TF treatment (36).

The TF involvement in the control of autoimmunity is also suggested by the TF effect on autologous rosette formation mentioned above.

Clinical data: Human serum shows TF activity when applied in the mouse rosette inhibition assay described above (24). We have not yet performed detailed studies on the biochemical characteristics of human TF, but it is already established that human TF behaves like mouse or pig TF for diafiltration through Amicon membranes of various molecular weight cut-offs; it also binds to CM cellulose at pH 6.3 and not to DEAE cellulose at pH 7.3.

Human TF disappears from the serum after thymectomy in myasthenic patients (24) with a half-life of less than 6 hours. As in the mouse, TF level depends on age. Serum TF is stable until the age of 15-20 years and declines progressively afterwards to become insignificant in most subjects over 30 years of age.

In systemic lupus erythematosus (50, 51), serum TF has consistently been found at a low level before any treatment in young patients under 25, an age where control subjects still show a high hormone level. This data is in keeping with the low TF level found in NZB mice and would suggest that a deficiency in TF secretion might play a role in SLE pathogenesis.

Conversely, normal or high TF levels have been found in *rheumatoid arthritis* (51), particularly in patients over 40, who showed a hormone level significantly higher than normal controls of the same age in 65 per cent of cases. In keeping with this data, T cells evaluated by sheep cell spontaneous rosette formation showed normal or high values in most cases with a correlation with TF level.

In *immunodeficiency states,* TF level was strictly normal in pure agammaglobulinemia (6 cases studied) but TF was undetectable (as in nude mice) in two cases of Di George's syndrome. Normal or decreased (but not zero) TF levels have been found in ataxia telangectasia and various immunodeficiencies with variable onset.

In *myasthenia gravis,* TF levels were normal in patients less than 20 years of age but tended to be high (although inconsistently) in older patients (24).

REFERENCES

1. Bach, J. F. & Dardenne, M. (1972) *Cell. Immunol.* **3**, 11.
2. Bach, J. F. & Dardenne, M. (1973) *Cell. Immunol.* **6**, 394.
3. Bach, J. F. & Dardenne, M. (1972) *Cell. Immunol.* **3**, 1.
4. Hudson, L., Greenberg, A. H., Roitt, I. M. & Bach, J. F. (1973) *Scand. J. Immunol.* **2**, 425.
5. Bach, J. F., Reyes, F., Dardenne, M., Fournier, C. & Muller, J. Y. (1971) *in*: Cell Interactions and receptor antibodies in immune responses. (O. Makela, A. Cross and T. U. Kosunen, ed.) Acad. Press. N.Y. p. 111.
6. Charreire, J., Dardenne, M. & Bach, J. F. (1973) *Cell. Immunol.* **9**, 32.
7. Bach, J. F., Muller, J. Y. & Dardenne, M. (1970) *Nature* **227**, 1251.
8. Bach, J. F., Dardenne, M. & Fournier, C. (1969) *Nature* **222**, 998.
9. Bach, J. F., Dardenne, M. & Davies, A. J. S. (1971) *Nature, New Biology* **231**, 110.
10. Bach, J. F., Dardenne, M., Goldstein, A. L., Guha, A. & White, A. (1971) *Proc. Nat. Acad. Sci.* (U.S.A.) **68**, 2734.
11. Dardenne, M. & Bach, J. F. (1973) *Immunology* **25**, 343.
12. Bach, J. F. & Dardenne, M. (1972) *Transpl. Proc.* **4**, 345.
13. Bach, J. F. & Dardenne, M. (1973) *Immunology* **25**, 353.
14. Dardenne, M., Papiernik, M., Bach, J. F. & Stutman, O. (1974) *Immunology* **27**, 299.
15. Dardenne, M. & Bach, J. F. - This volume.
16. Bach, J. F., Dardenne, M. & Bach, M. A. (in press) *Ann. N.Y. Acad. Sci.*
17. Bach, J. F., Dardenne, M. & Pleau, J. M. (1974) *C.R. Acad. Sci.* (Paris) **278**, 335.
18. Goldstein, A. L., Guha, A., Zatz, M. M., Hardy, M. A. & White, A. *Proc. Nat. Acad. Sci.* (Wash.) **69**, 1800.
19. Goldstein, G. (1974) *Nature* **247**, 11.
20. Trainin, N. This volume.
21. Bach, J. F., Dardenne, M. & Salomon, J. C. (1973) *Clin. Exp. Immunol.* **14**, 247.
22. Papiernik, M., Nabarra, B. & Bach, J. F. (1975) *Clin. Exp. Immunol.* **19**, 281.
23. Lacombe, M., Perner, F., Dardenne, M. & Bach, J. F. (1975) *Surgery.*
24. Bach, J. F., Dardenne, M., Papiernik, M., Barois, A., Levasseur, P. & Le Brigand, H. (1972) *Lancet* **2**, 1056.
25. Dardenne, M., Tournefier, A., Charlemagne, J. & Bach, J. F. (1973) *Ann. Immunol.* **124 c**, 465.
26. Dardenne, M., in press.
27. Bach, J. F., Duval, D., Dardenne, M., Salomon, J. C., Tursz, T. & Fournier, C. (1975) *Transpl. Proc.* **7**, 25.
28. Fournier, C. & Bach, J. F. (this volume).
29. Bach, M. A., Fournier, C. & Bach, J. F. (In press) *Ann. N.Y. Acad. Sci.*
30. Komuro, K. & Boyse, E. A. (1973) *Lancet* **i**, 740.
31. Papiernik, M. & Fournier, C. In preparation.
32. Bach, M. A. (1974) *C.R. Acad. Sci.* (Paris) **278**, 3023.
33. Bach, M. A. & Bach, J. F. (1973) *Eur. J. Immunol.* **3**, 778.
34. Bach, M. A. (1974) *Ann. Immunol.* **125 c**, 865.
35. Bach, M. A. & Bach, J. F. (1974) *in*: "Prostaglandin synthetase inhibitors" (H. J. Robinson and J. Vane eds.) Raven Press, N.Y.
36. Bach, M. A. & Niaudet, P. (In press)
37. Niaudet, P. & Bach, M. A. (Submitted to publication)
38. Micklem, H. S. & Anderson, N. (1972) *in*: Cell Interactions. 3rd. Lepetit Colloquim North Holland, Amsterdam p. 229.
39. Charreire, J. & Bach, J. F. (1974) *Lancet* **2**, 229.
40. Charreire, J. & Bach, J. F. (In press) *Proc. Nat. Acad. Sci.* (USA).
41. Charreire, J. & Bach, J. F., This volume.
42. Bach, J. F., Cantor, H., Roelants, G. & Stutman, O. (this volume).
43. Duval, D. (in preparation).
44. Charreire, J. & Bach, J. F. (submitted to publication).
45. Workshop Proceedings (this volume).
46. Doenhoff, M. J. & Davies, A. J. S. (1971) *Cell. Immunol.* **1**, 82.
47. Bach, J. F. (1973) *Lancet* **9**, 1320.
48. Monier, J. C., Thivolet, J., Beuvin, A. J., Czyba, J. C., Schmitt, D. & Salussola, D. (1971) *Path. Eur.* **6**, 357.

49. Dardenne, M., Monier, J. C., Biozzi, G. & Bach, J. F. (1974) *Clin. Exp. Immunol.* **17**, 339.
50. Bach, J. F. & Dardenne, M. (1972) *J. Urol. Néphrol.* **78**, 994.
51. Bach, J. F., Dardenne, M. & Clot, J. (In press) *in*: Proc. Intern. Symp. on Immunological Aspects of Rheumatological Diseases. (J. Clot and J. Samy, eds.).

Biological Activity of Thymic Hormones

T CELL SUBSETS: TERMINOLOGY PROBLEMS

JEAN-FRANÇOIS BACH*, HARVEY CANTOR**, GEORGES ROELANTS*** & OSIAS STUTMAN****

Several lines of evidence argue in favour of the existence of different T cell subpopulations which differ according to their markers and functions. That such subpopulations, as defined by a number of physical or biological properties and immune functions, do exist is now well established, although we cannot say as yet whether the T cell subsets defined by each group's assay are identical. Moreover, it is not clear whether the T cell subsets that have been described represent different stages in T cell maturation or whether they represent products of separate T cell lines (even if derived from a common precursor), although recent evidence (see Cantor & Boyse, this volume) suggests that "mature" subsets may represent products of different lines of maturation. The aim of this note is to briefly review the main pieces of evidence which have led to the notion of T cell heterogeneity and to discuss the relationships among the cells considered in each system as well as the terminology used by each author. It appears that there are striking similarities, but also clear-cut differences, among the various cell classifications. We shall not propose a new terminology here. Rather we shall set side by side in an explicative fashion the available terminologies. It should be emphasized that all of the data which will be discussed have been obtained in the mouse and that there is little evidence to justify their extrapolation to other species at present.

I. T CELL SYNERGY EXPERIMENTS

The idea of T cell subclasses was first introduced by H. Cantor and M. Raff (1, 2) and was based in part on synergy between T cells in the graft versus host reaction; this synergy was later confirmed in the mixed lymphocyte reaction and the cell-mediated lympholysis assay.

A. *Graft versus Host reaction* (GvH) data (3-6)

When newborn F_1 mice are injected with small doses of parental lymph node

* Hôpital Necker, Paris, France
** Children's Cancer Research Foundation, Boston, USA
*** Basel Institute for Immunology, Basel, Switzerland
**** Sloan Kettering Institute, New York, USA

cells or thymus cells alone, they do not experience a major GvH reaction (assessed by a spleen index). However, mixtures of small numbers of theta-positive lymph node cells and thymocytes induce a substantial GvH reaction which is not explained by a simple additive effect. This synergy is also seen when thymus cells are replaced by spleen cells (taken from ALS-treated animals) or when lymph node cells are replaced by peripheral blood lymphocytes. Cell dilution studies indicate that the effect is proportional to the number of thymus cells inoculated when a low number of lymph node cells is administered. These data suggested that the thymus cells might be the effector cells, a notion also suggested by further studies in which a mixture of C57BL/6 thymus cells and BALB/c lymph node cells were injected into (C57BL/6 $\times$ BALB/c) F_1 mice. When spleen cells of the recipient F_1 mice were subsequently injected into BALB/c or C57BL/6 newborn parental recipients, only recipients allogeneic to the donor of the thymocytes suffered GvH reactions. Based on these synergistic effects and the effects of adult thymectomy, Cantor and Raff designated thymus cells as T_1 cells and lymph node cells as T_2 cells (1, 2). It is relevant to considerations concerning the relationship of these two interacting T cells that recovery from ALS treatment is noted earlier for T_1 cells than for T_2 cells (7).

B. *Mixed lymphocyte reaction* (MLR)

The MLR is essentially a T cell-mediated proliferative response (8), even if some B cells may be recruited in the course of the reaction (9). *In vitro* synergy between thymus cells and lymph node cells has been reported by Howe (10), Hayry (11), and Walford (12).

C. *Cell mediated lympholysis* (CML)

The CML reaction is the specific lymphocytotoxicity arising in MLR against the stimulating cells. Several workers have reported a synergy of thymus and lymph node cells in this reaction (13, 14). Again, thymus cells can be replaced in this synergy by ALS-treated mouse spleen cells (15). The thymic dependence of the two populations in question was assessed in these experiments by their inactivation after treatment with antitheta serum and complement and passage through nylon wool columns. The nature of the effector cells has been investigated using thymus and lymph node cells differing at the θ (14) or the θ and MLC locus (16) and studying the proportion of killer cells generated in MLC that bear antigens distinguishing the LN or thymus component. In the two studies (14, 16), the effector cells appeared to be descended from lymph node cells.

II. EARLY EFFECTS OF ADULT THYMECTOMY (ATX)

Adult thymectomy has been thought for many years to have little effect if any on the immune system, since more than 6 months elapse before major immune defects are apparent. However, data have recently been accumulated which indicate that ATX in fact induced very early effects on the lymphoid system which were apparent a few days after the operation. Five of the systems in which those effects have been demonstrated will be discussed in some detail.

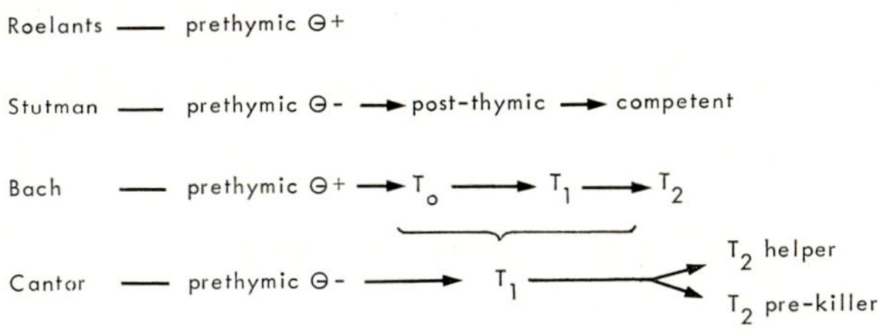

Fig. 1. Comparison of the terminologies used to define T cell subpopulations

A. *The mouse spontaneous sheep red cell rosette-forming cells*

A low percentage of lymphoid cells from unimmunized mice forms rosettes when mixed with sheep red blood cells (about 0.1 per cent in the spleen, 0.04 per cent in lymph nodes, 0.02 per cent in the thymus; all located in the steroid-resistant cell pool). These spontaneous rosette forming cells (sRFC) include antigen-sensitive cells, since their removal induces specific unresponsiveness as tested by transfer experiments (16). Theta-positive RFC, as defined by rosette inhibition after *in vitro* incubation with antitheta serum and complement, include several subsets which are termed T_0, T_1, and T_2 (17). T_0 RFC are inhibited only at high antitheta serum (AθS) concentration (e.g. 1/20) but the inhibition is still θ-specific; they are found in normal bone marrow. T_1 RFC are inhibited by low AθS concentration (e.g. 1/1000), and are present in spleen and thymus. T_2 RFC are inhibited by low AθS concentrations (e.g. 1/200), although significantly higher than those acting on T_1 RFC and are present in lymph nodes. Azathioprine, a purine analogue, inhibits theta-positive RFC and is inactive on theta-negative RFC (18). Interestingly, there is a ranking of azathioprine sensitivity from 1 μg/ml for T_1 RFC, 50 μg/ml for T_2 RFC to 500 μg/ml for T_0 RFC expressed in minimal inhibiting concentrations (19). Radioautography experiments have shown that both T_1 and T_2 RFC have a lifespan longer than 30 days (19).

Adult thymectomy suddenly decreases the spleen RFC sensitivity to azathioprine on day 5 postthymectomy (18, 20), a decrease completely corrected by *in vitro* or *in vivo* treatment with low amounts of thymic extracts or of purified circulating thymic factor (21, 22). However, adult thymectomy does not alter lymph node T_2 RFC AθS- or azathioprine sensitivity. Conversely, short term ALS *in vivo* treatment depletes lymph node T_2 RFC but not spleen T_1 RFC. (18)

The normalization of spleen RFC azathioprine sensitivity by thymic hormones is also obtained in neonatally thymectomized and nude mice but 10-20-fold higher concentrations of the hormone are needed in the latter case than after ATX (22). One may also note that T_0 RFC seen in nude mice have a small but significant amount of θ-antigen as detected by AθS rosette inhibition (18).

B. *Autologous Rosette Forming cells (ARFC)*

A small percentage of normal lymphoid cells bind autologous erythrocytes forming rosettes (23, 24). ARFC predominate in the thymus, but are also found in the spleen and to a lesser extent in lymph nodes. ARFC levels are increased 10-20-fold within 6 weeks after ATX (24-26) (a significant increase being observed as soon as 6 days after thymectomy). Such increase in ARFC levels is corrected by injection of thymic hormone (thymosin or circulating TF) (25, 26). ARFC are also increased in aged mice and nude mice, but much less so than in adult thymectomized mice. ARFC belong to the less dense cells of the spleen, they adhere to nylon and are essentially steroid-sensitive in the thymus (26).

C. *Theta antigen*

We have already mentioned the early effects of adult thymectomy on θ positive spleen RFC (as soon as 7 days postthymectomy). Adult thymectomy is also followed within 3-4 weeks by a decrease in the number of θ positive cells when assessed by cytotoxicity tests or immunofluorescence tests (1, 27, 29). As found for θ positive RFC, adult thymectomy does not alter the lymph nodes as much as it alters spleen cells (1, 29).

D. *MLC-CML*

Adult thymectomy has been reported to depress the MLR in the mouse (30) and in the rat (31, 32). Adult thymectomy can also depress CML responses, even when the T cell number in the cultures is fixed by filtration on nylon columns (33). However, early after ATX (3 weeks), Cantor finds that both MLC and CML responses are enhanced (34). The reasons for this difference are not clear, but may involve the different intervals after ATX and differences in cell culture conditions.

E. *Antibody responses* (1, 2, 34).

Studies of the effect of ATX on the antibody response to BSA indicate that the ability to generate helper (T) memory is significantly impaired within one month after surgery (2). At this time, the primary helper activity is completely intact.

F. *Contrasting effects of ATX and short-term in vivo ALS treatments*

It is interesting that most of the effects mentioned above for adult thymectomy are not induced by ALS, which mainly affects recirculating T lymphocytes as found in the peripheral blood. In fact, ALS has been shown to deplete lymph node T_2 RFC rather than T_1 RFC (18), to deplete lymph node as well as spleen theta-positive cells (28), to deplete primary antibody responses but not the development of immunologic memory (34), and to deplete prekiller cells (15). These are all functions which are relatively resistant to ATX.

G. *Conclusions*

Taken together, the above studies suggest the existence of two subsets of T cells. One cell type is sensitive to the short-term effects of ATX, bears large amounts of θ antigen, and is involved in MLC and CML reactions as well as in the development of immunologic memory. A second cell type, also θ^+, is resistant to the short-term effects of ATX but sensitive to ALS and is fully competent. Analogies with the T cell synergy experiments mentioned above indicate a similarity between the ATX-sensitive cell and Cantor's T_1 cell on the one hand, and between the ALS-sensitive cell and Cantor's T_2 cell on the other hand

III. RESTORATION OF THE IMMUNOCOMPETENCE OF THYMECTOMIZED MICE

T cell differentiation is probably associated with different maturation stages, the knowledge of which might be relevant to the concept of T cell subsets. In other words, one may wonder whether some of the T cell heterogeneity discussed above might not be explained by cells at different stages of maturation. Experiments by O. Stutman, A. L. Goldstein and N. Trainin have shed some light in that regard.

A. *Relative restorative capacity of embryonic and newborn cells* (35-38).

After the age of 45 days, neonatally thymectomized mice lose their capacity to recover immunocompetence in the presence of a thymus graft. However, when the thymus graft is supplemented with early embryonic cells (yolk sac or 14-day-old fetal liver), restoration of immunocompetence can be demonstrated by mitogen responses, helper effects in antibody production, MLC, and GvH reactivity. No such restoration is obtained if the thymus is grafted within a cell-impermeable Millipore chamber. However, 45-day-old neonatally thymectomized mice injected with newborn (and still incompetent) spleen cells plus thymus in Millipore chambers or functional epithelial thymomas are immunologically reconstitued. This difference in sensitivity to thymic humoral function relates to the stage of T cell differentiation: 14-day-old fetal cells (prethymic cells) need the thymic microenvironment to differentiate while newborn or adult cells (postthymic cells) need only the thymic humoral function. The maturation of the prethymic to the postthymic cells probably involves direct contact with the thymus epithelium, as suggested by studies using chromosome markers showing the migration of 14-day fetal cells to the thymus.

Moreover, there is no immunological reconstitution of nude mice which lack postthymic cells by a thymus in a Millipore chamber. The relationship of postthymic cells to mature peripheral T cells is suggested by studies using chromosome markers where purified newborn postthymic precursor cells grafted in neonatally thymectomized mice became competent T cells under the influence of antigenic stimulation of after exposure to thymus in diffusion chambers.

Systematic study of the postthymic cells (38) has shown that they are present in newborn bone marrow, spleen, and liver and in adult bone marrow or spleen of normal and neonatally thymectomized animals. Postthymic cells disappear 40-50 days after adult thymectomy, but are not altered by short-term *in vivo* treatment with ALS. They adhere to nylon, have a low density in BSA gradient, and large volume in velocity sedimentation at unit gravity; they are rapidly dividing and not recirculating. These cells bear some θ antigen and are essentially nonimmunocompetent (no response to PHA or Con A; no responsiveness in MLC or GvH).

B. *Immunological effects of thymic extracts*

Several *in vitro* and *in vivo* effects of thymic extracts on immune responses have been reported. A. Goldstein's "thymosin" allows neonatally thymectomized mice to reject skin allografts (39) and to induce a GvH reaction (40); N. Trainin's "thymic humoral factor" induces GvH reactivity *in vitro* and *in vivo* in spleen cells from neonatally thymectomized mice and stimulates thymus cells (but not bone marrow cells) in a Claman's type of bone marrow - thymus synergy experiment for anti-SRBC antibody responses (41). Both thymosin and thymic humoral factor have been shown to stimulate MLC response in thymocytes (41, 42), but not in the spleen. Lastly, we may mention the decrease in anti-PVP antibody formation obtained in NZB mice after treatment with J.-F. Bach's circulating thymic factor (44) which is suggestive for suppressor T cell restoration. Note, however, the absence of data bearing on nude mice in these functional assays.

IV. ALLOANTIGENIC MARKERS (HETEROGENEITY, EFFECTS OF THYMIC HORMONES)

The *theta antigen* is not uniformly distributed in all T cells. There is some suggestion from immunofluorescence and absorption data that lymph node cells bear less theta antigen than do thymus cortical cells. For example, low concentrations of anti-θ serum more readily deplete PHA-responsive cells than MLC-responsive cells (45). Discontinuous BSA density gradients allow the separation of low density cells with less than 10 per cent θ-positive cells and high density cells rich in θ-positive cells (46, 47, 48).

Thymic hormones can induce the theta antigen expression in spleen RFC from adult or neonatally thymectomized or nude mouse RFC which naturally have a small amount of θ antigen (see above). Similarly, Komuro & Boyse have shown that incubation of low density fractions from normal spleen cells, separated on a BSA gradient, with thymic extracts increased the number of θ positive cells (47). This effect was also obtained with nonthymic extracts at higher concentrations, which indicates that induction of theta may be achieved nonspecifically (49). This reservation applies less to the rosette assay where adequate controls, including serum from thymectomized animals, have always proved to be negative, eventually in blind studies (50, see this volume).

The existence of a cell population with a small amount of θ antigen in nude mice, as discussed above for spleen RFC, has been recently confirmed and extended by Roelants and Loor, (51, 52). In brief, these cells which represent up to 20 per cent of nude spleen cells are characterized by a low membrane density of the θ and TL antigens, the absence of surface immunoglobulin, and a slow electrophoretic mobility which is similar to that of thymocytes but not of peripheral T cells. They are absent in the thoracic duct and have a rapid turnover (1-2 days). They bear, like sRFC, antigen-specific receptors. Interestingly, these cells disappear rapidly after thymus grafting, also when the graft is placed within a Millipore diffusion chamber, which is suggestive of their dependence on a thymic hormone.

Ly antigens - Recent experiments by Cantor & Boyse (see this volume) indicate that Ly antigens are not equally distributed among T cell subsets. Thus, in C57BL/6 mice, the ATX sensitive T_1 subset bears Ly-1.2, 2.2, 3.2 antigens, whereas T_2 cells bear either the Ly-1.2 or Ly-2.3/3.2 antigen. Ly-1.2^+ cells are "programmed" to mediate helper function for both antibody production and for the production of cell-mediated responses, whereas Ly-2.3/3.2^+ cells are programmed to express killer activity upon contact with antigen. From a number of observations, it is likely that both "mature" subsets, termed T-2^h and T-2^k are the descendents of a common progenitor - the Ly-123^+ T_1 cell.

CONCLUSIONS (Fig. 1 and Table I)

It is still impossible to reconcile all of these data, although many similarities have been shown. It appears that there exists a T cell subset with little or no immunocompetence (Stutman's postthymic cell; Bach's T_0 cell) which can be converted under the influence of thymic humoral function to a population of more competent cells still relatively immature, short lived, and nonrecirculating (Cantor's and Bach's T_1 cell). Bach has suggested that the T_0-T_1 transformation may be reversible (22, 53, 54) and under the control of cyclic AMP (48), which is itself regulated by thymic hormones, and that T_0 and T_1 represent different metabolic states of the same cell. At the two extremes, there would be a very immature cell (called a prethymic cell) which would need direct contact with the thymic microenvironment (perhaps to find high levels of

TABLE I: Comparison between the characteristics of T cell subsets

	O. Stutman		
	Prethymic	*Posthymic*	*Ma T c*
Main location in normal mice	*Yolk sac, fetal liver (14 d), newborn spleen*	*Lymphohemopoietic organs including normal BM and newborn spleen*	*Per phe lym orga*
Appearance in ontogeny	9 d	birth	7–1
NTX mice spleen (early after TX)	+	+	—
Nude spleen	+	—	—
Functional sensitivity to Ad. TX	0	+ (↘)	0
Induction with thymic humoral function	0	+ (↗)	?
Sensitivity to ALS *in vivo*	?	0	
Sensitivity to high dose of steroids *in vivo*	?	?	?
Density	low	low	hig
Adherence to nylon	?	+	—
Volume (velocity sedimentation)	medium	"large"	sma
Lifespan	?	30–45 d	2 m
Traffic	?	Spleen seeking	LN ing
Recirculation	?	No	Yes
Proliferative rate	high(?)	high	low
Markers			
Alloantigen-θ (cytotoxicity with C)	—	—	+
θ (by function inactiv.)	—	+	+
θ (Ag. binding inhibition)	?	?	?
θ (Immunofluorescence)	?	?	?
TL	?	+ ?	—
Ly (1.2, 2.2, 3.2)	?	?	?
Mitogens response: PHA	—	—	+
Con A	—	—	+
Functions			
GVH (splenomegaly)	—	—	+
MLC (to MHC differences)	—	—	+
Primary antibody response (helper function)	?	?	?

humoral factors) and a totally mature and competent T cell (Cantor's and Bach's T_2 cell and Stutman's competent T cell). Lastly, recent data from Cantor (see above) indicate that mature and T_2 cells may be divisible into subsets based upon Ly antigens and different immunologic function.

REFERENCES

1. Cantor, H. (1972) in *Proceedings of the 2nd Lepetit Colloqium*, North-Holland, Amsterdam, p. 73.
2. Raff, M. C. & Cantor, H. (1971) *Progress in Immunology* **4**, 93.
3. Cantor, H. (1972) *Cell. Immunol.* 3, 461.
4. Cantor, H. & Asofsky, R. (1970) *J. Exp. Med.* **131**, 235.
5. Cantor, H. & Asofsky, R. (1972) *J. Exp. Med.* **135**, 764.

oor and elants	*J. F. Bach*				*H. Cantor*		
ϑ+weak hymic)	*Prethymic*	T_0	T_1	T_2	T_1	T_2h (*helper*)	T_2k (*prekiller*)
		BM AT x *Spl*	*Thymus spleen*	*L. nodes blood*	*Thymus*	*Lymph nodes, peripheral blood*	*Blood, lymph nodes*
	?	?	?	?	Early	late	late
	+	+	–	–	+	–	–
	+	–	–	–	–	–	–
	0	+ (↗)	+ (↘)	0	+(↘)	0	0
	0	– (↘)	+ (↗)	0	?+	?	?
	?	0	0	+ (↘)	±	+	+
	?	?	0	0	?	?	?
	?	low	?	high			
	?	+	?	–	?	no	no
um	?	?	?	?			
	?	?	>30 d	>30 d	<30 d	> 90d	>90 d
					Spleen seeking	LN seeking	LN seeking
					∓	++	++
l 24 h							
	?	?	+	+			
	?	?	+	+	++	++	++
	+	+	+	+			
					+++	++	++
luoresc.)					?+	–	–
					Ly-1, 2, 3+	Ly-1+	Ly-2,3+
				+			
				+	Precursor of effector cell	Amplifier	
			+	+	+	+	+
					Early precursor	Pre-Helper	Pre-Killer
					Precursor	Pre-Helper	

6. Asofsky, R., Cantor, H. & Tigelaar, R. E. (1971) *Progress in Immunology* **1**.
7. Morse, H. C. III, & Asofsky, R. (1974) *Cell. Immunol.* **11**, 19.
8. Festenstein, H., Davies, A. J. S., Leuchars, E., Wallis, V. J. & Doenhoff, M. J., in: "Lymphatic tissue and Germinal Centers in Immune response", eds. L. Fiore-Donati & M. G. Hannea Jr. Plenum Publ. Corp. N.Y. p. 121.
9. Piguet, P. F. & Vassali, P. (1972) *J. Exp. Med.* **136**, 962.
10. Cohen, D. & Howe, M. L. (1973) *Proc. Nat. Acad. Sci. USA* **70**, 2707.
11. Hayry, P. & Andersson, L. C. (In press).
12. Tittor, W., Gerbase-Delima, M. & Walford, R. L. (1974) *J. Exp. Med.* **139**, 1488.
13. Andersson, L. & Hayry, P. (1974) in *Proc. 8th Leuk. Cult. Conf.* eds. K. Lindahl & O. Osoba Acad. Press. New York p.
14. Wagner, H., Rollinghöf, M. & Nossal, G. (1973) *Transpl. Rev.* **17**, 4.
15. Cantor, H. & Simpson, E. (1975) Submitted for publication.
16. Bach, J.-F., Muller, J. Y. & Dardenne, M. (1970) *Nature* **227**, 1251.
17. Bach, J.-F. & Dardenne M. (1972) *Cell. Immunol.* **3**, 11.
18. Bach, J.-F. & Dardenne, M. (1973) *Cell. Immunol.* **6**, 394.

19. Martin-Taieb, C., Guy-Grand, D., Griscelli, C. & Bach, J.-F. (1974) *Cell. Immunol.* **11**, 325.
20. Bach, J.-F., Dardenne, M. & Davies, A. J. S. (1971) *Nature New Biol.* **231**, 110.
21. Bach, J.-F., Dardenne, M., Goldstein, A. L., Guha, A. & White, A. (1971) *Proc. Nat. Ac. Sci.* **68**, 2734.
22. Bach, J.-F. & Dardenne, M. (1973) *Immunology* **25**, 353.
23. Micklem, H. S. & Anderson, N. (1972) in *Proceedings of the 3rd Lepetit Colloquium*, North Holland, Amsterdam, p. 229.
24. Charreire, J. & Bach, J.-F. (1974) *Lancet* **2**, 229.
25. Charreire, J. & Bach, J.-F. (this volume).
26. Charreire, J. & Bach, J.-F. (1975) *Proc. Nat. Acad. Sci.* (In press)
27. Schlesinger, M. & Yron, I. (1972) *J. Immunol.* **104**, 798.
28. Raff, M. C. & Wortis, H. H. (1970) *Immunology* **18**, 931.
29. Fournier, C. (In preparation).
30. Bach, M. A. & Bach, J.-F. (1972) *Transpl. Proc.* **4**, 165.
31. Schwarz, R. & Robson, L. C. (1971) *Transplantation* **5**, 1046.
32. Folch, H. & Waksman, B. (1972) *J. Immunol.* **5**, 1046.
33. Andersson, L. C., Hayry, P., Bach, M. A. & Bach, J.-F. (1974) *Nature* **252**, 252.
34. Simpson, E. & Cantor (1975) (Submitted for publication).
35. Stutman, O. (This volume).
36. Stutman, O., Yunis, E. J. & Good, R. A. (1970) *J. Exptl. Med.* **132**, 583.
37. Stutman, O., Yunis, E. J. & Good, R. A. (1970) *J. Exptl. Med.* **132**, 601.
38. Stutman, O. (In press) *Ann. N.Y. Acad. Sci.*
39. Goldstein, A. L., Guha, A., Zatz, M. M., Hardy, M. A. & White, A. (1972) *Proc. Nat. Acad. Sci.* **69**, 1800.
40. Goldstein, A. L., Asanuma, Y., Battisto, J. R., Hardy, M. A., Quint, A. & White, A. (1970) *J. Immunol.* **104**, 359.
41. Trainin, N. *et al.* (This volume).
42. Goldstein, A. L. (This volume).
43. Umiel, T. (This volume).
44. Bach, J.-F., Dardenne, M., Bach, M. A., Fournier, C., Charreire, J. & Pleau, J. M. (This volume).
45. Howe, M. & Cohen, L. (1974) in Proc. 8th Leuk. Cult. Conference. (K. Lindahl, K. Essling & D. Osoba, eds.) Acad. Press. N.Y., p. 611.
46. Stobo, J. D., Rosenthal, A. S. & Paul, W. E. (1973) *J. Exp. Med.* **138**, 71.
47. Komuro, K. & Boyse, E. A. (1973) *J. Exp. Med.* **138**, 479.
48. Bach, M. A., Fournier, C. & Bach, J.-F. (In press) *Ann. N.Y. Acad. Sci.*
49. Scheid, M. P., Hoffmann, M. K., Domuro, K., Hammerling, U., Abbott, J., Boyse, E. A., Cohen, G. H., Hooper, J. A., Schulof, R. S. & Goldstein, A. L. (1973) *J. Exp. Med.* **138**, 1027.
50. Dardenne, M., Papiernik, M., Bach, J.-F. & Stutman, O. (1971) *Immunology* **27**, 299.
51. Loor, F. & Roelants, G. E. (1974) *Nature* **251**, 229.
52. Roelants, G. E. & Loor, F. (This volume).

Biological Activity of Thymic Hormones

DISCUSSION

WHITE, Palo Alto

My comments and questions are directed only toward ascertaining the degree to which there may be several different molecules that produce similar biological effects. This is one of the major objectives of this Workshop and Symposium. Certain of the biological effects that Dr. Bach has described for his thymic humoral factor have been produced by Dr. Trainin's factor and by the thymosin preparation isolated by Dr. Goldstein and myself, and about which he will be speaking later. From Dr. Trainin's described molecular weight of THF and particularly its amino acid composition, it is quite unlikely that thymosin and THF are the same molecule, nor can thymosin be an aggregate of Dr. Trainin's factor because of the marked differences in amino acid composition of the two proteins. Thymosin contains a cysteine residue, as Dr. Goldstein will report later, and Dr. Trainin's factor contains no cysteine. Thus, I believe that an aggregation phenomenon is ruled out as an explanation of the larger molecular weight of thymosin even though there is a heat step in the thymosin fractionation procedure.

I might direct attention, however, to the fact that acidic proteins do aggregate when lyophilized in the presence of a trace of phosphate buffer (Chilson, O. P., Costello, L. A. & Kaplan, N. O. (1965), *Biochemistry, 4,* 271; Everse, J. & Stolzenbach, F. E., In "Methods in Enzymology," ed. W. B. Jakoby, vol. XXII, pp. 33-38, Academic Press). Indeed, we have been able to convert thymosin, molecular weight 12,500 to a molecule of molecular weight approximately 70,000 by lyophilization in the presence of 0.001 M sodium phosphate buffer. Therefore, as indicated in my presentation this morning, artifacts may enter into protein purification and isolation. These are well-known and have been described (c.f. references above). However, in our laboratory, homogeneous thymosin as isolated has a molecular weight of 12,500. Moreover, the question is open as to whether smaller molecules, with thymosin-like activity, can be "separated" from thymosin of molecular weight 12,500.

If Dr. Bach will provide the amino acid composition of his product from pig serum, it may be possible to decide whether or not thymosin is a polymerized form of his TF factor.

BACH, Paris

I have no slides on that particular topic. The reason for this is that, having a very small amount of material as we have (a few μg), there is a certain degree of imprecision in the amino acid analysis, so that the only thing I can say is that our data are not incompatible with a close similarity between TF and THF.

WHITE, Palo Alto

I believe that what you have stated previously rules out the possibility that thymosin is an aggregate of the pig serum thymic humoral factor.

SWART, Rijswijk

It is unlikely that Bach's hormone can be polymerized to Allan Goldstein's because the isoelectric point of TF is 7.4 and that of thymosin is 4, so there must be a categoric difference in amino acid composition.

TRAININ, Rehovot

In my ignorance as a biochemist, I used to tease Dr. White on a few occasions saying that, probably because he is such an excellent biochemist, he uses very sophisticated ways to prepare his materials and that is the reason why he got a bigger molecule. By using the acetone step and the heat step, he probably denaturated the molecule or produced an aggregate of the true simple molecule of the hormone. In any case, the fact is that, by using the simple procedure that we have described today, we arrived at a level on which the differences cannot be explained by simple aggregation of molecules. So, I think that after this meeting I will not tease you any more about this problem.

BACH, Paris

Can I make one comment and ask one question? I would firstly agree with what you said; there is little argument in favour of aggregation. I just put forward this possibility as a formal one. Now the question is to Nathan: do you know what is the active concentration in protein of your most purified fraction in the GvH assay?

KOOK, Rehovot

We are using it in between 5 to 10 or 20 micrograms, so we haven't done any dilution studies; that is what I was asking. We are saving these studies for the adenyl cyclase kinetic experiments and the MLC, which is much more quantitative.

GOLDSTEIN, Galveston

I agree with what Dr. White has said; it is unlikely, based upon amino acid composition, that Bach's molecule is a monomer of the larger thymosin molecule or that thymosin is an aggregate. I think the amino acid composition rules out that possibility. Now with regard to the Trainin molecule, I would make the same comment. Fraction 8 is the first peptide we have purified; it has a molecular weight of 12,000 and is one of 3 peptides that we have now purified from fraction 5. We know that the molecular weights of the peptides in fraction 5 range from about 1,000 to about 15,000. It is still possible that one of these peptides will be identical to the molecules reported by Bach and Trainin. I have 3 questions regarding the chemistry of the Trainin molecule. One, was the gel electrophoresis of your fraction run at an acid pH or alkaline pH? Secondly, do you know the isoelectric point? Thirdly, at what wave length do you measure the optical density of your fractions?

KOOK, Rehovot

This gel electrophoresis is an isoelectric focusing. The pH ranges between 4 and 8.7, the isoelectric point is about 5.6, and the reading of absorbancy is done at 280 or 230 nm. At 230, we get better reading, and at 280 very small readings.

Biological Activity of Thymic Hormones

THYMOSIN: CHEMISTRY, BIOLOGY, AND CLINICAL APPLICATIONS

ALLAN L. GOLDSTEIN, GARY B. THURMAN, GERALDINE H. COHEN & JOHN A. HOOPER

I. INTRODUCTION

Advances in immunobiology point to a major role for the endocrine thymus in the ontogenesis, function, and senescence of the immune system (Goldstein & White 1973, Trainin 1974). Ongoing studies indicate that impaired production and/or secretion of the thymic hormone, thymosin (and possibly of other thymic factors), may underlie many of the immunological deficiencies observed in animals after experimental thymectomy (Asanuma *et al.* 1970, Goldstein *et al.* 1970) or in humans with thymus dysgenesis (Goldstein *et al.* 1974, Goldstein *et al.* 1975, Sakai *et al.* 1975, Wara *et al.* 1975).

In this paper, we discuss recent advances in our knowledge of the chemistry and biology of thymosin and present a hypothesis for a mechanism of action of thymosin. In addition, we describe several of the new biological assays that are being used to measure thymosin activity *in vitro* and *in vivo* and explore the prospects for use of thymosin in the clinic to treat diseases associated with thymic malfunction.

The emerging appreciation of the breadth of endocrine influence of the thymus on homeostatic processes opens up a gamut of new approaches involving the use of thymosin for therapeutic manipulation of the immune system in patients with immune deficiencies associated with cancer, autoimmune disorders, and aging.

II. HISTORICAL BACKGROUND

A. *Critical Evidence Establishing the Thymus as an Endocrine Gland*

One prerequisite for establishing the endocrine function of an organ is the demonstration that cell-free extracts of the organ will replace, in whole or in part, the specific biological functions of that organ (White & Goldstein 1968). This criterion has now been amply satisfied for the thymus gland. Reconstitu-

Division of Biochemistry, Department of Human Biological Chemistry and Genetics, University of Texas Medical Branch, Galveston, Texas 77550
This research supported, in part, by National Cancer Institute Grants DHEW 5R01 CA 15419-02 and DHEW 2R01 CA 14108-03 and The John Hartford Foundation, Inc.

tion studies show that crude and partially purified thymic extracts from various animal sources restore many of the immunological deficiencies brought about by removal of the gland (Asanuma *et al.* 1970, Goldstein *et al.* 1970, Goldstein *et al.* 1972).

A second prerequisite for establishing an endocrine function for an organ is the demonstration that a secreted product of that organ circulates in the blood. The presence of a thymic specific serum factor (TF) with thymosin-like activity detected in the blood of animals and humans by means of a sheep RBC rosette bioassay has now been demonstrated by Bach *et al.* (1973). In mice, this activity disappears rapidly from the circulation following thymectomy (Bach *et al.* 1971).

Our own studies, which have included the development of a radioimmunoassay for bovine and human thymosin, provide further evidence that circulating thymosin can be detected in the blood of several mammalian species (Schulof

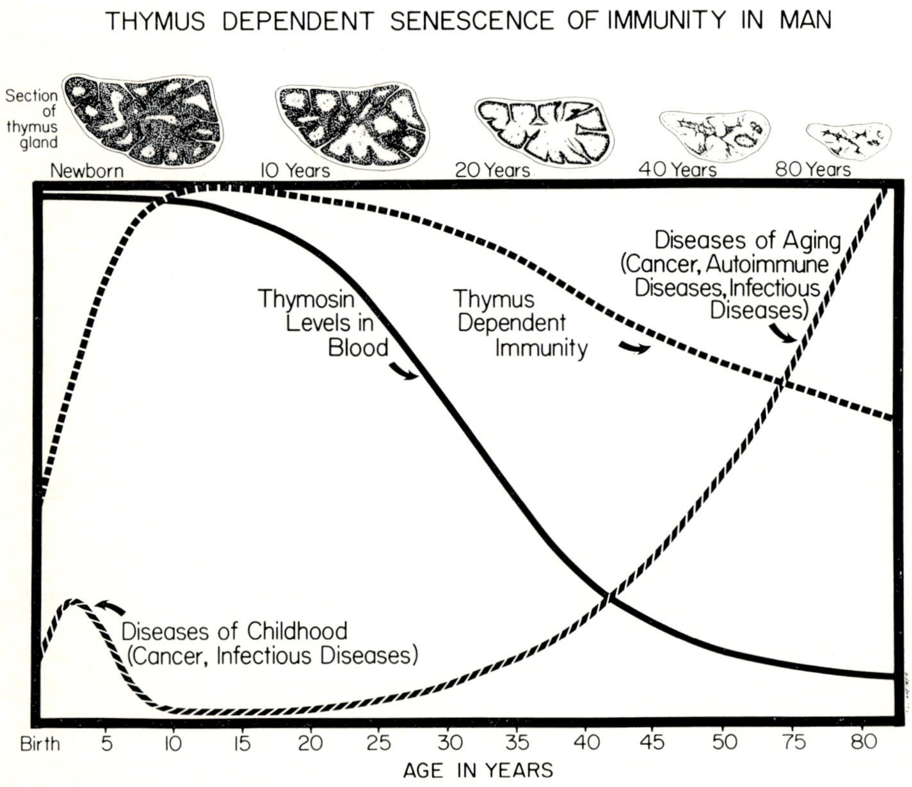

Fig. 1. Schematic diagram outlining the changes in thymosin levels, thymus dependent immunity, and histology of the thymus gland with age. There appears to be a direct correlation between the diseases of childhood and aging and the senescence of thymus-dependent immunity.

1972, 1973, Goldstein *et al.* 1974). Using the rosette assay and the RIA, we have observed that levels of circulating thymosin decrease with age in man and in other mammals and preliminary studies indicate that thymosin levels may be altered in patients with specific immunodeficiency diseases or cancer. The diminution of immunological function with age in man, no doubt associated with the observed atrophy of the thymus and decreased thymosin or "thymosin-like" activity in the blood, is schematically represented in Fig. 1.

The presence of thymosin in the blood strengthens the hypothesis that the thymus, in addition to influencing the maturation of lymphoid stem cells *in situ* as they transverse the gland, may also affect the maturation of immature lymphoid cells belonging to discrete populations located peripheral to the thymus gland. In addition to thymosin, several thymic factors have been reported that have biological activity *in vitro* and *in vivo* (c.f. reviews of thymic factors by Goldstein & White 1971, 1973, Trainin 1974). The biological and chemical properties of two of these factors (THF and TF) are reviewed in othei chapters of this book. Suffice it to say, there is evidence that the thymus gland contains and/or secretes several biologically active factors, some of which may play a physiological role in the expression of immunity.

B. *Biological Studies with Thymosin in Animals*

Our own efforts have contributed to the elucidation of the endocrine function of the thymus gland in the development of host resistance. Thymosin was first detected as a lymphocytopoietic factor in mouse and rat thymus extracts in 1965 (Klein *et al.* 1965, 1966). The preparation of a stable, acetone powder form of the biologically active fraction (thymosin) from a variety of sources including thymus tissue of the mouse, rat, calf, rabbit, and human was achieved in 1966 (Goldstein *et al.* 1966). The purification to homogeneity of one thymus protein manifesting thymosin biological activity was achieved in 1972 (Goldstein *et al.* 1972). When administered to neonatally thymectomized mice, it was shown that partially purified thymosin: a) reduces the incidence of wasting and death (Asanuma *et al.* 1970, Goldstein *et al.* 1972); b) stimulates lymphocytopoiesis (Klein *et al.* 1965, 1966, Goldstein *et al.* 1966, White *et al.* 1969, Goldstein *et al.* 1970, White & Goldstein 1970, Miller *et al.* 1973); and c) restores or amplifies cell-mediated immunity and enhances tumor rejection in several types of immunologically deficient animals (Goldstein *et al.* 1970, Zisblatt *et al.* 1970, Hardy *et al.* 1971, Goldstein *et al.* 1972, Khaw & Rule 1973, Gershwin *et al.* 1974). In addition, it was found to enhance immunity in normal mice (Hardy *et al.* 1968, Thurman *et al.* In press) and in aged mice (Strausser *et al.* 1971). *In vitro* studies also demonstrate that thymosin can convert immature mouse lymphoid cells into cells bearing more mature T cell characteristics and function (Wolf & Erb 1970, Goldstein *et al.* 1971, Bach *et al.* 1971, Scheid *et al.* 1973). Using ficoll-hypaque separated lymphocytes from patients with primary and secondary immunodeficiency diseases, it was recently found that short-term incubation with thymosin *in vitro* increases significantly the number of T cells detected as E-rosettes (Wara & Ammann 1975, Goldstein *et al.* 1974, Sakai *et al.* 1975, Wara *et al.* 1975).

C. *Purification and Chemical Characterization of Thymosin*

The method for purification of thymosin (Goldstein *et al.* 1966, 1972) has been modified (Hooper *et al.* 1974) and scaled up to increase the yield of purified thymosin. Standard precautions against bacterial contamination are taken and preparations are routinely checked for pyrogenicity by both the limulus endotoxin assay (Cooper *et al.* 1973) and the rabbit pyrogenicity assay (McClosky *et al.* 1971). Pyrogen-free sterile water is used throughout; the procedures are performed at 4 °C unless stated otherwise.

The purification procedure is outlined in Fig. 2.

Thymus tissue is thawed and trimmed free of adipose tissue and is processed in batches of 5 kg. The thymus tissue is homogenized in three volumes of 0.15 M NaCl and 1 per cent octyl alcohol (v/v) in a Waring blender for 3 min at top speed. The homogenate is centrifuged at 14,000 × g to sediment the nuclear materials and 2 liter portions of the supernatant are heated with stirring to 80 °C in a boiling water bath. The voluminous precipitate of heat-denatured protein is removed by filtration through Miracloth. The clear yellow filtrate is cooled to 4 °C and added slowly, with stirring, to 5 volumes of acetone at −10 °C. The precipitate is collected on a large Buchner funnel, washed with several volumes of cold (−10 °C) acetone, and dried in a dessicator under reduced pressure. The white powder obtained by this procedure is suspended in 10 volumes of 10 mM $NaPO_4$, pH 7.0, and stirred at room temperature for 1 h. A small amount of insoluble residue is removed by centrifugation at 15,000 × g and the sample is adjusted to a protein concentration of 25 mg/ml as determined by the Lowry procedure (Lowry *et al.* 1951). Saturated ammonium sulfate solution adjusted to pH 7.0 with NH_4OH is added (33.3 ml to each 100 ml of solution), and the solution is stirred for 1 h. The precipitate is removed by centrifugation and the supernatant is adjusted to pH 4.0 with 10 per cent acetic acid. Solid ammonium sulfate (14.6 g/100 ml) is added and the suspension is stirred for 1 h. The precipitate is collected by centrifugation, dissolved in 10 mM Tris-HCl (pH 8.0) at a concentration of 10 mg/ml protein, and subjected to ultrafiltration at room temperature in an Amicon DC-2 hollow fiber system (concentration mode, H1DP10 membrane cartridge). The filtrate is collected at 4 °C, concentrated by rotary evaporation under reduced pressure, and desalted on a 5 × 80 cm column of Sephadex G-25 (fine) equilibrated with deionized water. The protein peak which elutes in advance of the salt and nucleotide peak is pooled, concentrated by rotary evaporation, and dried by lyophilization.

Further purification is achieved by column chromatography and preparative polyacrylamide gel electrophoresis. One gram of the lyophilized protein is dissolved in 100 ml of 10 mM mercaptoethanol in 50 mM Tris-HCl, pH 8.0, and the solution is percolated through a 2 × 40 cm column of DEAE cellulose

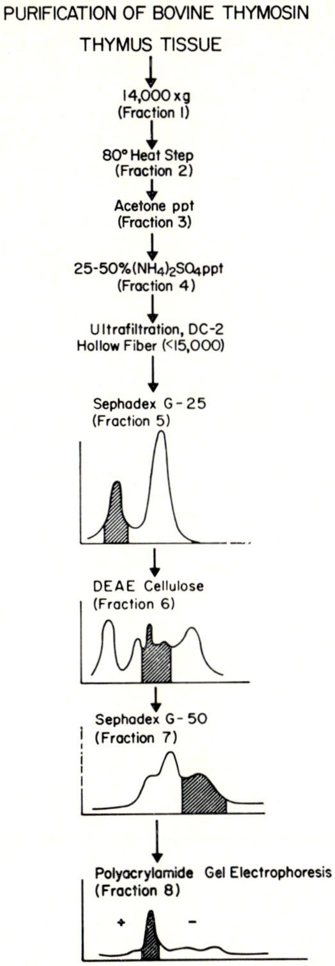

Fig. 2. The purification of bovine thymosin fraction 8. From Hooper *et al.* (1975).

(Whatman DE-32) equilibrated with the same buffer. After washing the column with one bed volume of starting buffer, the chromatogram is developed with a linear gradient formed by 800 ml of 10 mM mercaptoethanol in 50 mM Tris-HCl, pH 8.0, as the starting buffer and 800 ml of 10 mM mercaptoethanol and 0.8 M NaCl in 50 mM Tris-HCl, pH 8.0, as the limit buffer. The thymosin-containing fractions are pooled and subjected to gel filtration on a 3.8×150 cm column of Sephadex G-50 (fine) equilibrated with 0.2 M KCl and 10 mM mercaptoethanol in 10 mM Tris-HCl, pH 8.0. The active fractions are desalted by gel filtration on G-25 and subjected to preparative polyacrylamide gel electrophoresis. This procedure utilizes a 15 per cent polyacrylamide gel (6 cm high) that has been preelectrophoresed with 5 mmoles of cysteine as a free

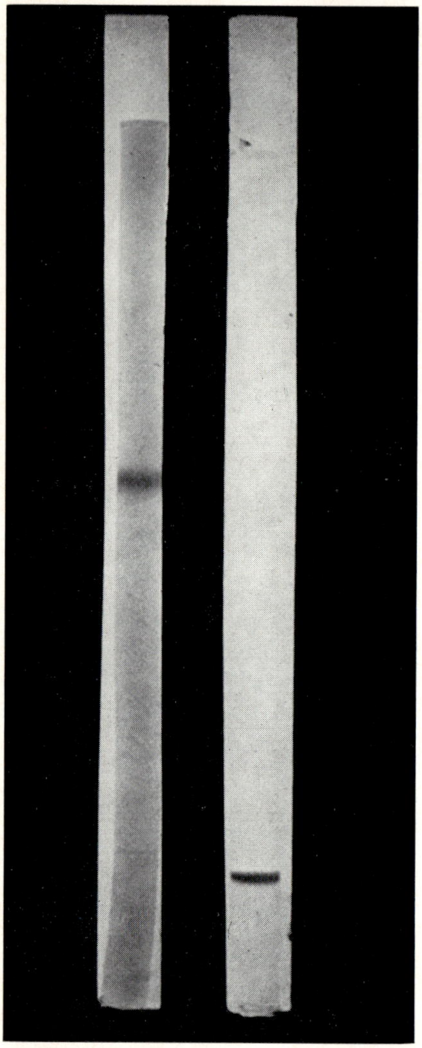

Fig. 3. Acrylamide gels of thymosin at pH 8.3 (right) and pH 2.9 (left). Thymosin fraction 8 (100 μg) was applied to basic and acidic gels (5 × 125 mm). From Hooper *et al.* (1975).

radical scavenger. The sample (150-200 mg) is electrophoresed at 100 milliamps using a standard pH 8.3 Tris-glycine buffer system, and the first protein peak eluted from the bottom of the gel, which contains a single protein component, is designated as thymosin fraction 8.

Thymosin fraction 8 isolated by the procedure outlined in Fig. 2, migrates as a single band on 15 per cent polyacrylamide gels at pH 8.3 and 2.9, as shown in Fig. 3. Fraction 8 is essentially free of carbohydrate, lipid, and nucleotide and contains no cyclic AMP.

TABLE I

AMINO ACID COMPOSITION OF BOVINE THYMOSIN FRACTION 8

Amino acid	*Residues/ molecule*	*Amino acid*	*Residues/ molecule*
Lysine	4	Alanine	7
Histidine	1	Cysteine[b]	1
Arginine	2	Valine	5
Aspartic acid	22	Methionine[b]	2
Threonine[a]	4	Isoleucine	3
Serine[a]	5	Leucine	6
Glutamic acid	32	Tyrosine	1
Proline	5	Phenylalanine	2
Glycine	6	Total	108

The data are presented as assumed numbers of residues per molecule. The molecular weight is approximately 12,200. A separate analysis for tryptophan was performed.

[a] Extrapolated to zero time from 24, 48 and 72 h hydrolysates.

[b] Determined as cysteic acid and methionine sulfone by performic acid oxidation.

From Hooper *et al.* (1975)

As shown in Table I, amino acid analysis reveals that thymosin fraction 8 is a protein with a molecular weight of approximately 12,200 and contains 108 amino acid residues. Fifty-percent of the residues are acidic and no unusual amino acids are observed. The molecule contains one residue of histidine, one of cysteine, and no tryptophan. Reduction and S-carboxymethylation of thymosin fraction 8 followed by gel filtration on a Sephadex G-50 column equilibrated with 6 M guanidinium chloride in 10 mM Tris-HCl, pH 7.5, results in the detection of smaller sub-units (Hooper *et al.* 1975). Studies are presently in progress to determine the sequence of the smaller subunits and their relation to the intact thymosin fraction 8 molecule.

As yet we do not know whether all of the biological activity observed with thymosin fraction 5 can be ascribed to a single molecular species (fraction 8) or whether multiple thymic factors must act in concert to endow the host with the normal complement of immunity. Thymosin fraction 5 contains at least 11 other heat-stable acidic polypeptides as well as thymosin fraction 8. Their molecular weights range from 1,200 to 14,000. Isolation and characterization of these substances is in progress. The suggestion that other biologically active factors are present in fraction 5 comes from our recent observations that not all preparations of thymosin fraction 8 are as active as cruder fractions when tested in some of the *in vitro* systems presently under investigation (Hooper *et al.* 1975). This decreased specific activity may reflect chemical modification of the molecule or removal of an active component or cofactor during the purification procedure.

Some of the bioassays that are presently being used to measure thymosin activity *in vitro* and *in vivo* are listed in Table II.

TABLE II

BIOASSAYS FOR THYMOSIN

IN VITRO
- Spontaneous mouse rosette assay (Bach *et al.* 1971)
- Human E-rosettes [spontaneous (Wara & Ammann 1975); activated (Wybran *et al.* In press)]
- Cytotoxicity [expression of theta and TL] (Scheid *et al.* 1973)
- Mitogens [bone marrow conversion and amplification of T cell responses] (Woody *et al.* 1971, Touraine *et al.* 1974)
- MLR [$T_1 \rightarrow T_2$ and amplification of T cell responses] (Cohen *et al.* 1974)
- RIA [calf and human] (Schulof 1972, Schulof *et al.* 1973, Goldstein *et al.* 1974)
- Antibody formation (Wolf & Erb 1970, In press)
- Helper function (Miller *et al.* 1973)
- GVH (Lowenberg *et al.* 1973)

IN VIVO (Murine Models)
- Neonatally thymectomized (Asanuma *et al.* 1970, Goldstein *et al.* 1970, 1972); adult thymectomized (Bach *et al.* 1971, Goldstein *et al.* 1972)
- Nude (Thurman *et al.* 1974)
- Immunosuppressed (Goldstein *et al.* 1970, Hardy *et al.* 1971, Zatz *et al.* In press)
- NZB (Dauphinee *et al.* 1974, Gershwin *et al.* 1974)
- Normal (Goldstein *et al.* 1966, Hardy *et al.* 1969, Thurman *et al.* 1975)
- Casein-induced amyloidosis (Scheinberg *et al.* In press)
- Tumorogenesis [spontaneous (Khaw & Rule 1973, Waksal *et al.* 1974); viral induced (Zisblatt *et al.* 1970, Hardy *et al.* 1971); cell transfer (Praeger *et al.* In preparation]
- Aging (Strausser *et al.* 1971, Thurman *et al.* 1975)

III. BIOASSAYS FOR MEASURING THYMOSIN ACTIVITY *IN VITRO* AND *IN VIVO*

A. *New* in vitro *Mixed Lymphocyte Assay*

In our laboratory, two bioassays are routinely used to monitor biological activity of thymosin-containing fractions. The first is a one-way mixed lymphocyte reaction (MLR) developed by G. Cohen (Cohen *et al.* In press). The second is a mitogen bioassay developed by G. Thurman (Thurman *et al.* In press) which measures the capacity of lymph node cells from thymosin-treated mice to respond to T cell mitogens. The methodologies for both assays are described in detail in other chapters of this text.

An example of the effect of thymosin on responder thymocytes or spleen cells from CBA/J mice in a one-way MLR is shown in Fig. 4. The one-way mixed lymphocyte reaction by CBA thymocytes cultured with mitomycin-C-blocked spleen cells is markedly enhanced by thymosin fraction 5 (Fig. 4, left panel). This enhancement cannot be explained simply as increased survival of the treated thymocytes, since the MLR of the syngeneic cell cultures does not increase with added thymosin. Moreover, we have never observed a thymosin-induced mitogenic effect on thymocytes cultured alone for 5 days.

In contrast to the effects of thymosin on responder thymocytes, thymosin addition results in a depressed MLR by responder spleen cells, although cell densities are adjusted for an optimal baseline (thymosin-free) response (Fig. 4,

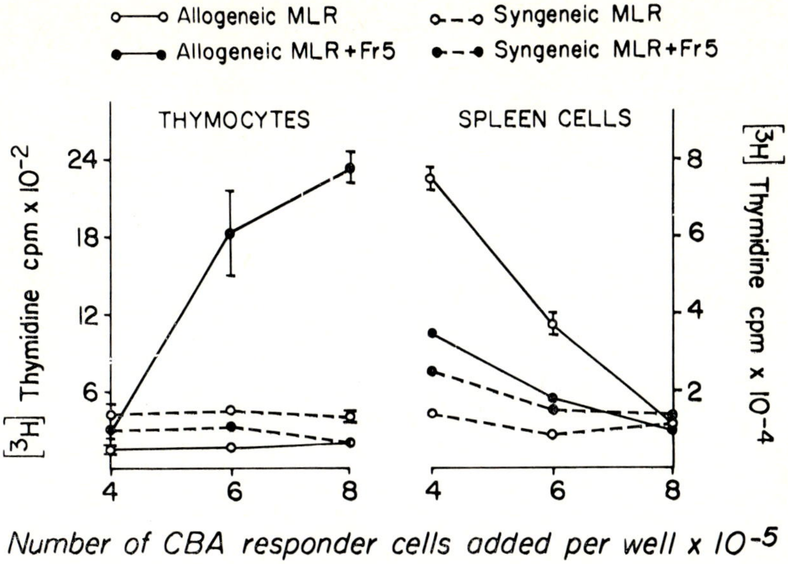

Fig. 4. Stimulatory and suppressive effects of thymosin fraction 5 on mixed lymphocytee reaction. Details of the methods are presented by Cohen and Goldstein elsewhere in this book. In allogeneic cultures, 4×10^5 mitomycin-C blocked C57BL/6J spleen cells per microtiter well were used, while, in the syngeneic cultures, 4×10^5 mitomycin-C treated CBA/J spleen cells per microtiter well were used. The one-way MLR by various numbers of responder CBA thymocytes incubated in the presence or absence of thymosin fraction 5 is shown in the left panel. Solid circles indicate presence of thymosin throughout the culture time. Open circles indicate absence of thymosin. Solid lines denote allogeneic cell combinations. Broken lines denote syngeneic cell combinations. From Cohen *et al.* (1975).

right panel). A similar depression of the MLR response is seen following addition of thymosin to responder lymph node or bone marrow cells. The dramatic effect of thymosin on thymocytes suggests that a major action of the hormone may be to convert immunologically immature thymocytes (T_1 cells) into more mature T cells (T_2 cells) which then have the capacity to respond in a MLR. With this assay, it is possible to observe a dose-related response. We have found that other calf tissue extracts prepared in a manner identical to the preparation of thymosin fraction 5 contain some thymocyte MLR-enhancing activity as does LPS (endotoxin) and mercaptoethanol (2-ME). The tymosin-like activity in fraction 5 preparations obtained from nonthymic tissue has been noted previously in our laboratory in other bioassays (Goldstein *et al.* 1970, Goldstein *et al.* 1971). Other molecules such as cyclic AMP, dibuteryl cyclic AMP, bovine serum albumin, or erythropoitin present throughout the 5-day culture period do not enhance this thymocyte MLR.

Before we can obtain meaningful data from the MLR bioassay, fractions must be measured for endotoxin content in the limulus lysate bioassay. Nonspecific enhancement with mercaptoethanol (ME) necessitates the removal by gel filtration of this reducing agent from fractions extracted in the presence of 2-ME.

TABLE III

BIOASSAYS FOR THYMOSIN: RESPONSIVENESS TO MITOGENS OF LYMPH NODE LYMPHOCYTES FROM C57/BL/6J MICE TREATED DAILY FOR 14 DAYS WITH THYMOSIN OR A VARIETY OF CONTROL FRACTIONS

Fraction	*μg/ injection*	*Mean incorporation of ³H-TdR (cpm ± standard error)*				
		Control	*PHA-P*	*Con A*	*PWM*	*LPS*
Saline	–	1,680 ± 136	7,272 ± 555	15,486 ± 184	2,238 ± 251	851 ± 50
Thymosin Fr 5	100	1,681 ± 209	14,465 ± 446	64,289 ± 8,070	4,488 ± 254	1,491 ± 64
Spleen Fr 5	100	1,764 ± 123	10,620 ± 555	38,044 ± 6,315	3,147 ± 154	1,194 ± 82
Brain Fr 5	100	2,158 ± 284	9,578 ± 108	35,107 ± 7,184	4,533 ± 572	2,032 ± 200
BSA[a]	5,000	2,279 ± 9	8,291 ± 1,198	17,167 ± 1,310	2,899 ± 370	964 ± 36
BSA	100	1,841 ± 175	5,337 ± 1,043	14,637 ± 79	2,794 ± 295	914 ± 73
LPS[b]	1	2,040 ± 377	9,813 ± 335	21,284 ± 418	2,319 ± 91	778 ± 10
2-ME[c]	1	2,427 ± 103	9,501 ± 236	8,149 ± 4,449	13,571 ± 2,728	8,113 ± 628

[a] BSA: Bovine Serum Albumin
[b] LPS: *E. coli* lipopolysaccharide
[c] 2-MF: 2-mercaptoethanol

From Thurman *et al.* (In press)

B. *New* in vivo *Mitogen Assay*

Data obtained from the newly-developed T cell mitogen assay for thymosin is shown in Table III. Normal or adult thymectomized 12-week-old C57BL/6J mice are injected daily for 2 weeks with thymosin. On day 15, the mice are sacrificed and lymph nodes are removed and prepared for use in microcultures. The lymph node lymphocytes are cultured with phytohemaglutinin (PHA), Concanavalin A (Con A), pokeweed mitogen (PWM), or *E. coli* lipopolysaccharide (LPS) and, at 72 h of culture, the amount of ^{3}H-thymidine incorporated during the last 8 h of the culture period is determined. The data shown in Table III is derived from studies of normal C57BL/6J mice injected daily with thymosin fraction 5, spleen fraction 5, brain fraction 5, bovine serum albumin, LPS, 2-mercaptoethanol, or saline for 14 days. On the 15th day, the mice were sacrificed and lymphocyte microcultures were prepared from the lymph nodes of the treated animals. The lymphocytes from the thymosin-treated mice show the greatest increase in responsivity to Con A. Spleen fraction 5 and brain fraction 5 also induced a significant, but smaller, increase in lymphocyte responsiveness to Con A; BSA, LPS, and 2-mercaptoethanol are not significantly effective in increasing the responsiveness of lymphocytes to Con A. In comparison to the Con A response, the responses to other mitogens were much less affected by administration of thymosin. It is not known whether the ability of spleen fractions or brain fractions to generate biological activity in this and other assays reflects the presence of a depot form of thymosin which is dependent on the presence of an intact thymus in the donor animal or whether the activity is attributable to tissue-specific molecules bearing molecular and/or antigenic features common to all agents which trigger T cell maturation.

The effect of thymosin on the responsiveness of lymph node cells to Con

A may provide an important clue to unravelling some of the secrets of T cell differentiation. For example, it is known that murine thymocytes respond well to the mitogen Con A, but poorly to PHA. The potent effect of thymosin in increasing Con A responsiveness may reflect thymosin-induced maturation of a subpopulation of pre-T cells that reside in the lymph nodes. Alternatively, thymosin may induce the maturation of stem cells elsewhere in the body and signal their migration to the lymph nodes.

In other studies, it has been observed that the increase in the Con A responsiveness of lymph node cells following thymosin treatment is coupled with, at higher thymosin doses, a decrease in the response to Con A of lymphocytes residing in the spleen (Thurman *et al.* 1975). The reason for this decrease in the spleen cell response after high thymosin doses is not well understood at present. It is known that a population of short-lived, cortisone-sensitive, immature T cells migrate to and are present in the spleen (Raff & Cantor 1971). Accordingly, the thymosin-induced increase in Con A responsiveness by a population of lymph node cells (Table III) suggests that, under the influence of thymosin, less mature lymphoid cells leave the spleen and "home" to the lymph node. This interpretation is supported by preliminary studies showing that removal of the spleen prior to treatment of mice abrogates the thymosin-induced increase in Con A responsiveness of the lymph node cells (Thurman & Goldstein, in preparation). These observations also suggest that thymosin-induced maturation occurs prior to migration.

C. In vivo *Studies in NZB Mice*

In the first 16 weeks of life, New Zealand Black (NZB) mice develop an autoimmune and lymphoproliferative disease similar in many ways to human systemic lupus erythematosus and lymphoid malignancy. Although the etiology of the human autoimmune disease has yet to be determined, recent studies of the NZB mouse suggest that the primary defect may be attributable to the decreased production of thymosin (Bach & Dardenne 1972, Dauphinee *et al.* 1974, Gershwin *et al.* 1974).

TABLE IV

MEAN GRAFT SURVIVAL OF C57BL/6 SKIN IN THYMOSIN-TREATED 7-MONTH-OLD NZB/W FEMALE MICE

Treatment	*Mice*	*MGS ± S.E.M.*
Thymosin[a]	6	11.6 ± 0.6[b]
Control[c]	6	14.0 ± 0.4[b]

[a] Thymosin, 250 μg, was given i.p. for 5 days ending 1 day prior to grafting.
[b] $p < 0.01$, Student's t-test.
[c] Saline, 0.1 ml, was given i.p. for 5 days ending 1 day prior to grafting.
From Gershwin *et al.* (1974)

TABLE V

INDUCTION OF MLR IN LYMPH NODE CELLS OF 7-MONTH-OLD NZB/W MICE BY THE *in vivo* INJECTION OF THYMOSIN

Treatment[a]	*Stimulator*	*Responder*	*Uptake of ^{3}H-TdR*
			cpm $\pm$ S.E.
Saline		NZB/W	589 $\pm$ 53
Saline	C_3H	NZB/W	121 $\pm$ 46
Saline	C_3H	NZB/W	911 $\pm$ 85
50 μg/day	C_3H	NZB/W	2,139 $\pm$ 101[b]
250 μg/day	C_3H	NZB/W	10,887 $\pm$ 854[b]
50 μg/day		NZB/W	774 $\pm$ 85
250 μg/day		NZB/W	1,011 $\pm$ 127

[a] NZB/W mice received 0.1 ml saline, 50 μg/day thymosin or 250 μg/day thymosin intraperitoneally five times per week for 3 weeks.

[b] $p<0.01$ compared with saline-treated controls, Student's t-test.

From Gershwin *et al.* (1974)

In contrast to other strains, NZB mice exhibit a significant decrease in the number of spontaneous rosette-forming cells within the first few weeks post-birth, and this drop is preceded by a significant decrease in serum thymosin-like activity. Bach & Dardenne (1973) found that rosette-forming cells in NZB mice could be reconstituted *in vivo* by thymosin administration (Bach *et al.* 1973). Based on these studies, we have looked at the effect of thymosin in young and old NZB mice. As diagrammed in Fig. 5, we have found that thymosin fraction 5 can correct an abnormal DNA synthetic (i.e., proliferative) response of spleen- and lymph-node-seeking thymocytes which appears at 8 weeks of life (Dauphinee *et al.* 1974). Additional studies have shown that thymosin can reconstitute other defective immune responses in older (6-8

TABLE VI

SPLENIC DIRECT PLAQUE-FORMING CELL (PFC) RESPONSE TO PRIMARY IMMUNIZATION WITH 2×10^{8} SRBC IN THYMOSIN-TREATED 7-MONTH-OLD NZB/W FEMALE MICE

Treatment	*No. of mice*	*PFC/spleen Geometric mean*	*PFC/10^6 spleen cells Geometric mean*	*$Log_{10}\pm$S.E.M.*
Thymosin[a]	5	19,020	141	2.1484 $\pm$ 0.10[b]
None	8	1,023	18	1.2582 $\pm$ 0.25[b]

[a] Each mouse received 250 μg thymosin i.p. for 5 days and 1 day later they were immunized with SRBC, i.p.

[b] $p<0.01$, Student's t-test.

From Gershwin *et al.* (1974)

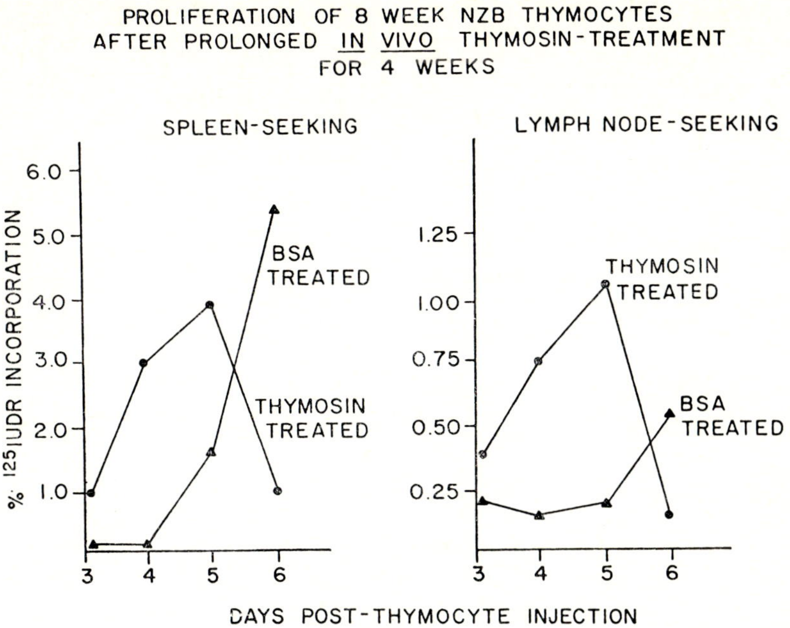

Fig. 5. Proliferation of 8-week NZB thymocytes after prolonged *in vivo* thymosin treatment for 4 weeks. Incorporation of [^{125}I-]IdU by spleen-seeking and lymph-node-seeking thymocytes from thymosin-treated or albumin (BSA)-treated NZB donors. Treatment was started at 28 days; each mouse received 3 intravenous injections per week of either 0.1 mg of thymosin or bovine serum albumin in 0.1 ml. From Dauphinee *et al.* (1974).

months old) NZB mice after onset of the autoimmune syndrome (Gershwin *et al.* 1974). Administration of thymosin for 2 weeks restores and enhances the capacity of these anergic NZB mice to reject skin allografts (Table IV), to respond in the MLR (Table V), and to make antibodies in response to injection with sheep RBC (Table VI). The thymosin-induced restoration of the proliferative pattern of spleen and lymph-node-seeking NZB thymocytes injected into lethally-irradiated histo-incompatible hosts is consistent with the hypothesis that thymosin induces generation of suppressor T cells capable of shutting off *in vivo* the thymocyte proliferative response in the spleen and lymph node.

These studies in NZB mice suggest that thymosin acts either to induce the appearance of new T cells with suppressor-like characteristics or to exert a more direct influence on aberrant T cells causing them to revert to more normal modes of function. From the results observed in NZB mice, it appears that an endocrine disturbance may underly many immunological abnormalities associated with autoimmunity and lymphoid malignancy in New Zealand mice and, possibly, in humans.

D. In vivo *Studies in Genetically Thymusless (Nu/Nu) Mice*

We have recently found that thymosin fraction 5 and thymosin fraction 8 can stimulate lymph node lymphocytes of nude mice to respond to T cell mitogens such as PHA-P and Con A. Thymosin fraction 5 given 5 times a week intraperitoneally at a dose of 100 μg per injection for 3 weeks enhances the capacity of lymph node cells cultured in microculture to respond to T cell mitogens *in vitro* (Fig. 6). These data suggest that thymosin has the capacity to convert pre-T cells into cells with more mature T cell characteristics. Alternatively, the data of Wortis *et al.* (1974) suggest that nude mice possess theta-bearing cells, and thus thymosin may act on T_1-like lymphocytes to amplify their capacity to mature *in vivo*.

E. In vivo *Studies in Experimentally Induced Amyloidosis in Mice*

Most recently, we have found that thymosin fraction 5 can significantly reduce the incidence of casein-induced amyloidosis in the spleens of CBA/J mice (Scheinberg *et al.* In press) (Table VII). A spleen preparation equivalent to fraction 5 given in the same concentrations as thymosin was not effective. These studies suggest that abnormal T cell function may be related to the etiology of amyloidosis. Support for this suggestion comes from the recent observations of Scheinberg & Cathcart (In press). These investigators have found that the

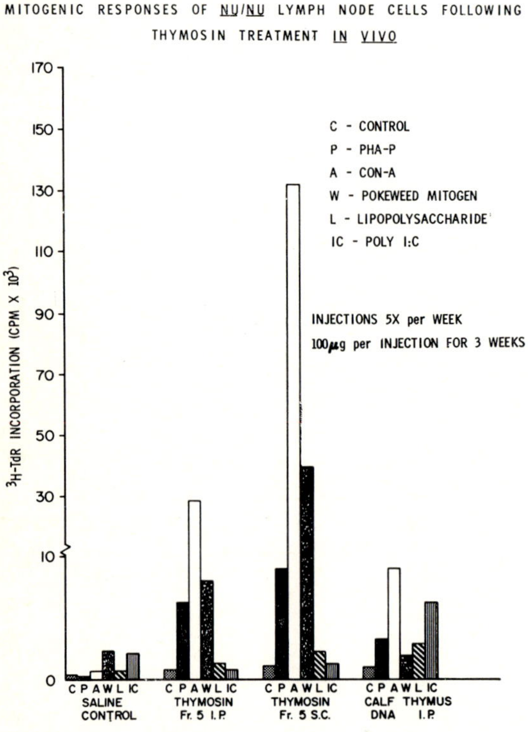

Fig. 6. Mitogenic responses of (Nu/Nu) lymph node cells following thymosin treatment *in vivo*.

TABLE VII

THYMOSIN-INDUCED REDUCTION IN AMYLOIDOSIS IN MICE

	No. of mice	*Amyloid score (percent)* 0	1	2	3	4	*Mean amyloid score*
Casein[a]	20	5	25	5	35	30	2.6[c]
Casein + Spleen, Fraction 5[b]	10	10	10	10	–	70	3.11
Casein + Thymosin, Fraction 5[b]	18	44	6	28	22	–	1.3[c]

[a] 20 daily injections
[b] 500 μg every other day
[c] t = 3.14
$p < 0.01$

From M. Sheinberg *et al.* (In press)

lymphocytes obtained from the spleens of mice in the early stages of casein-induced amyloidosis respond abnormally to T cell mitogens. They also observed that at the same time the response to B cell mitogens such as LPS, Poly I-Poly C, and dextran are either normal or enhanced (Scheinberg & Cathcart 1974). Additional recent studies of mice during casein-induced amyloidosis show that the capacity to make antibodies to sheep RBC is also depressed (Scheinberg & Cathcart. In press).

The decreased T cell responses seen during the development of amyloidosis are similar to the depressed T cell responses seen in the aged NZB mouse (Gershwin *et al.* 1974, Good & Yunis 1974) or with the aging process in man (Good & Yunis 1974). Our studies suggest that autoimmune disease, amyloidosis, and other diseases of aging may share a common etiology.

IV. FIRST CLINICAL TRIALS WITH THYMOSIN

A. In vitro *Studies*

The observation that the number of E-rosettes (a T cell indicator) formed by peripheral blood lymphocytes of some immunodeficient patients can be increased *in vitro* by addition of thymosin has led to the development of an assay for thymosin as well as for the identification of patients with thymosin-dependent immunodeficiency diseases in man (Wara & Ammann, 1974). The methods for this E-rosette bioassay of thymosin are presented in Fig. 7.

Representative studies of human E-rosettes in patients with primary immunodeficiency diseases conducted in the laboratories of Drs. Wara and Ammann at the University of California Medical Center at San Francisco, Dr. Richard Hong, University of Wisconsin Medical Center at Madison, and Dr. John Montgomery at Baylor Medical Center in Houston are outlined in Table VIII.

Thymosin has no detectable effect on the numbers of total E-rosettes if the lymphocytes are obtained from normal individuals (Table VIII). These data show that thymosin increases the number of E-rosettes formed by lymphocytes

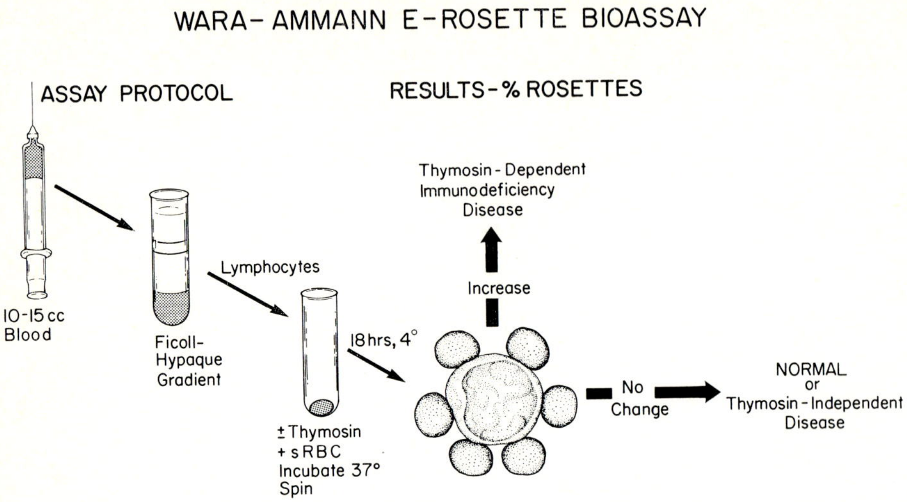

Fig. 7. Peripheral blood lymphocytes are isolated by ficollhypaque gradient centrifugation. The isolated lymphocytes are adjusted to a concentration of 4 × 10^6 cells per ml of Hanks medium. Sheep red blood cells (SRBC) are washed and a 1 per cent suspension is prepared. Lymphocytes in a volume of 0.25 ml are incubated with 0.25 ml of the sheep RBC suspension. Bovine thymosin fraction 5 is added to the cell suspension at concentrations of 50 to 500 μg/ml. Following the addition of thymosin, the suspensions are incubated for 5 min to 1 h at 37 °C, centrifuged for 5 min at 200 × g, and incubated overnight for 18 h at 4 °C. Triplicate wet cell preparations are examined by phase microscopy and the percentage of lymphocytes binding 4 or more SRBC is determjned.

TABLE VIII

EFFECT OF THYMOSIN (FRACTION 5) ON HUMAN T-CELL ROSETTES OF IMMUNODEFICIENT PATIENTS

Investigators (Institute)	*Disease*	*Baseline*	*Thymosin treated*	*Significant increase*
D. Wara and A. Ammann	Normal	56%	61%	−
(University of California	Thymic Hypoplasia	20%	45%	+
Medical Center)	Varient DiGeorge	25%	49%	+
	Thymic Hypoplasia and Successful Thymus Transplant	32%	38%	−
	Ataxia Telangiectasia	27%	43%	+
	Possible Autoimmune Disease	30%	53%	+
	Combined Immunodeficiency	17%	20%	−
R. Hong	Normal (4)	43–76%	46–60%	−
(University of Wisconsin	DiGeorge	30%	54%	+
Medical Center)	Lupus Erythematosus	59%	75%	+
	Cartilage Hair	10%	20%	+
J. Montgomery	Normal	66%	68%	−
(Baylor Medical School)	Combined Immunodeficiency	10%	8%	−

from patients with thymic hypoplasia and DiGeorge syndrome as well as those from patients with lupus erythematosis and ataxia telangiectasia. The capacity of thymosin to increase *in vitro* the number of total E-rosettes from patients with other known or suspected primary and secondary immunodeficiency diseases including lupus erythematosis, assorted malignancies, and other immunodeficiency diseases has now been documented by a number of additional laboratories. Thymosin does not appear to influence the number of E-rosettes from patients with severe combined immunodeficiency disease, where the defect is apparently at the level of the stem cells. Of special interest in Table VIII is data from a patient with thymic hypoplasia who had previously received a successful thymic transplant. Thymosin had no effect on the number of peripheral blood E-rosettes in this cases. As discussed below, the Wara-Ammann E-rosette assay has been particularly useful in identifying patients with cellular immunodeficiency diseases that may respond to thymosin therapy. The increase

TABLE IX

In vitro EFFECT OF THYMOSIN (FRACTION 5) ON E-ROSETTES IN PATIENTS WITH PRIMARY AND SECONDARY IMMUNODEFICIENCY DISEASES

Age	*Clinical diagnosis*	*E-Rosettes Baseline*	*Thymosin treatment*	*Significant increase*
54	Lung Cancer (Undifferentiated Adenocarcinoma)	24%	42%	+
32	Hodgkin's Disease, Stage IV–B	34%	47%	+
22	Acute Lymphocytic Leukemia	35%	52%	+
40	Acute Myelomonocytic Leukemia	23%	54%	+
47	Disseminated Melanoma	23%	37%	+
69	Stem Cell Leukemia[a]	71%	74%	—
66	Endometrial Carcinoma[b]	61.5%	70%	—
56	Acute Myelogenous Leukemia	2%	17%	+
Normal Adults	(n=8)	34–71%	43–72%	—

[a] Complete remission
[b] No metastasis found

From Sakai *et al.* (1975)

in the number of E-rosettes with thymosin *in vitro* appears to reflect a thymosin-dependent immunodeficiency disease. The failure to change the number of E-rosettes with thymosin *in vivo* seems to indicate that the patient is either normal or has a thymosin-independent disorder (e.g., stem cell deficiency).

A representative *in vitro* study of the effects of thymosin fraction 5 on E-rosette number in patients with secondary immunodeficiency diseases is shown in Table IX. The cancer patients evaluated included those diagnosed as having lung carcinoma, Hodgkin's disease IVB, acute lymphocytic leukemia, acute myeloblastic leukemia, disseminated melanoma, endometrial carcinoma, or stem cell carcinoma. Following *in vitro* incubation of their peripheral blood lymphocytes with thymosin, there were significant increases in numbers of E-

TABLE X

In vitro EFFECT OF THYMOSIN (FRACTION 5) ON E-CELL ROSETTES OF SEVERELY BURNED PATIENTS

Age	*Type of burn*	*Days post burn*	*E-cell rosettes Baseline*	*Thymosin treatment*	*Significant increase*
3 yr.	33%, 3rd degree	2	25%	N.T.*	
		22	15%	19%	—
		29	6%	10%	—
		36	16%	54%	+
		43	58%	59%	—
5 yr.	72%, 3rd degree	15	12%	21%	+
		22	6%	13%	+
		29	0%	0%	—
		36	13%	24%	+
		50	21%	53%	+
		64	45%	43%	—
2 yr.	31%, 3rd degree	8	20%	N.T.	
		15	13%	27%	+
		22	31%	67%	+
		29	54%	53%	—
6 yr.	60%, 3rd degree	4 hr.	10%	18%	+
		7	22%	53%	+
		21	15%	26%	+
		28	59%	55%	—
Normal controls	(n = 18)		35–69%	22–75%	—

* N.T. = not tested

From Goldstein *et al.* (1975)

rosettes for most of the patients in this group. There were two exceptions: a patient with endometrial carcinoma without known metastasis who had a high baseline (thymosin-free) number of E-rosettes (62 per cent) and one with stem cell carcinoma who also had a high baseline number of E-rosettes and was in a state of complete remission at the time of testing. Again, there was no significant effect by thymosin on the total E-rosettes obtained from normal adults. The observation that the peripheral lymphocytes of cancer patients in remission do not respond to further thymosin treatment *in vitro* suggests that the *in vitro* E-rosette assay may also be a useful indicator to evaluate the state of remission as well as the potential for effectiveness of thymosin therapy *in vivo*.

We have recently initiated a study of T cell function in severely burned children. The *in vitro* effect of thymosin fraction 5 on the number of E-rosettes obtained from severely burned patients is shown in Table X. Lymphocytes from patients with third degree burns covering 31-72 per cent of their bodies were studied. The number of E-rosettes circulating in the blood following a severe burn is markedly depressed (Table X). The total number of endogenous T cells in these patients increases with time during recovery. It is noteworthy, however, that incubation of lymphocytes with thymosin *in vitro* at specific times post-burn markedly elevates the number of E-rosettes. As the patients'

TABLE XI

SUMMARY OF SALIENT FEATURES OF WARA-AMMANN E-ROSETTE BIOASSAY

1. Thymosin increases T cell rosettes in a dose response relationship in many primary and secondary immunodeficiency diseases.
2. "Stem cells" or "precursor T cells" are required in the lymphocyte population for an increase in T cell rosettes following thymosin incubation *in vitro*.
3. The total T cell rosettes obtained from normal individuals do not increase further when incubated with thymosin.
4. One can obtain from the blood of normal individuals subpopulations of lymphocytes, so called "active" and "null" cells which can and do respond to thymosin *in vitro*.
5. An increase in T cell rosettes following incubation with thymosin *in vitro* may predict which patients will respond to thymosin therapy *in vivo*.

levels of E-rosettes rise to control values (4-9 weeks later), the *in vitro* effect of thymosin diminishes. Earlier studies by Rappaport and colleagues (Rappaport *et al.* 1964) and by Sakai and associates (Sakai *et al.* 1972) have shown that cell-mediated immunity and general T cell function are impaired in patients who have sustained severe burns. Our studies suggest that these defects may result from depletion of thymosin-induced T cells or insufficient production and/or release of thymosin by the thymus gland after severe burns (Goldstein *et al.* 1974). The most salient features of the E-rosette assay reported to date are summarized in Table XI.

Taken together, the above *in vitro* studies suggest that a defect in thymosin production by the thymus may exist in individuals with these disorders and that a population of lymphoid cells dependent upon thymosin for their differentiated state circulates in the blood. Although the origin of this thymosin-sensitive cell is not known, it does not appear to be present in patients with combined immunodeficiencies (reported here and elsewhere). This suggests that this cell type may play an important role in the early stages of maturation of the immune system as well as in later stages of life when it circulates in the blood. The possibility that the thymosin-responsive "precursor" cell originates in the bone marrow compartment of man is suggested by the very recent reports of Touraine and associates (Touraine *et al.* 1974) who were able to induce expression of T cell surface markers on cells from subpopulations of human bone marrow with thymosin. Previous studies of mouse models in our laboratory have similarly identified a population of thymosin-responsive bone marrow cells (Goldstein *et al.* 1971, Bach *et al.* 1971).

B. In vivo *Studies*

The first clinical trial of thymosin was initiated in April 1974 by Dr. Arthur Ammann and Dr. Diane Wara at the University of California Medical Center in San Francisco (Wara *et al.* 1974). The patient was a 5-year-old female with thymic hypoplasia and hyperimmunoglobulinemia A. There was no family history of immunodeficiency disease. The patients' history included gastrointestinal tract salmonellosis at age 10 months, chronic malabsorption syndrome, Candida sepsis at age 2 years, growth failure, recurrent pneumonia, recurrent otitis media, and recurrent skin infections. A thymic shadow was absent on X-ray. A lymph node biopsy revealed no corticomedullary differentiation, lack of both plasma cells and lymphocytes, and a predominance of reticular cells. The patient's total lymphocyte count was depressed as was the *in vitro* lymphocyte mitogenic response to PHA. Delayed hypersensitivity skin tests were negative. Hyperimmunoglobulinemia A was diagnosed because of elevated IgA, decreased IgG and normal IgM titers, and a lack of antibody production following immunization with polyvalant pneumococcal polysaccharide and keyhole limpet hemocyanin. The per cent E-rosettes varied from 10 to 20 per cent over a 2-year period. The patient received 2 units of transfer factor at age 3-1/2 and 3-3/4 years without subsequent clinical improvement. Because of the failure to respond clinically to transfer factor and the observed increase in percent E-rosettes following *in vitro* incubation with thymosin (from 15 per cent to 48 per cent), thymosin therapy was initiated.

One week after initiation of daily thymosin injections (1 mg/kg/day), the percent of endogenous E-rosettes (i.e., without thymosin incubation *in vitro*) increased to 40 per cent; by two weeks, endogenous E-rosettes increased to 50 per cent; and by 3 weeks to 55 per cent. Delayed hypersensitivity skin test reactivity to mumps and Candida became positive, resulting in indurations of 10 and 5 mm respectively by the end of therapy. The patient's subnormal *in vitro* lymphocyte response to PHA and responsiveness in an MLC remained unchanged. The patient improved clinically, showing increased appetite, decreased diarrhea, and a 1.5 kg weight gain. Shortly after termination of thymosin therapy, her E-rosette number dropped and her clinical condition deteriorated. Thymosin therapy was resumed and again her per cent E-rosettes immediately increased and her clinical condition improved. Weekly subcutaneous injections of thymosin fraction 5 (1 mg/kg/week) are sufficient to maintain an E-rosette level greater than 45 per cent. The patient is now 10 months post-initiation of thymosin therapy and continues to do well clinically while receiving weekly thymosin injections. Her percent of endogenous E-rosettes remains between 45 and 50 per cent and delayed hypersensitivity skin tests remain positive.

A second child, one with a sex-linked combined immunodeficiency disease, has been studied by Dr. Goldman and colleagues at the University of Texas Medical Branch (unpublished observations). The child had low levels of endogenous E-rosettes (1 per cent) which did not change after *in vitro* incubation with thymosin (2 per cent). In spite of the lack of response *in vitro*, it was felt that thymosin therapy should be initiated. Thymosin was administered in doses of up to 300 mg per m^2 (skin surface area) per day for 21 days. There was no change in the total number of E-rosettes circulating in the blood nor in the immunological status of the patient, nor were there side effects after administering extremely high doses of thymosin.

Most recently, phase I trials in cancer patients have been initiated here at the University of Texas Medical Branch and at the M. D. Anderson Hospital and Tumor Institute in Houston. The objectives of the phase I studies are: 1) to determine the maximum tolerable dose of thymosin administered subcutaneously; 2) to determine the quantitative and qualitative toxicity of thymosin administered subcutaneously; 3) to determine if thymosin administered subcutaneously affects the constitution of immunodeficiency disease associated with malignancy; and 4) to determine if thymosin produces a response rate in dissiminated malignancy. To date, 22 patients have received one or more doses of thymosin ranging from 50 mg/m^2 to 300 mg/m^2 per day for 7 days.

Although the number of individuals treated is too small for statistical reliability and it is too preliminary in the study to say anything about the effects of thymosin on disseminated malignancy, the following points are worth noting: 1) thymosin, in the majority of patients, has been tolerated well and there is no indication of toxicity; 2) there have been no systemic reactions, no change in a variety of routine laboratory tests, and no fever response attributed directly to thymosin; 3) the majority of the patients treated to date have responded to thymosin therapy with a significant increase in number of T cells (E-rosettes) in the blood and a general tendency for conversion of skin tests from negative to positive. The most consistent finding has been the increase in E-rosettes during thymosin treatment.

Table XII depicts the changes in the number of E-rosette-forming cells in one patient with Hodgkin's IVB before, during, and after administration of thymosin *in vivo*. Four days after the initiation of thymosin therapy, the E-rosette-forming capacity in this patient approached normal levels. Further increases in E-rosettes were observed on the 7th day of injection. Of interest is the fact that the lymphocytes obtained from this patient were no longer responsive, with respect to E-rosette forming ability, to the *in vitro* addition

TABLE XII

INCREASE IN NUMBER OF E-ROSETTES IN A PATIENT WITH HODGKIN'S DISEASE, STAGE IV-B, DURING TREATMENT WITH THYMOSIN

	Before treatment with thymosin	*In vivo* *Days of treatment with thymosin*[a] 4	7
Total WBC (cells/mm^3 of blood)	3,300	3,300	3,300
Lymphocyte numbers (cells/mm^3 of blood)	495	792	384
E-rosettes-patient			
without thymosin	9.5%	43%	54%
with thymosin	38%	57%	65%
E-rosettes-control			
without thymosin	58%	81%[b]	51%[b]
with thymosin	50%	76%[b]	44%[b]

[a] 1 mg Fraction 5/kg
[b] Without *in vivo* administration of thymosin

From Sakai *et al.* (1975)

of thymosin, suggesting that the E-rosette assay may be a useful indicator to evaluate the effectiveness of thymosin therapy *in vivo*.

Based upon the encouraging results from early phase I studies, large-scale clinical trials are imminent at a number of clinical centers in which it will be determined whether thymosin is effective in enhancing T cell functions in patients with known or suspected T cell deficiencies, including those associated with cancer, autoimmune diseases, and other terminal immunodeficiency diseases.

V. MECHANISM OF ACTION OF THYMOSIN

Although the basic mechanism of thymosin action has not been defined, data from several laboratories suggest that thymosin activates lymphoid stem cells via an adenylate cyclase mechanism (H. Pollard, personal communication, Webb, personal communication). Under appropriate conditions, this activation and/or derepression of genetically programmed lymphoid stem cells by thymosin results in the rapid maturation of precursor T cells (pre-T) into immunologically competent T lymphocytes.

As shown in Fig. 8, pre-T cells can be induced by thymosin, cAMP, or other factors (specific and nonspecific) to express T cell surface antigens (θ, T1) (Bach *et al.* 1971, Scheid *et al.* 1973) and functional characteristics such as azathioprine sensitivity (Bach *et al.* 1971, Goldstein *et al.* 1972), MLR reactivity (Cohen *et al.* In press), PHA responsivity (Woody *et al.* 1972), antibody production (Wolf & Erb 1971, Wolf 1974 In press) and *in vitro* GVH responsiveness (Löwenberg *et al.* 1972).

In vitro studies indicate that thymosin can also act on immature thymocytes

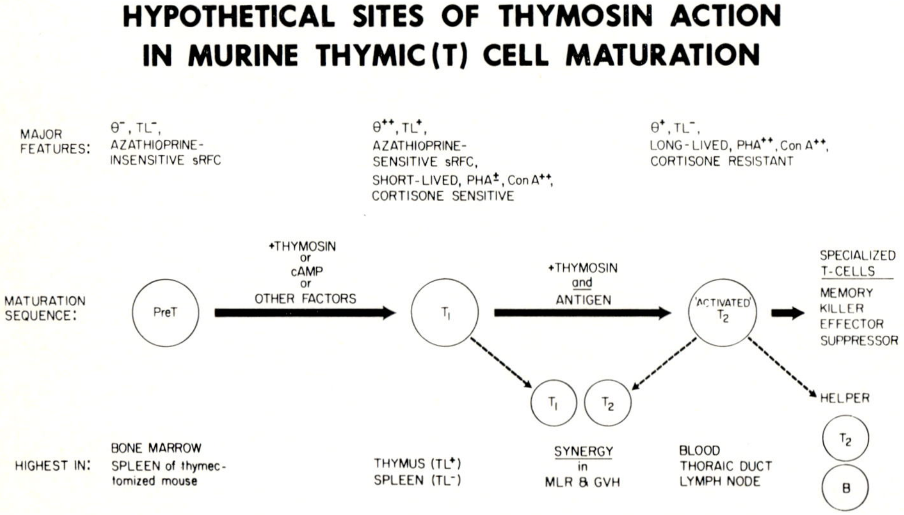

Fig. 8. Hypothetical sites of thymosin action. See text for explanation. From Cohen *et al.* (1975).

(T_1-cells) in the presence of antigens, facilitating their differentiation toward full immunological function as more mature T_2 cells (Cohen *et al.* In press). One subclass of these mature specialized T cells, the so-called "suppressor" or "regulator" T cell, is dependent upon thymosin for its maturation. These suppressor cells apparently exert the fine control over other subpopulations of T and B lymphocytes. Studies showing depressive or suppressive effects by thymosin on the capacity of murine spleen or lymph node cells to respond in the MLR (Cohen *et al.* In press) have led us to propose that the enhancement or suppression of an immunological response may depend upon the ratio of less mature T_1 cells to the more mature T_2 cells in close contact at the time of antigenic challenge. Thus, the so-called "suppressor" cells may not represent a qualitatively different class of T cells but may represent the end result of the excessive generation of T cells whose development is dependent upon thymosin. It may be that hyperthymic function results in thymosin overproduction, which in turn could lead to formation of excessive numbers of T cells which then suppress other T and B cell functions. Most recently, Waldmann and his associates (Waldmann *et al.* 1974) have documented that the immunodeficiency disease, common variable hypogammaglobulinemia, actually results from excess production of "suppressor" T cells.

Hypothymic function, as occurs in aging, may result in the secretion of less thymosin which in turn leads to a decrease in the optimal number of "suppressor" T cells formed. The lack of suppressor T cells in this case might result in the loss of regulation over other T and B cell populations and perhaps lead to the appearance of maverick "autoaggressive" lymphoid cells and eventually to autoimmune disease. The studies by Dauphinee and associates (Dauphinee *et al.* 1974) on NZB mouse in which "suppressor" cell disappearance is related to deficient levels of circulating thymosin support this hypothesis.

Loss of "suppressor" cell function may also lead to excessive proliferation of other T and B cells and thus may be a factor in the development of certain malignancies and/or "blocking antibodies."

Studies designed to elucidate the mechanism by which thymosin induces the maturation of T cells and maintains immune function at the cellular and molecular levels are presently underway in several laboratories. An increased understanding of these basic control mechanisms would be greatly relevant to clinical areas where it now appears that thymosin has a promising future for bolstering the immune responses of patients with thymic malfunction.

BIBLIOGRAPHY

Asanuma, Y., Goldstejn, A. L. & White, A. (1970) *Endocrinology* **86**, 600.
Bach, J.-F., Dardenne, M. & Davies, A. J. S. (1971) *Nature, Nvw Biology* **231**, 110.
Bach, J.-F. & Dardenne, M. (1972) *Cellular Immunol.* **3**, 11.
Bach, J.-F., Dardenne, M. & Bach, M. A. (1973) *Transplant. Proc.* **5**, 99.
Bach, J.-F., Dardenne, M. & Salomon, J. C. (1973) *J. Clin. Exper. Immunol.* **14**, 247.
Cohen, G. H., Hooper, J. A. & Goldstein, A. L. (1975) *Ann. N.Y. Acad. Sci.* **249**, 145.
Cooper, J. F., Levin, J. & Wagner, H. H. (1973) *J. Lab. Clin. Med.* **78**, 138.
Dauphinee, M. J., Talal, N., Goldstein, A. L. & White, A. (1974) *Proc. Nat. Acad. Sci.* **71**, 2637.

Gershwin, M. E., Ahmed, A., Steinberg, A. D., Thurman, G. B. & Goldstein, A. L. (1974) *J. Immunol.* **113**, 1068.
Goldstein, A. L., Slater, F. D. & White, A. (1966) *Proc. Nat. Acad. Sci.* **56**, 1010.
Goldstein, A. L., Asanuma, Y., Battisto, J. R., Quint, J., Hardy, M. A. & White, A. (1970) *J. Immunol.* **104**, 359.
Goldstein, A. L. & White, A. (1970) *In* G. Litwack, ed., "*Biochemical Actions of Hormones*", pp. 456-502, Academic Press, Inc., New York.
Goldstein, A. L. & White, A. (1971) In R. Levine and R. Luft, eds. *Advances inrMetabolic Disorders*, 5, pp. 149-182, Academic Press, Inc., New York.
Goldstein, A. L., Guha, A., Zatz, M. M., Hardy, M. A. & White, A. (1972) *Proc. Nat. Acad. Sci. (USA)* **69**, 1800.
Goldstein, A. L. & White, A. (1973) *In* A. J. S. Davis and R. L. Carter, eds., *Contemporary Topics in Immunobiology*, 2, pp. 339-350, Plenum Publishing Co., New York.
Goldstein, A. L., Hooper, J. A., Schulof, R. S., Cohen, G. H., Thurman, G. B., McDaniel, M. C., White, A. & Dardenne, M. (1974) *Fed. Proc.* **33**, 2053.
Goldstein, A. L., Wara, D. W., Ammann, A. J., Sakai, H., Harris, N. S., Thurman, G. B., Hooper, J. A., Cohen, G. H., Goldman, A. S., Costanzi, J. J. & McDaniel, M. C. (1975) *Transplant. Proc.* **7**, Suppl. I.
Good, R. A. & Yunis, E. S. (1974) *Fed. Proc.* **33**, 2040.
Hardy, M. A., Quint, J., Goldstein, A. L., State, D. & White, A. (1968) *Proc. Nat. Acad-Sci.* **61**, 875.
Hardy, M. A., Zisblatt, M., Levine, N., Goldstein, A. L., Lilly, F. & White, A. (1971) *Transplant. Proc.* **III**, 926-928.
Hooper, J. A., McDaniel, M. C., Thurman, G. B., Cohen, G. H., Schulof, R. S. & Goldstein, A. L. (1975) *Ann. N-Y. Acad. Sci.* **249**, 154.
Khaw, B. A. & Rule, A. H. (1973) *Br. J. Medicine* **28**, 28.
Klein, J. J., Goldstein, A. L. & White, A. (1965) *Proc. Nat. Acad. Sci.* **53**, 812.
Klein, J. J., Goldstein, A. L. & White, A. (1966) *Ann. N-Y. Acad. Sci.* **135**, 485.
Lowrey, O. H., Rosenbrough, N. J., Farr, A. L. & Randall. R. J. (1951) *J. Biol. Chem.* **193**, 265.
Löwenberg, B., Nieuwerkerk, H. T. M. & Van Bekkum, D. W. (1972).
Miller, H. C., Schniege, S. K. & Rule, A. (1973) *J. Immunol.* **111**, 1005.
Raff, M. & Cantor, H. (1974) *In* B. Amos, ed., *Progress in Immunology*, pp. 83-93, Academic Press, New York.
Rappaport, F. T., Converse, J. M., Horn, L., Ballantyne, D. L. & Mulholland, J. H. (1964) *Ann. Surg.* **159**, 390.
Sakai, H., Daniels, J. C., Lewis, S. R., Lynch, J. B., Larson, D. L. & Ritzmann, S. E. (1972) *J. Reticuloendothelial Soc.* **11**, 19.
Sakai, H., Costanzi, J. J., Loukas, D. F., Gagliano, R. G., Ritzmann, S. E. & Go!dstein A. L. (1975) *Cancer*.
Scheid, M. P., Hoffman, M. K., Komuro, K., Hammerling, U., Abbott, J., Boyse, E. A., Cohen, G. H., Hooper, J. A., Schulof, R. S. & Goldstein, A. L. (1973) *J. Exp. Med.* **138**, 1027.
Scheinberg, M. A. & Cathcart, E. S. (1974) *Clin. Res.* **22**, 428.
Scheinberg, M. A., Cathcart, E. S. & Goldstein, A. L. In press, *Clin. Res.*
Schulof, R. (1972) *Tex. Rep. Biol. Med.* **30**, 195.
Strausser, H. R., Bober, L. A., Bucsi, R. A., Shillcock, J. A. & Goldstein, A. L. (1971) *Exp. Geront.* **66**, 373.
Thurman, G. B., Ahmed, A., Strong, D. M., Gershwin, M. D., Steinberg, A. D. & Goldstein, A. L. (1975) *Transplant. Proc.* **7**, Suppl. I, 299.
Thurman, G. B., Silver, B. B., Hooper, J. A., Giovanella, B. C. & Goldstein, A. L. (1974) *In* J. Rygaard & C. O. Poulsen, eds., *Proceedings of the first International Workshop on Nude Mice*. Gustav Fischer Verlag, Stuttgart, pp. 105-117.
Trainin, N. (1974) *Physiol. Rev.* **54**, 272.
Touraine, J. L., Touraine, E., Incefy, G. S. & Good, R. A. (1975) *Ann. N.Y. Acad. Sci.* **249**, 335.
Waksal, S. D., Barker, G. & St. Pierre, R. L. (In press) *Ann. N.Y. Acad. Sci.*
Waldmann, T., Broder, S., Durm, M., Blackmann, M., Blaese, R. M. & Strober,rW. (1974) **2**, 1573.
Wara, D. W. & Ammann, A. J. (In press) *Ann. N-Y. Acad. Sci.*
Wara, D. W., Goldstein, A. L., Doyle, W. & Ammann, A. J. (1975) *New England J. of Med.* **292**, 70.

White, A. & Goldstein, A. L. (1968) *Prespect. Biol. Med.* **11**, 475.
White, A., Goldstein, A. L., Banerjee, S. & Asanuma, Y. (1968) In *Proc. 3rd Intl. Congress of Endocrinology*, 1228.
White, A. & Goldstein, A. L. (1970) *In* G. E. W. Wolstenholme and J. Knight, eds., *Control processes in Multicellular Organisms*, Ciba Foundation Symposium, J. A. Churchill, Ltd. London, 210-237.
White, A. & Goldstein, A. L. (1971) *In* E. Mihich, ed., *Regulation of Cell Metabolism; Organizational Aspects of the Molecular Level*, Academic Press, Inc., New York.
Wolf, B. (1975) *Ann. N.Y. Acad. Sci.* **249**, 278.
Wolf, B. & Erb, S. D. (1970) In *Proc. Ann. Leukocyte Cult. Conf.*, 4th.
Wortis, H. H., Anderson, H. R. & Dresser, D. W. (1974) *Nature* **234**, 1250.
Wybran, J., Levin, A. S., Fudenberg, H. H. & Goldstein, A. L. (1975) *Ann. N.Y. Acad. Sci.* **249**, 300.
Zisblatt, M., Goldstein, A. L., Lilly, F. & White, A. (1970) *Proc. Nat. Acad. Sci.* **66**, 1170.

Biological Activity of Thymic Hormones

DISCUSSION

ROTTER, Rehovot

I would like to ask you, what is your definition of a suppressor T cell as related to the maturation stage?

GOLDSTEIN, Galveston

Our studies suggest that the suppressor T cell is an immature lymphoid cell that has seen a thymic humoral influence. These cells are probably cortisone-sensitive, home to the spleen in preference and to lymph nodes, and are lost very rapidly after adult thymectomy. They probably represent virgin T cells that have not been corrupted by their environment.

ROTTER, Rehovot

So how could you explain that our THF, which we now consider as a factor which causes maturation of cells, would induce suppressor activity? I mean, you would expect the opposite. With thymus hormones, you increase the maturation stages of cells. So, it is expected that, once you have more THF, you would have mature cells that are not suppressor T cells, according to your definition.

GOLDSTEIN, Galveston

Yes, that's right.

ROTTER, Rehovot

So, are these suppressor cells?

GOLDSTEIN, Galveston

No! I am saying that the suppressor capacity may really represent just a change in the ratio between T_1 and T_2 cells and that what we call suppressor T cells may really represent just a less mature T cell population. Depending upon how many T_1 to T_2 cells you have, you can either get a synergism or suppression.

ROTTER, Rehovot

So, if you have less thymus hormone, you would expect a better T suppressor function?

GOLDSTEIN, Galveston

No! For example, in the NZB mouse, when the thymosin levels decrease in the serum, you loose the suppressor T cells and the mice develop autoreactive cells.

KRUISBEEK, Rijswijk

Allan, we know that you are concerned as to the effect of endotoxin in the various bioassays. Could you tell us what the effect of endotoxin is on the human E rosettes?

GOLDSTEIN, Galveston

We haven't looked, and we would doubt that endotoxin would specifically increase E rosettes.

HONDIUS-BOLDINGH, Oss

Dr. White told us something about a modified procedure without the heat treatment and the acetone precipitation. Did it change anything in the characteristics or recovery of the final product?

GOLDSTEIN, Galveston

I am sure we are going to find several ways to prepare biologically active molecules, some probably better than those presented at this workshop. But, certainly, thymosin is heat-stable. Dr. Trainin's THF is also heat-stable. The only factor today that is not heat-stable is Bach's factor, which is very unusual for a peptide with a molecular weight of 1000. I suspect it is actually also heat-stable, but that it is taken out of solution with some other contaminating serum component during heating.

HONDIUS-BOLDINGH, Oss

And the other two substances from your fraction 5. Are they also biologically active?

GOLDSTEIN, Galveston

In the MLR system, they are. We have yet to put them in other critical assays.

LUCKEY, Columbia

I would like to comment that our LSH_h is heat labile and, except for that, I would presume it to be very similar to your thymosin (MW 12,000) because it is 15,000 MW. And, being heat-labile, you can very easily use the material as your inactive control by heating it. So that you should add that to your list of heat-labile thymic protein hormones.

VAN BEKKUM, Rijswijk

I thank you very much for this comment. Thank you, Allan, for this masterful presentation. You gave us also much hope for the application of the thymus hormone.

Biological Activity of Thymic Hormones

ANALYSIS OF HORMONE PREPARATIONS FROM NORMAL AND IRRADIATED CALF THYMUS AND CONTROL PREPARATIONS BY SODIUM DODECYL SULPHATE ELECTROPHORESIS

A. C. W. SWART*, E. J. VAN DEN HENDE-TIMMER* &
D. W. VAN BEKKUM**

The preparations used during this workshop have been prepared by different procedures and the molecular weight assigned to the biologically active moiety in them by the producers varies widely: 1000 for Bach's; 3000 for Trainin's; and 12000 for Goldstein's preparation.

It was, therefore, of interest to analyse these hormones and to check the preparations for their molecular weight distribution.

In addition, three fractions prepared by us were analyzed, one from normal calf thymus and two from thymocyte-depleted calf thymus tissue obtained from irradiated animals.

Unfortunately, the Bach preparations were not available in sufficient quantity to allow analysis.

MATERIALS AND METHODS

Thymic humoral factor (THF) and an inactive control preparation extracted from calf thymus and spleen, respectively, by a published procedure (1) were supplied by Dr. N. Trainin and co-workers.

Thymosin fraction 5 and an inactive control preparation obtained from calf thymus and spleen, respectively, as described by Hooper *et al.* (2) were supplied by Dr. A. L. Goldstein and co-workers.

The three fractions prepared by us were isolated according to the method of Goldstein (2) for thymosin fraction 5: one from normal calf thymus (thymosin fraction 5_s) and two from thymus tissue of two irradiated calves, thymosin $5_{irr\,1}$ and $5_{irr\,2}$.

The calves were each exposed to 500 rad whole body γ-irradiation from a ^{137}Cs source at a dose rate of 100 rad/hour. They were sacrificed 48 h after irradiation. Histological examination showed that the thymus was severely depleted of thymocytes; according to rough calculation, less than 10 per cent of the normal content of small lymphoid cells was present in these glands.

Sodium dedecyl sulfate (SDS) gel electrophoresis was performed on 15 per

* Institute for Experimental Gerontology-TNO, 151, Lange Kleiweg, Rijswijk (ZH), The Netherlands and
** Radiobiological Institute-TNO, 151, Lange Kleiweg, Rijswijk (ZH), The Netherlands

cent acrylamide gels in 10 cm long tubes of 6 mm inner diameter. All solutions were as described in reference 2. Samples were boiled with mercaptoethanol and SDS before application. Electrophoresis was carried out for 15 h at 3 mA per tube.

Carbonic anhydrase (MW 29,000), myoglobin (MW 17,000) and lysozyme (MW 14,000) were used as both external and internal references. A linear relationship between log MW and mobility was assumed for the calculation of molecular weights. Calculations are based on only myoglobin and lysozyme as references.

RESULTS AND DISCUSSION

The figures show that all preparations were very heterogeneous. Both preparations of Trainin contain material of molecular weight 11,000 and higher. A heavy band at MW 15,000 in the spleen extract (Fig. 1) probably represents chains of hemoglobin, because the spleen extract was faintly red in color. THF, which is reported to have a molecular weight of 3,000, is not visible (Fig. 1),

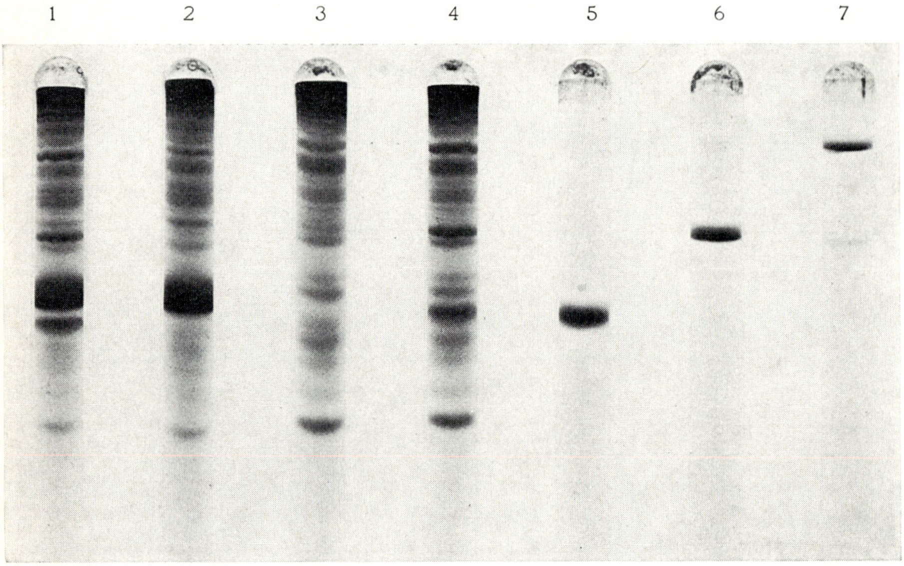

Fig. 1. SDS gel electrophoresis of Trainin's preparations.

1. Spleen extract, 240 μg, with references, each 20 μg.
2. Spleen extract, 240 μg.
3. THF, 260 μg.
4. THF, 260 μg, with references, each 20 μg.
5. Lysozyme, 20 μg.
6. Myoglobin, 20 μg.
7. Carbonic anhydrase, 20 μg.

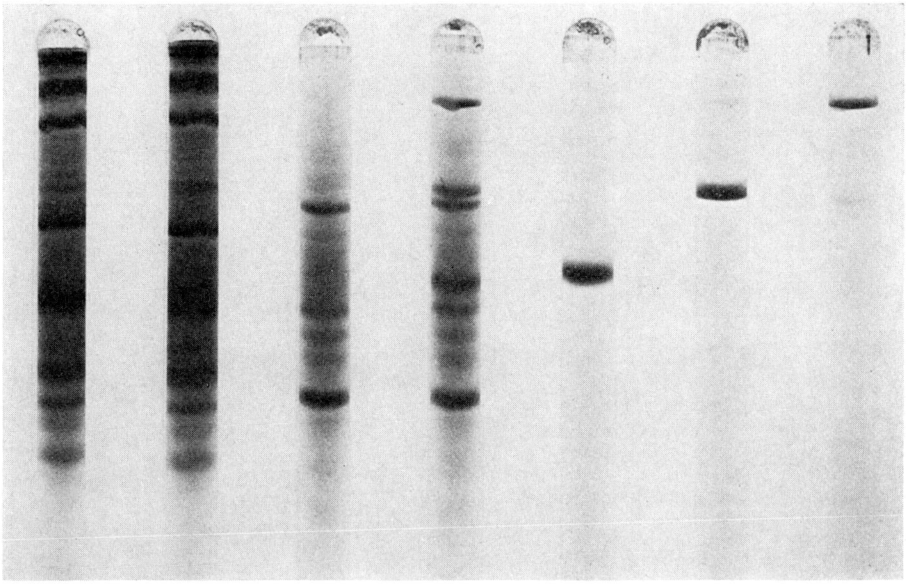

Fig. 2. SDS gel electrophoresis of Goldstein's preparations.

1. Spleen extract, 250 μg, with references, each 20 μg.
2. Spleen extract, 250 μg.
3. Thymosin fraction 5, 250 μg.
4. Thymosin fraction 5, 250 μg, with references, each 20 μg.
5. Lysozyme, 20 μg.
6. Myoglobin, 20 μg.
7. Carbonic anhydrase, 20 μg.

either because the amounts were too low to be detected or because it was lost during the staining and destaining procedure.

Goldstein's spleen extract (Fig. 2) contains material of MW 9000 and higher and thymosin fraction 5 (Fig. 2) contains material of MW 8000 and higher, although almost all of it is between 11,000 and 17,000.

A thick band at MW 11,000 in Goldstein's thymosin fraction 5 and in our fraction 5_s (Fig. 3) seems to be a likely candidate for thymosin, which is reported to have a molecular weight of 12,200 (2). It should be noted that this band is absent or almost absent in fractions $5_{irr\,1}$ and $5_{irr\,2}$ (Fig. 3).

The biological activity of fractions $5_{irr\,1}$ and $5_{irr\,2}$ was kindly assayed by 3 participants in the present workshop, using concentrations similar to those employed for thymosin fraction 5. Both fraction $5_{irr\,1}$ and $5_{irr\,2}$ showed some activity in the adenyl cyclase assay (+) (Dr. A. Kook), were fully active in the *in vitro* GvH assay (++) (Dr. M. Small), but inactive (—) in the *in vitro* azathioprine rosette inhibition assay (Dr. M. Dardenne).

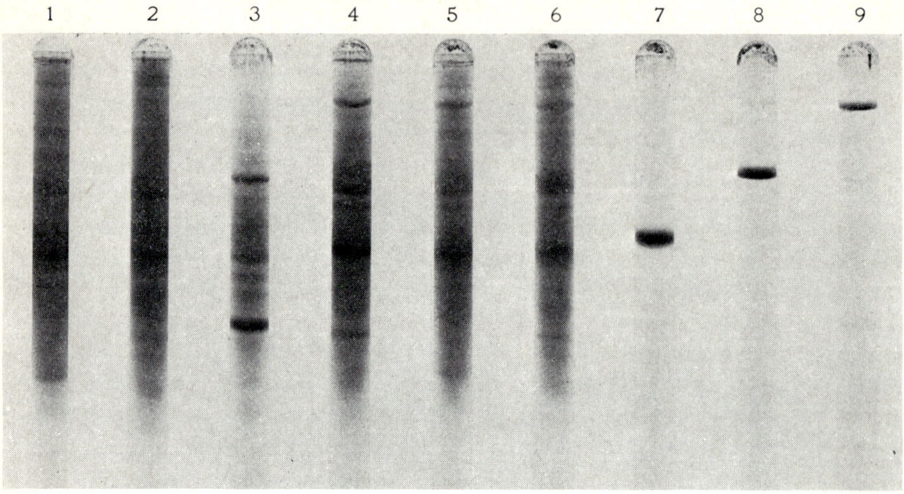

Fig. 3. SDS gel electrophoresis of fractions prepared in Rijswijk, compared to Goldstein's thymosin fraction 5.

1. Thymosin fraction 5_{irr-1}, 260 µg.
2. Thymosin fraction 5_{irr-2}, 260 µg.
3. Goldstein's thymosin fraction 5.
4. Thymosin fraction 5_s
5. Thymosin fraction 5_{irr1} with references, each 20 µg.
6. Thymosin fraction 5_{irr2}
7. Lysozyme, 20 µg.
8. Myoglobin, 20 µg.
9. Carbonic anhydrase, 20 µg.

REFERENCES

1. Trainin, M. & Small, M. (1970) *J. Exp. Med.* **132**, 885.
2. Hooper, J. A., McDaniel, M. C., Thurman, G. B., Cohen, G. H., Schulof, R. S. & Goldstein, A. Z. (1974) *Annals of the New York Acad. Sci*.

Biological Activity of Thymic Hormones

DISCUSSION

KOOK, Rehovot

I have only one suggestion to make, that is: if you are going to run it next time, you should also run a couple of samples which are not boiled with SDS prior to application on the polyacrylamide gels. The reason is that I am afraid that boiling leads to aggregation. I do believe that THF is a subunit of Allan Goldstein's thymosin and that the complex of several subunits that he gets is due to the heating step in his preparative procedure.

SWART, Rijswijk

We have also run our first fraction 5, prepared according to A. Goldstein non-boiled and we obtained exactly the same results as with boiling.

KOOK, Rehovot

Did you study the effect of boiling the electrophoresis samples in the case of THF?

SWART, Rijswijk

No, we didn't.

COHEN, Galveston

In the SDS gel technique, the boiling in the presence of SDS and mercapto-ethanol is required for maximum disaggregation and denaturation of protein into subunits.

SWART, Rijswijk

I agree, this is generally accepted as the best procedure.

VAN BEKKUM, Rijswijk

Well, I think that it is at least satisfactory to us that Dr. Kook has expressed himself as being "anti-kooking".

Biological Activity of Thymic Hormones

SUMMARY OF THE RESULTS OF THE WORKSHOP

ADA M. KRUISBEEK

The results of the Workshop are summarized in the accompanying Table. Detailed descriptions of the assays listed here can be found elsewhere in this book.

The results should not be interpreted without taking the following points into account:

1. The hormone concentrations used were selected after extensive discussions with all participants. Every assay has been optimalized for only one of the

TABLE I

QUANTITY OF THYMIC HORMONES USED DURING THE WORKSHOP

	THF	*Thymosin*	*TF*
Adenylcyclase (thymus)	40 μg	100 μg	100 ng
In vitro GvH	20 μg	20 μg	100 ng
Rosette inh. (*vitro*)	200 μg*	200 μg	1000 ng
Rosette inh. (*vivo*)	(1×) 100 μg	(1×) 100 μg	(1×) 500 ng
Autologous Rosette (*vivo*)	(2×) 100 μg	(2×) 100 μg	(2×) 500 ng
θ induction (*vivo*)	(2×) 100 μg	(2×) 100 μg	(2×) 500 ng
Cycling CFU (*vitro*)	50 μg	100 μg	60 ng
Mitogens thymus (*vitro*)	20 μg*	100 μg*	100 ng*
Mitogens spleen (*vitro*)	20 μg*	100 μg*	100 ng*
MLC spleen (*vitro*, tubes)	20–80 μg	100 μg	100 ng
MLC thymus (*vitro*, tubes)	20–80 μg	100 μg	100 ng
MLC spleen (*vitro*, microtitre)	20–80 μg	100 μg	100 ng
Mitogens (*vivo*)	(14×) 100 μg	(14×) 100 μg	(14) × 500 ng
MLC thymus (*vitro*)	100 μg*	100 μg*	75 ng
Popliteal LN (*vivo*)	(3×) 1 mg	(3×) 1 mg	n.d.

Explanation:
* Serial dilutions of this quantity have been tested; the quantity listed represents the highest dose employed. In *in vitro* assays the quantity mentioned is the concentration of hormone per ml cell suspension; cell suspensions contain 1×10^6 to 10×10^6 uncleated cells per ml (variations from assay to assay).
In *in vivo* experiments the quantity mentioned is a daily injection, the number of days is placed in parentheses. Control preparations (i.e. spleen extracts) are used in the same quantity as the maximal thymic hormone concentration.

Institute for Experimental Gerontology, Lange Kleiweg 151, Rijswijk (ZH), The Netherlands

TABLE II

SUMMARY RESULTS INTERCOMPARISON THYMIC HORMONE PREPARATIONS

	THF *hormone*	*control*	*Thymosin* *hormone*	*control*	*TF* *hormone*	*control*	*other* *control*
Adenylcyclase (thymus)	++	—	++	—	—	—	—
In vitro GvH	++	—	++	+	+	—	
Rosette inh. (*vitro*)	+	—	+	—	++	—	
Rosette inh. (*vivo*)	+	—	+	—	++	—	
Autologous Rosette (*vivo*)	++	—	++	—	++	—	
θ induction (*vivo*)			(inconclusive results)				
Cycling CFU (*vitro*)	++		±		±		—
Mitogens thymus (*vitro*)	++	—	++	—	±	n.d.	—
Mitogens spleen (*vitro*)	++		±		++		—
MLC spleen (*vitro*, tubes)	++	—	—	—	+	++	
MLC thymus (*vitro*, tubes)	+		+		n.d.		
MLC spleen (*vitro*, microtitre)	+		+		n.d.		—
Mitogens (*vivo*)			(technical errors)				
MLC thymus (*vitro*)			(technical errors)				
Popliteal LN (*vivo*)			(inconclusive results)				

Explanation of signs: scores made by performer of assay within the limits of 4 marks:
++ very active (values as in own laboratory); + active; ± dubious; — negative n.d. = not done
Thymosin isolated from irradiated calf thymus was negative in Rosette inhibition test (*vitro*) and positive in the *in vitro* GvH assay.

three hormones; therefore, possible negative or dubious results can be due to incorrect concentrations. The time available for the Workshop, however, did not permit extensive dose-effect studies. Where several different doses were tested, this is indicated in the Table by an asterisk.

2. The expression "inconclusive results" has been used to indicate suggestive but inconsistent results; these assays apparently need further adaptation prior to being used as bioassays for thymic hormone activity.

3. The control preparations for THF and thymosin were spleen extracts prepared according to the same procedure as was used for the THF or thymosin preparation. The control for TF was an inactive fraction eluted prior to the hormone fraction from Sephadex G 25 (i.e., inactive in the assays performed by the group of J.-F. Bach).

4. In the mitogen assays (after *in vitro* treatment), the Con A response always peaks at lower concentrations of THF than does the PHA response.

ASSAYS

Adenyl cyclase:	Activation of adenyl cyclase activity by THF - A. Kook
In vitro GvH:	*In vitro* Graft versus Host - M. Small

Rosette inh. (*vitro, vivo*):	Rosette inhibition after *in vitro* treatment with hormone or with serum from *in vivo* treated animals - M. Dardenne
Autologous Rosettes:	Decrease in autologous Rosette formation after *in vivo* treatment - J. Charreire
θ induction:	θ induction (measured in cytotoxicity assay) after *in vivo* treatment - C. Fournier
Cycling CFU:	Activation of cycling of colony forming units after *in vitro* treatment - D. Zipori
Mitogens thymus, spleen:	Mitogen stimulation after *in vitro* treatment - V. Rotter
MLC thymus, spleen:	Mixed lymphocyte reaction after *in vitro* preincubation - T. Umiel
Mitogens (*vivo*):	Mitogen stimulation in lymph node and spleen cells after *in vivo* treatment - G. Thurman
MLC thymus (*vitro*):	Mixed lymphocyte reaction in *in vitro* treated cells - G. Cohen
Popliteal LN (*vivo*):	Popliteal lymph node assay (rats) after *in vivo* treatment - S. Knaan

Biological Activity of Thymic Hormones

DISCUSSION

BACH, Paris

On behalf of the French group, I would first like to compliment the organizers of the Workshop on their remarkable achievement. I also would like to say that I agree in principle with the way the data are presented. I would like in addition to make 3 comments on our own results.

The first is about the theta induction assay. It is true that somewhat inconclusive results were obtained, perhaps it is more interesting to say that the six preparations were negative in this assay with the possibility of a ± for one or two preparations. This is a minor comment, but is is important because of the discussion on the specificity of the cytotoxicity assay.

The second comment concerns our own preparation; it is interesting to see (and I realized that better when I looked at that slide) that our preparation is mainly active on spleen cells and that all tests on thymus cells were negative, which is not surprising in views of our conception of the action of our product. However, concerning the negative findings with adenyl cyclase, I should mention that these results bear on two experiments which is always difficult to interpret.

I would *lastly* like to emphasize the fact that, in my mind, if all tests were of interest, some of them are more likely to be used as screening assays for chemical work than others. Thus, it is obvious that the *in vitro* GvH assay, the sheep red cell rosette assay, and the autologous rosette assay gave clear-cut and very discriminating results. However, autologous rosette can only be used so far *in vivo*, which is a weakness. From what we heard on Monday, all other tests gave some erratic results with positive controls from time to time, which makes them difficult to use as screening assays.

GOLDSTEIN, Galveston

I'm glad that so many assays worked well and that there is reasonable agreement on the action of preparations that were supposedly active or inactive. Many dose-response-curves are bell-shaped. Due to this, preparations that are in reality very potent could seem inactive in some assays.

Biological Activity of Thymic Hormones

POSSIBLE SITE OF ACTION OF THE VARIOUS THYMIC HORMONE PREPARATIONS

I. BETEL

As a biochemist by training, I have been involved in the isolation and purification of enzymes. It strikes me that the participants in this Workshop seem to entertain the idea that the success of their specific method of isolating the active principle from the thymus gland can be measured by the number of assays in which a positive response is obtained with that particular preparation. As it is hardly likely that all assays employed in this Workshop measure responses by the same target cell, the finding that a preparation elicits universally positive responses would either mean that the "thymus hormone" acts on a number of distinct target cells, or that the preparation is rather impure in that it contains a number of different active principles.

Since that is the only information to be gained from the results obtained with THF at this Workshop; we have to compare the results obtained with thymosin and TF, each of which yielded positive as well as negative results. The important finding is that these differences do *not* run parallel in the various assays. If the negative responses were due to the lower specific activity of a preparation, one might expect the negative and the positive results to appear in the same assays with both thymosin and TF. Since this is not so, the alternative explanation, namely that thymosin and TF contain different active principles as far as their main activity is concerned, becomes more likely. If we more closely inspect those assays which show a decisively different response to thymosin as compared to TF (bold type in Table I), it seems that TF is more active in the assays with spleen cells than in the assays employing thymus cells and that the reverse is true for thymosin. Taking into account the viewpoints of Cantor, Stutman, and others concerning T cell populations, this might indicate that TF is acting more specifically on a more mature population of cells and thymosin on a more immature population and, finally, that THF would combine both properties. This is as far as I would like to go, with the restriction that this interpretation of the results is only a speculation, since the differences observed during this Workshop may well be due to other factors. I hope that such speculations will stimulate efforts to investigate the more purified hormone preparations, that each group now seems to have in the same range of assays to see if the differences in response become more pronounced or perhaps disappear.

Radiobiological Institute-TNO, Lange Kleiweg 151, Rijswijk (ZH), the Netherlands.

TABLE I

RESULTS INTERCOMPARISON OF THYMUS HORMONE PREPARATIONS

WITH INDICATIONS OF DIFFERENCES IN BIOLOGICAL ACTIVITY BETWEEN THYMOSIN AND TI

	THF		*Thymosin*		*TF*		*other*
	hormone	*control*	*hormone*	*control*	*hormone*	*control*	*control*
Adenylcyclase (thymus)	++	—	++	—	—	—	—
In vitro GvH	++	—	++	+	+	—	
Rosette inh. (*vitro*)	+	—	+	—	++	—	
Rosette inh. (*vivo*)	+	—	+	—	++	—	
Autologous rosette (*vivo*)	++	—	++	—	++	—	
θ induction (*vivo*)			(inconclusive results)				
Cycling CFU (*vitro*)	++		±		±		—
Mitogens thymus (*vitro*)	++	—	++	—	±	n.d.	—
Mitogens spleen (*vitro*)	++		±		++		—
MLC spleen (*vitro*, tubes)	++	—	—	—	+	++	
MLC thymus (*vitro*, tubes)	+		+		n.d.		
MLC spleen (*vitro*, microtitre)	+		+		n.d.		—
Mitogens (*vivo*)			(technical errors)				
MLC thymus (*vitro*)			(technical errors)				
Popliteal LN (*vivo*)			(inconclusive results)				

Explanation of signs: scores made by performer of assay within the limits of 4 marks:
++ very active (values as in own laboratory); + active; ± dubious; — negative

Biological Activity of Thymic Hormones

DISCUSSION

ZIPORI, Rehovot

I would like to specify, that the material which we used here for measuring cycling of colony forming cells is a crude thymus extract. At home, we used material after passing through the G25 column and it worked very similarly. I do not know if the completely purified material will work the same, but this is going to be tested in the near future.

BACH, Paris

There is a point which has not yet been raised, which is, the amount of material which has been injected or added *in vitro* (ng levels for TF; μg levels for thymosin and THF). I would like to ask Allan Goldstein what is the degree of purification of the fraction 5 he has given us, expressed in terms of pure thymosin? What is the percentage of thymosin present in the preparation you gave us?

GOLDSTEIN, Galveston

It is hard to give an exact figure. The biological activity found depends on the assay. We find an identical pattern of thymosin fraction 5 on SDS gels as was just shown to you. There are at least 10 components and we do not know how many of them stimulate or inhibit responses.

VAN BEKKUM, Rijswijk

I am very glad that this question was raised about the doses employed for both the *in vitro* and the *in vivo* experiments. The doses were arrived at following a compilation of the best guesses by both the producers of the hormones (reasoning from the experience they have in their own tests and trying to extrapolate to the other people's tests) and by the authors of the individual assays. Needless to say that these guesses may have been wrong after all. It is certainly striking to everybody who had a look at the concentrations used that TF is being used at much lower concentrations than the other two substances. And what that means, we do not know.

TRAININ, Rehovot

I want to comment on Dr. Betel's statements. Contrary to his suggestions, I feel that, in analogy with other hormones, e.g., the estrogens or testosterone, it is more likely for the thymus hormone to have several different target cells than a single one. This idea would fit our results excellently.

LUCKEY, Columbia

Dr. Bach's question made my mind turn over. Seeing those gels, and we have just worked on assays using those gels, a very rough estimate of that heavy band, which I thought was thymosin, has to be 75 per cent or 90 per cent of the total; and then Allan's remarks made me ask the question, what is thymosin? I mean, I automatically went to that heavy band, but I do not think he will automatically do that. Can you tell me what thymosin is now?

GOLDSTEIN, Galveston

I wish I could clear up all the remaining problems that we have in terms of chemical and biological characterization. I think it is going to be a family of thymosins. The rapidly moving band on the SDS gels consists of 3 acidic molecules. All of them seem to have biological activity.

KOOK, Rehovot

I think I would like to add one more point about the structure of the hormone. There are papers that I came across recently which suggest that there exists a large degree of heterogeneity in hormone families. Thus you can have two molecules which have the same structure, one has biological activity and the other does not.

You can have other molecules which have the same biological activity but have a different structure. This might be the case in our situation. Secondly, I want to indicate that all three preparations contain a significant proportion of the same acidic amino acids, which are glutamic and aspartic acids. I don't know if we can really say that we have completely pure molecules in our hands, but I think that each one of us may have a preparation containing the active site of the hormone. As far as I can see, there is no real difference between our preparation and Allan Goldstein's preparation when compared on the basis of biological activities. So, maybe the whole discussion between us is not relevant.

VAN BEKKUM, Rijswijk

That is certainly a very sobering thought, Dr. Kook.

LUCKEY, Columbia

Dr. White suggested that, when you lyophilize the 12,000 molecular weight thymosin, you go up towards 70,000 and you alluded to it 2 or 3 times in conversation and 70,000 is not changed by SDS treatment. What do you think, Allan?

GOLDSTEIN, Galveston

The fraction that we sent here was a lyophilized fraction. There is no aggregation due to lyophilization of fraction 5.

PART TWO

Materials and Methods of Various Bioassays for Thymic Hormone

Biological Activity of Thymic Hormones

ACTIVATION OF MEMBRANAL ADENYL CYCLASE OF LYMPHOID CELLS BY THYMIC PREPARATIONS

ABRAHAM I. KOOK

Spleen cells from neonatally thymectomized (NTx) mice are incapable of responding in the *in vitro* GvH assay (Trainin *et al.* 1969). Incubation with the thymus hormone restores the ability of these cells to respond in the *in vitro* GvH test (Trainin *et al.* 1969, Trainin & Small 1970). We found that small quantities of dibutyryl cAMP or of theophylline (a known inhibitor of cyclic nucleotide phosphodesterase) (Sutherland & Robinson 1968) can be substituted for THF in the above assay (Kook & Trainin 1974). These results indicated that cellular cAMP plays a role in the induction of immunocompetence in spleen cells from NTx mice and suggested a hormonal mechanism of activation of lymphoid cells mediated via cAMP. Indeed, we were able to demonstrate that THF increases significantly the activity of adenyl cyclase in spleen cells from either normal or NTx mice, and that intracellular levels of cAMP increase following short exposure of thymocytes to the thymus hormone (Kook & Trainin 1974).

Other agents known to stimulate cAMP production in lymphoid cells were tested for their capacity to induce GvH activity in spleen cells from NTx mice. PGE_2 was shown both to stimulate cAMP production and to induce GVH activity in our *in vitro* GvH assay. The PGE_2-induced intracellular increase in cAMP could be blocked by flufenamic acid. Under these conditions, PGE_2 lost its ability to induce GvH activity in spleen cells from NTx mice (Kook & Trainin 1974).

These results indicate that the increment in cAMP levels induced by THF is an *obligatory step* in the pathway leading to induction of immunocompetence by THF. In consequence, in the present experiments, we aim to test the activity of various thymic preparations by means of their capacity to stimulate adenyl cyclase activity in lymphoid cells. The assay is based on the conversion of ^{3}H-ATP to ^{3}H-cAMP by adenyl cyclase following the procedure of Krishna *et al.* (1968). Cells tested are incubated in Eagle's medium (E.M.) and exposed to thymic hormone for specified periods of time. Following incubation the cells are washed, homogenized and the membranes collected by centrifugation. ^{3}H-ATP is added as a substrate for the enzyme and the ^{3}H-cAMP which is gen-

Department of Cell Biology, The Weizmann Institute of Science, Rehovot, Israel

erated in then isolated by chromatography on Dowex 50-H^+ columns, and measured.

Thirty $\times 10^6$ thymocytes or other lymphoid cells (spleen cells from normal or neonatally thymectomized (NTx) mice) in 30 ml of E.M. are incubated in the presence of THF for a specified time interval at 37 °C in a shaking water bath. Periods of incubation used by us varied from 5 to 60 min. The concentrations of THF used range from 20-130 μg protein/ml of incubation medium. After incubation the cells are centrifuged at 5 °C 1500 rpm for 5 min, and washed in excess of cold saline and recentrifuged. One half ml of incomplete reaction mixture (24 μmoles of Tris-HCl, pH 7.5; 198 μmoles of $MgSO_4$; 3 μmoles of phosphenol pyruvate; 6 μmoles of Cleland's reagent and either 3 or 6 μmoles of theophylline-ethylendiamine) are added to the cell pellet. The cells are suspended with a Pasteur pipette, frozen in liquid air, and thawed at room temperature. The disrupted cells are transferred to glass homogenizer tubes and ground for a total of 30 strokes with teflon pestles. The cell debris are transferred to centrifuge tubes. The glass homogenizer tubes are washed with another 0.5 ml of incomplete reaction mixture and the washing is added to the centrifuge tubes. The suspension is then centrifuged for 20 min at 0 °C (Spinco, Type 40 rotor; 14,500 rpm). The supernatant is discarded. The pellet is resuspended in 0.4 ml of incomplete reaction mixture, 0.1 ml of a solution containing 6 μmoles of NaF, 0.02 ml of a solution containing 50 μg pyruvate kinase and 0.1 ml of ^{3}H-ATP solution containing 1.2 μmoles of ATP having a specific activity of 1 μCi/1 μmole. This suspension is then incubated for 20 min at 30 °C in a shaking water bath. One tenth ml of water containing 0.5 mg of cAMP is added and the reaction is terminated by boiling for 3 min in a water bath. The mixture is then centrifuged at 2000 rpm for 10 min and the supernatant collected. 0.03 ml of water solution containing 15 μg of ATP is added to the supernatant and this is chromatographed on Dowex 50-H^+ columns, Bio Rad 50W-x 4 200-400 mesh (the columns are prepared by packing 6 ml of 50 per cent v/v suspension of the cation exchanger and water. The cation exchanger is washed extensively with water to eliminate material which absorbs U.V. light).

The columns are eluted with water and 1.3 ml fractions are collected at a 3 min interval in a fraction collector. The fractions are read at 260 μm. ATP is eluted first, cAMP second and AMP last. The cAMP peak is collected and an aliquote is counted in Bray's solution for maximum ^{3}H-efficiency. Usually, 2 ml of water solution is counted in 20 ml of Bray's solution. The results are expressed as ^{3}H-cAMP cpm/30 $\times 10^6$ cells. Alternatively, it could be expressed per protein.

In our experience the cAMP peak is collected over 8-10 tubes, i.e. in a total volume of 9-12 ml. The minimum number of columns per experiment is two, one for the control preparation and one for the material tested. The two columns should preferably be attached to one fraction collector and the rate of flow controled by the same peristaltic pump which can accommodate 2-4 channels. With one fraction collector the maximum number of columns that could be handled per day is 6. If one chooses to run 6 columns a day the following schedule is suggested: one column of normal cells, one of control preparation (spleen extract, lymph node extract, etc.) and one of the thymic preparation tested; each in duplicates.

Dose effect curves were clearly observed with increasing concentration of THF when measured both by the above assay of adenyl cyclase activation and when intracellular cAMP was measured by the Gilman procedure (Kook & Trainin 1974). The dose response curve is characterized by a plateau reached after a certain concentration of the THF tested. This is expected to vary between different preparations of THF.

Induction of immunocompetence is dose dependent on cAMP levels (Kook & Trainin 1974). It still should be taken into consideration that higher concentrations of THF could produce elevated levels of adenyl cyclase activity which are on the plateau while being already inhibitory in an immune assay.

The specificity of this test is based on the fact that extracts of other organs of the lymphoid system such as spleen and lymph nodes prepared by an identical way and used at the same concentrations were totally inactive. The effect of THF could be mimicked by DBcAMP, theophylline and prostaglandin E_2.

Possible target cells are thymocytes and thymus derived cells which could be found in spleens of NTx mice as well as in spleens from normal mice.

REFERENCES

1. Trainin, N., Small, M. & Globerson, A. (1969) *J. Exp. Med.* **130**, 765.
2. Trainin, N. & Small, M. (1970) *J. Exp. Med.* **132**, 885.
3. Sutherland, E. W. & Robinson, G. A. (1968) *Circulation* **37**, 279.
4. Kook, A. I. & Trainin, N. (1974) *J. Exp. Med.* **139**, 193.
5. Krishna, G., Weiss, B. & Brodie, B. B. (1968) *J. Pharm. Exp. Therap.* **163**, 379.

Biological Activity of Thymic Hormones

THF IN THE MLC BIOASSAY

TEHILA UMIEL

The mixed lymphocyte culture (MLC) is a model which represents the recognition phase of the *in vivo* homograft or of the graft versus host reactions (1).

In the one way MLC stimulator target cells are inactivated by pretreatment with mitomycin-C, thus the one way MLC provides a model to study the behaviour of responding cell to antigenic stimulation. It has been established that the responding cells in the MLC reaction are T cells (2, 3).

Since Thymic Humoral Factor (THF) plays a role in the process leading to the maturation of T cell populations, it was assumed that THF may increase the reactivity of T cells participating in the MLC reaction. It was indeed found, that 1 h preincubation of responding T cells from various sources (such as spleen of intact or thymectomized mice or thymus cells) with THF led to a significant increase of reactivity of these cells in a one way MLC response.

The MLC response is performed as follows: 2-3 month old C57BL/6 intact, neonatally or adult thymectomized mice and intact (C3H/eb × C57BL/6) F_1 mice are used as a source of responding and stimulating cells. Spleen, thymus or lymph nodes are aseptically removed and the organs are gently pressed through a stainless steel mesh. Then the cells are suspended in RPMI-1640 medium (Grand Island Biological Company, Chicago, Ill.) buffered with sodium bicarbonate and supplemented with penicillin, 100 units/ml. Streptomycin 100 μg/ml and 10 per cent inactivated Rehatuin fetal bovine serum (FBS) (Reheis Chemical, Chicago, Ill.). The cells are washed twice in RPMI-1640 and the pellet resuspended in RPMI-1640 containing 10 per cent FBS. Cells are counted in Turk sclution with a hemocytometer. Responding cells (spleen cells of intact or thymectomized mice of C57BL or F_1 source, or thymocytes) are incubated with THF (20 μg protein/ml) at 37 °C for 1 h in a shaking water bath. After incubation cells are washed twice in RPMI medium, centrifuged for 5 min and the pellets are resuspended in RPMI medium containing 10 per cent FBS. Cells are counted and adjusted to contain 10^6 cells/0.1 ml.

MLC experiments are carried out in Cook microtiter plates (M 220-29 ART, Cook Engineering Co.) containing 96 flat-shaped wells each of 0.275 ml volume. Stimulating spleen cells of F_1 origin (20×10^6/ml) are suspended in RPMI containing 10 per cent FBS, are incubated with mitomycin-C (m) (25 μg/ml) at

Department of Cell Biology, Weizmann Institute of Science, Rehovot, Israel

37 °C in a shaking water bath for 30 min. The cells are then washed twice in RPMI medium and counted. Cells are adjusted to contain 10^6 nucleated cells/0.1 ml. A volume of 0.1 ml of each responding and stimulating cells are distributed in each well, plates are covered with plastic lids and incubated at 37 °C in a humidified incubator in an atmosphere of 95 per cent air and 5 per cent CO_2. Seventy-two h following the initial time of incubation 2 μCi of tritiated thymidine are added in 50 λ of RPMI medium with 10 per cent FBS to each culture. Sixteen hours later cells are removed, washed with saline and precipitated with 5 per cent trichloroacetic acid and dried with methyl alcohol on a Whatman fiberglass filter. Filters are put in scintillation vials with simultaneous addition of 10 ml scintillation fluid and the counts per minute (CPM) are monitored. Triplicate cultures are used for each group in each experiment. In each single experiment it is necessary to set up syngeneic cultures ($F_1 \rightarrow F_1m$) and allogeneic cultures ($P \rightarrow F_1m$); this permits the use of an inner control for each individual experiment. The MLC stimulation index is calculated by deviding the mean CPM incorporated by allogeneic mixtures to the mean CPM incorporated by syngeneic mixtures.

Preincubation for 1 h in THF was shown to produce a marked elevation in the immunological competence of responding cells in the MLC reaction. These experiments also served to define more specifically the target cells for THF activity. Indeed lymphoid cell populations essentially devoid of T cells such as bone marrow derived spleen cells (B cells) and cells from nude mice were not activated by THF. On the other hand, lymphoid populations containing T cells such as spleen cells of intact or thymectomized mice and thymocytes were found to contain target cells for THF activity. Moreover, the maturation step under the influence of THF was strongly suggested by the MLC assay, since mature lymphoid cell populations such as cortison resistant thymocytes or lymph node lymphocytes were found to be unresponsive to THF treatment.

REFERENCES

1. Wilson, D. B., Blyth, J. L. & Nowell, P. C. (1968) *J. Exp. Med.* **128**, 1157.
2. Wilson, D. B., Silvers, W. V. & Nowell, P. C. (1967) *J. Exp. Med.* **126**, 655.
3. Valentine, F. T. (1971) *Cell-mediated immunity in vitro correlates*, ed. J. F. Revillard, Karger, Basel.

Biological Activity of Thymic Hormones

THE EFFECT OF THF ON THE REACTIVITY OF LYMPHOID CELLS TO PHA AND CON A

VARDA ROTTER

The end product of THF activity is expressed by an increase in immunocompetence of T cells. Indeed, immunomaturation of T cells mediated by THF restores the cellular GvH reactivity of neonatally thymectomized mice (1) and increases the competence of normal spleen and thymus cell populations in MLC reactions (2). On the basis of these observations it was expected that THF could also modify the response of T lymphocytes to T mitogens (3). Therefore, cells stimulated by PHA and Con A were submitted to the effect of THF during different periods of the reaction. It was found that while a considerable inhibition of the mitogenic reaction was observed when THF was present throughout the reaction, a striking increase occurred when cells were preincubated in THF for 24 h and then stimulated by the mitogens (4).

Since it is known that THF acts through an increase of intracellular cAMP (5) while T lectins raise intracellular cGMP (6), it was assumed that the inhibition in the mitogenic response observed by simultaneous exposure of the lymphoid cells to both agents (THF and T mitogens) was a result of an antagonism between these mechanisms. A long preincubation in THF for 24 h increases the mitogenic reactivity of lymphoid cells to PHA and Con A, since cell maturation is completed by then. The experiments were performed along the following steps: 6-8 weeks (C3H/eb $\times$ C57BL/6) F_1 female mice are used. Spleen or thymus cells are prepared in suspensions in cold RPMI-1640 (Gibco) by pressing the organs through a fine stainless steel mesh, washing twice in medium and filtering through a metal sieve. The cells are adjusted to 2×10^6 spleen cells/ml or 4×10^6 thymus cells/ml in RPMI-1640 enriched with 5 per cent heat inactivated fetal calf serum (Rehatuin NFS, Rehuis Chemical Co., Ill., USA). When thymus cell suspensions are tested 2×10^{-4} M mercaptoethanol is added.

These cell suspensions are distributed at 10 ml volume into glass test tubes and THF is added in decreasing amounts ranging from 40 μg/ml to 2.5 μg/ml. Cell suspensions containing different THF concentrations and cell suspensions containing spleen extract or PBS, are distributed into test tubes (Falcon 2001) 1 ml each. Cultures are incubated for 24 h at 37 °C in humidified air with 5 per cent CO_2. Thereafter, media containing THF or control preparations

Department of Cell Biology, Weizmann Institute of Science, Rehovot, Israel

are sucked off by vacuum and fresh medium is added. In each group of the different THF concentrations triplicate cultures were stimulated with PHA, Con A or PBS as control. Mitogens were added at a concentration of 3 μg/culture thymus cells and 1 μg/culture spleen cells. All cultures are incubated for 72 h at 37 °C in humidified air with 5 per cent CO_2.

Two hours before the end of the incubation period 2.5 μCi of tritiated methyl thymidine is added to each culture and the tube cultures are shaken for 2 h in 37 °C. The radioactive pulse is interrupted by placing the cultures in water-ice. The content of each culture is poured onto a fiberglass filter (Tamar, Israel) in a filtration system (Miles-Yeda, Rehovot, Israel) rinsed with saline, precipitated with 5 per cent trichloroacetic acid solution and dried in absolute ethanol, then the uptake of ^{3}H-thymidine is measured.

The results are represented by ΔCPM, CPM of mitogen stimulated cultures from which CPM of the control cultures is substracted.

These experiments indicate that THF acts on thymus derived cells at different stages of maturation. This effect is expressed by an increment in the mitogenic response of the target cells to PHA and Con A.

REFERENCES

1. Small, M. & Trainin, N. (1971) *J. Exp. Med.* **134**, 786.
2. Trainin, N., Kook, A. I., Umiel, T. & Albala, M. (In press) *Ann. N.Y. Acad. Sci.*
3. Andersson, J., Sjöberg, O. & Möller, G. (1972) *Transpl. Rev.* **11**, 131.
4. Rotter, V. & Trainin, N. (In press) *Cellular Immunol.*
5. Kook, A. I. & Trainin, N. (1974) *J. Exp. Med.* **139**, 193.
6. Hadden, J. W., Hadden, E. H., Haddov, M. K. & Goldberg, N. D. (1972) *Proc. Natl. Acad. Sci. USA.* **69**, 3024.

Biological Activity of Thymic Hormones

IN VITRO GRAFT-VERSUS-HOST ASSAY

MYRA SMALL

The capacity of lymphocytes to induce a graft-versus-host (GvH) response is a criterion used to measure their cell-mediated immunocompetence (1, 2). As in the *in vivo* GvH procedure performed by the method of Simonsen, splenomegaly can be measured *in vitro* and represents a counter-response of the "host" to challenge by immunocompetent "graft" cells. This *in vitro* assay is carried out by comparing the relative size of two matched spleen fragments: the test spleen explant challenged by nonsyngeneic lymphoid cells and the control spleen explant exposed to lymphocytes of syngeneic origin. This *in vitro* assay originally developed by Auerbach & Globerson (3) provides a sensitive test involving defined populations of cells. Induction of an *in vitro* allogeneic or semiallogeneic GvH response requires mature thymus-derived "graft" lymphocytes (4). Thus under our experimental conditions, spleen cells from neonatally thymectomized (nTx) parental mice do not induce enlargement of newborn F_1 spleen explants whereas the same number of spleen cells from intact parental donors consistently initiate a reaction of splenomegaly (4). The thymic humoral factor (THF) confers upon spleen cells from neonatally thymectomized donors the competence to induce this GvH response. This acquisition of competence can be achieved by injection of THF to NTx mice (5), or by direct *in vitro* interaction between THF and the spleen cells from these mice (4). This direct activation occurs both when thymic extracts are added to the culture medium surrounding the "graft" lymphocytes and the "host" spleen explants, or when "graft" dissociated spleen cells from neonatally thymectomized animals are preincubated in thymic extract for 1 h before antigenic challenge by the "host" tissue. By this technique the factor responsible for conferring competence on these lymphocytes has been demonstrated in extracts from thymus of syngeneic, allogeneic and xenogeneic origin (4, 5). No activity has been detected in control extracts prepared and tested in parallel from lymph node or spleen tissue of syngeneic, allogeneic or xenogeneic source (4, 5).

The relative enlargement of a (C3H/eb × C57BL/6) F_1 spleen explant challenged by parental cells as compared with a paired F_1 explant exposed to cells of syngeneic (C3H/eb × C57BL/6) F_1 origin reflects response to challenge by

Department of Cell Biology, Weizmann Institute, Rehovot, Israel immunocompetent lymphocytes. When 1×10^6 parental spleen cells are obtained from NTx C57BL mice no response is apparent in the absence of THF. Thus "graft" cells from a single NTx mouse are divided among cultures supplemented with THF, cultures supplemented with control extracts, or cultures without extract. Cultures of paired spleen fragments approximately $1.0 \times 1.0 \times 1.5$ mm in size are prepared from (C3H/eb × C57BL/6) F_1 mice less than 24 h of age. Cultures of paired spleen explants are maintained in filter wells consisting of Millipore filter paper 0.45 μ porosity and 25 μ thick glued to the underside of wells bored in strips of plexiglass (and sterilized by UV light followed by 70 per cent alcohol and two changes of sterile PBS). Each filter is placed in a Falcon organ culture dish (no. 3070) overlaying 1 ml of organ culture medium (OCM) consisting of Eagle's basal medium supplemented with 10 per cent horse serum (Difco no. 5357), 5 per cent chick embryo extract (prepared from 9-day embryos in an equal volume of Tyrodes solution), penicillin (100 u/ml) and streptomycin (100 μg/ml). Spleen explants are cut under sterile conditions, either by hand with two cataract knives or with the aid of a McIlwain tissue chopper (Mickle Laboratory Engineering Co.). Two spleen fragments of equal dimensions are explanted in each culture dish and they are checked after 1 day by measurement of the longest perpendicular diameters with an ocular micrometer at 10× magnification. Cultures are maintained in a 37 °C incubator in a water-saturated atmosphere of 90 per cent oxygen and 10 per cent CO_2. On day 0, suspensions of spleen cells from each NTx C57BL mouse and F_1 control are prepared by dispersing the cells through stainless steel meshes into OCM, and further dissociated by means of syringes with 27-gauge needles. Aliquots of cells are stained with Turks solution and nucleated cells counted in a hemocytometer, 1×10^6 cells in a volume of 5 μl is then added to each culture well with an orally controlled 5 μl micropipette, the well with the parental cells being marked, and cultures incubated for 4-4½ days. At the end of this time relative size of the cultures is determined again by measurement of the longest perpendicular diameters with the ocular micrometer. The calculated area of each test spleen explant is then divided by the corresponding area of its paired reference explant to provide a numerical index of splenomegaly. Since our results show that normal spleen cells consistently induce a response with an index ≥ 1.2, and the same number of cells from NTx donors only very sporadically evoke a response of this magnitude, we consider cultures reactive when the index of splenomegaly is 1.2 or more. Usually, 5 or more replicates are tested in each experimental group, and we express the results as the number of positive cultures per total number of cultures tested in each group. Thus the cells from a single neonatally thymectomized mouse are tested in 5 cultures without thymus extract and the same number of replicate cultures supplemented with each extract or fraction of thymic preparation to be tested. In this way, possible variation in the level of immune impairment of individual thymectomized mice do not affect the validity of the results.

In the case that genetic combinations other than that described are tested, preliminary work is required to determine the adequate number of cells for assay. The main limiting factor of this GvH assay is the all-or-none nature of the response which prevents quantitative comparisons. For this reason also, the effect of thymic hormones could be evaluated only on populations containing suboptimal numbers of immunologically competent lymphocytes. Thus, target cells have been found within the population of spleen cells from NTx mice (4, 5) in normal bone marrow (6) and in thymus (7). On the other hand, the GvH technique benefits from the advantage of detecting cumulative activity and of eliminating differences in physiologic properties of the lymphocyte populations tested.

REFERENCES

1. Elkins, W. (1971) *Prog. Allergy* **15**, 78.
2. Simonsen, M. (1962) *Prog. Allergy* **6**, 349.
3. Auerbach, R. & Globerson, A. (1966) *Exp. Cell. Res.* **42**, 31.
4. Trainin, N., Small, M. & Globerson, A. (1969) *J. Exp. Med.* **130**, 765.
5. Trainin, N. & Small, M. (1970) *J. Exp. Med.* **132**, 885.
6. Small, M. & Trainin, N. (1971) *J. Exp. Med.* **134**, 786.
7. Trainin, N., Levo, Y. & Rotter, V. (1974) *Eur. J. Immunol.* **4**, 634.

Biological Activity of Thymic Hormones

EFFECT OF THF ON CYCLING OF COLONY FORMING CELLS (CFU-S) FROM BONE MARROW OF THYMECTOMIZED MICE

DOV ZIPORI

The number of CFU-S in the bone marrow is reduced following neonatal thymectomy (1, 2). In addition, thymus deprivation is accompanied by changes in the rate of cycling of the bone marrow CFU-S population. Indeed, while about 25 per cent of these cells are in the S-phase of their cycle in normal mice, only 7 per cent are found in this phase in the bone marrow of thymectomized animals (3). Administration of THF either *in vitro* or *in vivo* reversed the suppressive effect of thymectomy on DNA synthesis in CFU-S. In the *in vitro* system, bone marrow cells from thymectomized mice were preincubated for half an hour in the presence of thymus hormone and exposed immediately after to the killing effect of ^{3}H-thymidine. The induction of cycling of CFU-S by THF is a fast process since it occurres within the short incubation period mentioned above (3). It, therefore, resembles from the kinetic point of view the effects of some hormones, drugs (4) and prostaglandin E_2 (5) on the cycling of CFU-S. The effect of THF is restricted, however, to CFU-S from bone marrow of thymectomized mice, while CFU-S from normal marrow and from fetal liver are not affected by this hormone (Unpublished results).

The minimal number of bone marrow CFU-S synthesizing DNA, i.e. cells in S phase was determined using the ^{3}H-thymidine "suicide" technique described by Becker *et al.* (6). This basic system was modified according to Löwenberg *et al.* (Personal communication). Female, 2-4 months old C3H/eb mice, thymectomized at 3 days after birth, were used throughout these experiments. In each experiment, bone marrow cells from 6-8 mice were pooled and cell suspension adjusted by dilution in phosphate buffered saline (PBS) to a concentration of 10^7 cells/ml. This suspension was distributed into plastic tubes, 2.0 ml each; and these samples were incubated with or without 100 μCi/ml of ^{3}H-thymidine (specific activity 22 Ci/mmol) for 30 min at 37 °C in a CO_2 (5 per cent) incubator. When thymus hormone is tested, a period of 30 min incubation in the presence of the hormone precedes the addition of ^{3}H-thymidine. The hormone is then added in a 50 μl volume. Saline, PBS or spleen extract served as controls. At the end of incubation cell suspensions are put in the cold, 10 ml cold PBS containing unlabelled thymidine (20 μg/100 ml) is added to each tube and the suspensions are centrifuged for 5 min at 1000 rpm.

Department of Cell Biology, Weizmann Institute of Science, Rehovot, Israel

The supernatant is then discarded, the cells are resuspended and washed again. They are then adjusted by dilution (in PBS) to a concentration of 8×10^4 cells/ml and 4×10^4 cells in 0.5 ml are injected i.v. into syngeneic 3 month old mice, 15 irradiated recipients in each group (1100 rad total body irradiation 1-2 h before bone marrow injection). Macroscopic spleen colony counts are performed 8 days later as described by Till & McCulloch (7). The proportion of CFU-S in S phase is calculated on the basis of loss of CFU-S in the bone marrow sample incubated with ^{3}H-thymidine, as follows:

$$\% \text{ CFU-S in S phase} = 1 - \left(\frac{\text{number of CFU-S with } ^3\text{H-thymidine}}{\text{number of CFU-S without } ^3\text{H-thymidine}}\right) \times 100$$

As the differences between the control and experimental groups is expected to be not more than 20 to 30 per cent, the significance of the experiments depends upon high survival rates of the recipients at 8 days post-irradiation. Increased mortality in any of the groups could blur the pattern of results.

The results reported here suggest that at least some of the CFU-S present in the marrow are under the control of thymus hormone.

REFERENCES

1. Trainin, N. & Resnitzky, P. (1969) *Nature* **221**, 1154.
2. Resnitzky, P., Zipori, D. & Trainin, N. (1971) *Blood* **37**, 634.
3. Zipori, D. & Trainin, N. (Submitted for publication).
4. Byron, J. W. (1973) *Nature New Biol.* **241**, 152.
5. Feher, I. & Gidali, J. (1974) *Nature* **247**, 550.
6. Becker, A. J., McCulloch, E. A., Siminovich, L. & Till, J. E. (1965) *Blood* **26**, 296.
7. Till, J. E. & McCulloch, E. A. (1961) *Radiat. Res.* **14**, 213.

Biological Activity of Thymic Hormones

THE SHEEP CELL ROSETTE ASSAY FOR THE EVALUATION OF THYMIC HORMONES

MIREILLE DARDENNE & JEAN-FRANÇOIS BACH

PRINCIPLE

Rosette forming cells (RFC) found in the spleen of adult thymectomized mice are less sensitive to azathioprine (AZ) than those present in normal mouse spleen; i.e., normal rosettes are inhibited by 1 μg/ml whereas it requires 70 μg/ml to inhibit rosettes of thymectomized animals. Thymic extracts confer on RFC from adult thymectomized mice a sensitivity to AZ identical to that of normal mouse RFC after a simple 75 min incubation at 37 °C. It is this property which has been used to establish a reproducible and quantitative bioassay for thymic hormones and more particularly for the circulating thymic factor (TF). The detailed data justifying this assay have been published (1, 2). Controls have shown that spleen extracts or serum from thymectomized mice are inactive, whereas serum from normal mice contains TF-like activity. Furthermore, inhibition is not 100 per cent, as a small number of rosettes are formed by B cells, and perhaps monocytes, which are not inhibited by AZ.

A. *Material*

1. Malassez cells with double chambers (Preciss from Verrefer, 75, rue St. Jacques - 75005 Paris) depth, 0.2 ml; volume, 1 mm^3.
2. Coverslips for Malassez chambers (22 mm × 32 mm; Gassalem, 8 rue de Richelieu, 75002 Paris).
3. Plastic tubes with round bottom: 5 ml hemolysis tubes (75 mm × 13 mm) and 40 ml tubes (97 mm × 30 mm; Labo Express Service, 4 rue de Seine, 91170 Viry-Chatillon).
4. Hanks' medium (Balanced Salt Solution with Sodium Bicarbonate: Serpasteur, 25, rue du Dr. Roux, Paris 15). Comment: phosphate buffer may be used instead of Hanks' medium (0.01 M, pH 7.2).
5. Azathioprine (AZ): solution for i.v. injection from Burroughs Wellcome; 50 mg lyophilized sodium salt. To be dissolved in distilled water (10 ml/flask).
6. Glass pipettes.
7. Apparatus for rosette suspension: rotating plateau from APELAB, 29 rue des Ecoles, 92 Bagneux; Rotating speed, 10 rpm; plateau inclination, between 0 and 30° from vertical axis; Radius, 10 cm.

INSERM U 25 Hôpital Necker, 161, rue de Sèvres, 75730 Paris Cedex 15, France

8. Potter from Thomas, Philadelphia, U.S.A. n°A. 1008: piston sold with Potter diameter appr. 0.5 mm less than the inside diameter of the Potter.

9. Sheep red blood cells (SRBC). SRBC are obtained from Pasteur Institute in preservative (Mayer buffer plus 1% formaldehyde). They are used as they are without further washing.

10. Turk's solution is used for the lymphocyte count (stock solution of "violet de gentiane" diluted at 10 per cent in distilled water. 1 ml of such solution is added to 0.5 ml of glacial acetic acid and 98.5 ml of distilled water).

B. *Mice*

C57Bl/6 mice from the Centre d'Elevage des Animaux de Laboratoire, Orleans, La Source, 45, France, aged 6-10 weeks, male or female, are used 1-8 weeks after thymectomy. It is desirable to check the quality of the thymectomy for each mouse at the time of spleen collection.

Thymectomy is performed by suction with a Pasteur pipette after anaesthesia with nembutal (1 mg for a 20 g mouse). The skin is cut, presternal fascia are dissected, and the superior part of the sternum is opened to give a better access to the thymus, which is removed by aspiration.

C. *Apparatus*

Microscope: All reading is done at 25× magnification for the objective and 10 (or 12) for the ocular.

Centrifuge: All centrifugations are performed in a refrigerated centrifuge at 4 °C. The rest of the manipulations is performed at room temperature between 15 and 30 °C according to season.

D. *Technique*

1. *Isolation of spleen cells*

Spleens are collected after bleeding the mice from the retro-orbital plexus and from the heart after opening the thoracic cage, until the death of the animal, in order to diminish the amount of red cells ultimately contaminating the preparation. All further manipulations are performed at 4 °C, the Potter and the tubes being placed in ice water. The spleen is placed, without being previously cut, at the bottom of a Potter in 3-4 ml of Hanks' medium where it is homogenized. For this homogenization, the piston is moved three to four times, pressing slightly on the bottom of the tube until the Hanks' medium, which is collected each time in a 40 ml plastic tube, is clear. Cells are then filtered on tergal (placed on a tea sieve) and washed twice in 40 ml plastic tubes filled with 30 ml of Hanks' medium. Each tube is filled with the content of one spleen. Washings are performed by centrifugation for 7 min at 1,200 rpm, that is 170 g (centrifuge with a 7 cm radius). Between the two washings and after the second one, the liquid is aspirated by vacuum through a tube fixed on a Pasteur pipette; 0.5 ml of Hanks' medium is then added. The tube is slightly agitated by hand and the cells are resuspended several times (about 10 times) in 0.5 ml medium with an 0.5 ml pipette. Once each spleen preparation has been resuspended in 0.5 ml of medium, the contents of the tubes are mixed after the second washing and the lymphocyte count is determined.

This count is performed in Malassez chambers after addition of Turk's solution which destroys red cells and stains nuclei of nucleated cells. The values found for the spleen are generally in the order of 80 to 120 millions nucleated cells, with quite significant variations according to mice. Hanks' medium is then added to fix the number of nucleated cells at 30,000/mm^3.

2. *Addition of the test sample and AZ*

The following solutions are mixed in a hemolysis tube:

a. 0.06 ml of Hanks' medium containing the serially diluted test sample. For very active fractions (active when diluted more than 1/5,000), the first dilution is generally made at 1/2,000 in the following way: 0.01 ml of the test sample is added to 2.5 ml of Hanks' medium and then to 0.015 ml of this mixture is added 0.105 ml of Hanks' medium, which gives a final dilution of 1/2,000 (250×8) in a volume of 0.12 ml which will be used to start serial dilutions In other cases, low dilutions are used directly.

b. 0.06 ml of AZ at 20 μg/ml (initial concentration). This preparation is obtained in the following way: 10 ml of distilled water are added to the flask containing the 50 mg of AZ. The flask is then agitated and 0.1 ml is collected and added to 4.9 ml of Hanks' medium in a hemolysis tube. 4 ml of Hanks' medium are added to 1 ml of this mixture, which makes a final dilution of 1/250, that is 20 μg/ml. Since AZ is only slightly soluble at low pH, it is necessary not to allow the pH to decrease below 7.0 (for example, by breathing in the tube which introduces large amounts of CO_2). If one has problems with this pH lowering, a phosphate buffer, instead of Hanks' medium may be used. Once prepared, the flask is kept for several days, but less than a week, and is discarded earlier if AZ crystals appear.

c. 0.05 ml of the cell suspension. To the mixture of the test sample and AZ (which contains cheracters the test sample diluted at 1/4000 final concentration in the example chose above and AZ diluted to 10 μg/ml), 0.05 ml of the cell suspension containing 30,000 cells per μl (1.5×10^6 cells) is added. Final concentration of the test sample is then 1/5600. Control tubes are prepared by replacing the test sample or AZ with a similar volume of Hanks' medium.

3. *Incubation*

The incubation is performed in an incubator at 37 °C for 75 min, after which sheep RBC are added.

4. *Addition of sheep RBC*

A SRBC suspension is prepared in the following way: 0.2 ml of the initial preparation (sold by the Pasteur Institute in a concentration of 15×10^6 cells/µl) is added to 15 ml of Hanks' medium (final concentration: 200×10^6 cells/ml). 0.06 ml of this suspension (12×10^6 cells) is added to the spleen cells.

5. *Rosette formation*

The cellular preparation thus obtained is centrifuged at 4 °C for 5 min at 1200 rpm (150 g). All tubes prepared for the day are centrifuged as soon as they are taken out of the incubator and sheep RBC are added to each tube. However, exceptionally, some tubes can be put in the refrigerator directly after taking them out of the incubator and can be maintained there for about 1/2 h before adding sheep RBC and centrifuging.

6. *Rosette resuspension*

Once centrifugation is completed, plastic caps are placed on the tubes. A first series of tubes is then resuspended according to the method described below. The other tubes which will not be read immediately in the first series are placed in the refrigerator at 4 °C.

The resuspension is made on the rotating apparatus for three minutes. At the completion of this resuspension, the contents of each tube are distributed into the two chambers of Malassez cells. This distribution is delicate and is performed at once for the tubes of the first series.

7. *Deposition of the cell suspension in the Malassez chamber*

It is crucial to act rapidly between the end of the resuspension and the collection of rosettes before they are deposited in Malassez chambers. In fact, rosettes which are heavier than the other cells have a spontaneous tendency to sediment in the tube and the collection of the supernatant of the preparation could then artificially be depleted of rosettes. This is the reason for which the liquid is collected in the tubes immediately after removing the tubes from the rotating apparatus. Most of the tubes' contents (60-80 per cent) is aspirated with a Pasteur pipette and then deposited on Malassez cells against the chamber which has been previously covered with a glass slide. The liquid then diffuses by capillarity into the chamber located immediately against the site where the cellular suspension has been deposited. The same procedure is repeated for the other chamber without waiting for the movement of the liquid to the second chamber. The lateral chambers are often filled spontaneously (*Comment:* another technique which consists of depositing the liquid in these lateral chambers can give erratic results, some preparations coming up badly in the chambers). Let us mention here again that is is crucial to act rapidly between the end of resuspension and the collection of the medium with the pipette, when the Pasteur pipette is held in hands before depositing the suspension, during the liquid deposition, and, lastly, between the two deposition times (one may prefer eventually to put the tubes back into the rotating apparatus before doing the second deposition in order to avoid sedimentation of the rosettes between the two depositions).

Before reading the rosettes, all Malassez chambers already filled are put on the table. One may leave the chambers at room temperature (between 15 and 25 °C) for 10 to 30 minutes before reading. It is, however, obvious that it is necessary to evaluate one's own reading capacity and not to prepare more chambers than it will be possible to read in the following 30 minutes.

8. *Rosettes reading*

For each tube, the content of two chambers is read, that is 2 μl (1 μl per chamber) or 6500 × 2 nucleated cells since 0.05 ml of the spleen cell suspension at 30,000/μl has been put in the medium to which has been ultimately added 0.18 ml of the other three solutions. It is useful, before having great experience with the test, to verify that the number of leukocytes in the chamber is about 6,500 or at least that it is the same in all tubes in order to be able to compare adequately the absolute rosette number from one tube to another.

Rosettes are defined as the agglutination of at least 4 red cells by nucleated cell. Another condition is the direct presence of a lymphocyte in the center of the rosettes, or in the absence of the lymphocyte in the center of the rosette, the perfect regularity of the morula with a size compatible with that of a rosette. In case of doubt, the reality of the rosette may be appreciated by verifying its volume by modifying the focussing (red cell clusters will often be seen only in the plane of red cells or by tipping the chamber slightly which will dissociate some nonspecific clusters). One should be aware of the fact that T cells are often the rosettes the least rich in red cells and the most fragile (3). It would be a mistake to be too strict and only count the more obvious B rosettes, since the assay is concerned with T rosettes. Fig. 1 gives the main aspects encountered with, in each case, the (sometimes arbitrary) decision of its belonging to rosettes. Let us mention that preparations of poor quality including numerous nonspecific clusters of leukocytes or erythrocytes or both will make very difficult, if not impossible, the reading of the rosettes.

9. *Interpretation and expression of the results*

In the absence of TF-like activity, the RFC contained in spleen cells from adult thymectomized mice are not inhibited by azathioprine at the concentration of 10 μg/ml. In the absence of azathioprine, the same RFC are not modified significantly by TF. These two controls are always included in the assay. When the test sample contains TF, RFC are inhibited by azathioprine and the maximum dilution of the sample giving rosette inhibition of more than 50 per cent is considered as the active dilution. One may thus express the results of this dilution in three ways.

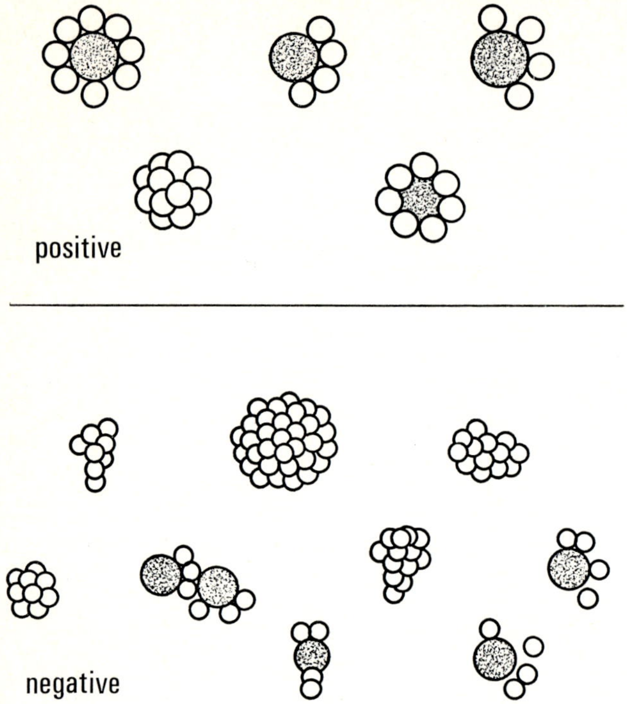

Fig. 1.

Example:

A preparation containing 10 μg/ml of proteins (assayed by amino acid analysis or Lowry's method) and serially diluted at 10^{-6} will be presented in one of the 3 following ways:

(1) $1/10^6$ for 10 μg/ml

(2) minimum active protein concentration
$10\ \mu g/ml \times 10^{-6} = 10$ pg/ml

(3) minimum absolute amount of proteins biologically active per tube $(0.06 \times 10\ \mu g) \times 10^{-6}$
i.e. 0.6 pg

CONCLUSION—GENERAL INTERPRETATION

The assay detects a biological activity present at high dilution in thymic extracts and normal serum and absent at the same concentrations in spleen extracts and in serum from thymectomized mice. Serum from normal mice concentrated 100 times on Amicon UM2 membrane is active at a dilution of 1/10,000, whereas serum from thymectomized mice or from nude mice concentrated under identical conditions remains always negative even at a dilution of 1/50.

One should, however, list the specificity limitations of the assay:

1. Other "immunoactive" products may be active in the assay. This is the case of cyclic AMP or of prostaglandins (4) which are thought to be possible intermediates in TF action. Cyclic AMP acts in synergy with TF on RFC and indomethacin, an inhibitor of prostaglandin synthetase, inhibits TF action. Moreover, we have recently described an allogenic factor secreted by T cells (not by epithelial cells of the thymus like TF) which is also active in the assay (5).

2. Some "toxic" samples (some buffers may be, for example, toxic) will sometimes inhibit the rosettes at low concentration which will make the results of the assay impossible to interpret (hence the importance of the control tube without azathioprine).

3. Some probably irrelevant products have been revealed to be active in the assay at high concentration (>10 µg/ml) (without any action on rosettes without azathioprine). This action without comparison to that of TF (which is active at 1 pg/ml, that is to say, concentrations 10^7 times lower) should, however, be known, even if it is ill-defined and poorly explained. It should prompt to be cautious when interpreting positive results obtained at high concentration of any product.

APPENDICES

APPENDIX 1: APPLICATION TO THE DETERMINATION OF THE CIRCULATING THYMIC HORMONE IN ANIMAL OR HUMAN BLOOD

A) *Conditions of blood collection*

Five ml of blood (in the human) or 0.5 ml (in the mouse) are collected in a hemolysis plastic tube in 2 per cent Liquemine (Roche) or heparin without preservative (0.1 ml Liquemine for 5 ml of blood). The Liquemine-containing tube is maintained in ice before blood collection and is left in ice until the blood sample is brought to the laboratory.

When the blood is collected in the hospital where the test is performed, the tube must be brought to the laboratory kept in ice. There, it is centrifuged at 4 °C and stored at −20 °C before being lyophilized.

When the blood is collected outside the hospital where the test is performed (but can be shipped there in ice), it is necessary to centrifuge the blood at 4 °C immediately. The plasma may then be stored at −20 °C for several days before being brought (still kept at −20 °C in dry ice) to the laboratory where the test is done.

It is also possible, and preferable, to lyophilize the sample and send it by ordinary mail, the hormone being stable once lyophilized (it is then important to note the volume of the initial sample).

B. *Assay*

The assay utilized for the determination of serum thymic hormone is essentially the same as that described above, with the exception that the test sample (ultrafiltered serum) is used instead of the thymic preparations and that, because of the relatively low levels, dilutions are made starting at TF 1/2 or 1/4. The serum sample has to be ultrafiltrated prior to use in the test, in order to remove all components with a molecular weight higher than 50,000. Briefly the ultrafiltration is performed as follows: CF 50 Amicon membranes (cone-shaped) are applied at the top of 40 ml plastic tubes. The serum is put at the bottom of the cone and then centrifuged for 30 minutes at 4 °C at 3000 rpm. The ultrafiltrate is tested in serial dilutions from 1/2 to 1/512.

APPENDIX 2: REPRODUCIBILITY. RESULTS PRESENTATION

Example of utilization of the sheep red cell rosette assay for the evaluation of thymic hormones. Three active thymic preparations (A. L. Goldstein's thymosin, N. Trainin's THF, and our TF) and 3 control preparations (A. L. Goldstein's spleen fraction V, Trainin's spleen extract, and a pig control serum fraction) were tested under code in three ways:

a. direct *in vitro* testing
b. *in vitro* testing of the serum of adult thymectomized mice injected with

TABLE I

In vitro AND *in vivo* TESTING OF THREE THYMIC AND CONTROL PREPARATIONS GIVEN UNDEI CODE. EACH VALUE REPRESENTS ONE SEPARATE DETERMINATION (ONE MOUSE OR ONE *in vivo* EXPERIMENT)

	A. L. Goldstein's		*N. Trainin's*		*J. F. Bach and M. Dardenne's*	
	Thymosin	*Spleen extract*	*THF*	*Spleen extract*	*TF*	*TF control*
In vitro testing						
Minimal active concentration	9 μg/ml	> 100 μg/ml	1.6 μg/ml	> 16 μg/ml	1.7 ng/ml	> 1 μg/ml
	25 μg/ml	> 100 μg/ml	1.6 μg/ml	> 100 μg/ml	15 ng/ml	> 1 μg/ml
In vivo testing (in ATX mice)	*100 μg*	*100 μg*	*100 μg*	*100 μg*	*500 ng*	*500 ng*
A - TF level in serum collected 2 hours after injection	1/100 1/100	1/16 <1/32	1/200	<1/16	1/1600	<1/16
	1/200 1/400	<1/100 <1/100	1/200	<1/16	1/6400	<1/16
	1/400	<1/100	1/800	<1/16	1/3200	<1/16
			150 μg:		*750 ng:*	
			1/800		1/12800	
			1/3200		1/12800	
B - Spleen RFC sensitivity to azathioprine	1.5 γ	100 γ	6 γ	> 100 γ	0.7 γ	100 γ
	0.7 γ	50 γ	6 γ	50 γ	0.3 γ	> 100 γ
	0.7 γ	50 γ	0.7 γ	50 γ	0.3 γ	> 100 γ
			150 μg:		*750 ng:*	
			3 γ		0.7 γ	
			1.5 γ		0.7 γ	

thymosin (100 μg), THF (100 and 150 μg), or TF (500 and 750 ng) or control preparations two hours earlier (single doses);

c. evaluation of AZ sensitivity of spleen RFC of the same mice 24 hours after the injection of the thymic or control preparation.

Table I gives the results obtained in this blind study. One may note the reproducibility and the discriminating potency of the three assays. It may happen, as for thymosin, that *in vivo* activity is better than could be expected from *in vitro* activity, a difference perhaps due to *in vivo* thymosin splitting and release of more active peptides.

REFERENCES

1. Bach, J.-F., Dardenne, M., Goldstein, A. L., Guha, A. & White, A. (1971) *Proc. Nat. Acad. Sci. USA* **68**, 2734.
2. Bach, J.-F. & Dardenne, M. (1973) *Immunology* **25**, 353.
3. Charreire, J., Dardenne, M. & Bach, J.-F. (1973) *Cell. Immunol.* **9**, 32.
4. Bach, M. A. & Bach, J.-F. (1973) *Eur. J. Immunol.* **3**, 778.
5. Bach, J.-F., Dardenne, M. & Pleau, J. M. (1974) *C.R. Acad. Sci.* **278**, 335.

Biological Activity of Thymic Hormones

THE EFFECT OF THYMIC HORMONES ON AUTOLOGOUS ROSETTE FORMING CELLS

JEANNINE CHARREIRE & JEAN-FRANÇOIS BACH

INTRODUCTION

A small percentage of mouse lymphocytes bind autologous or syngeneic erythrocytes with formation of rosettes (1, 2). These Autologous Rosette Forming Cells (ARFC) are found predominantly in the thymus and at lower percentages in the spleen (1). ARFC have elicited great interest because of their potential use as a model of self-recognition. We have recently shown that adult thymectomy dramatically increased the spleen ARFC level (3) and that thymic hormones corrected this increase after a short-term *in vivo* treatment (3). We propose here this new thymic hormone activity for a new *in vivo* assay for the hormone.

MATERIAL AND METHODS

Mice - Male and female CBA or C57B1/6 mice were used in all experiments except in some cases where nude mice (with the CBA background) were also utilized. When not specified, the mice were 6-8-weeks-old. Thymectomies were performed in 6-8-weeks-old mice by suction. "Thymus-deprived" mice were prepared by thymectomy followed by irradiation (850 r) and reconstitution by intravenous (i.v.) injection of 15×10^6 syngeneic bone marrow cells.

Thymic preparations - Purified thymic factor (TF) was obtained from pig blood and used bound to carboxymethyl cellulose to prolong its serum half-life (4). Thymosin (fraction V) was supplied by A. L. Goldstein (5).

Rosette test - The rosette method is basically the same as that described for sheep red cell rosettes (6) using autologous or syngeneic red cells instead of sheep red blood cells. In brief, it consisted of mixing lymphoid cells and erythrocytes (both washed 3 times) in various RBC/white cell ratios (from 4 to 128) in a total volume of 0.5 ml of Hanks medium. Material, apparatus, isolation of spleen cells, rosette formation and resuspension, deposition of cell suspension in the Malassez chamber, and rosette reading were performed as

INSERM U 25, Hôpital Necker, 161, rue de Sèvres, 75730 Paris Cedex 15

described in detail elsewhere in this volume (6) for the sheep red cell assay. However, in order to allow easy reading of the rosettes, an optimal cell density was obtained by maintaining the total cell number around 150,000/μl in a total volume of 0.25 ml. It was verified that the rosette numbers depended only on lymphocyte-erythrocyte ratios and not on cell density. Rosettes defined by the agglutination of at least 3 red cells per lymphocyte were read in 2 μl Malassez hemocytometer (instead of the 1 μl chamber used for the sheep red cell rosettes). Macrophages were routinely eliminated by preincubation of the lymphoid cells for 90 min at 37 °C in plastic tubes before adding erythrocytes. "Autologous rosettes" were formed with erythrocytes obtained from the mice from which the lymphoid cells had been obtained. "Syngeneic rosettes" were formed with erythrocytes from mice of the same strain as that of the lymphocyte donor. Identical results were obtained for syngeneic and autologous RFC. All erythrocyte preparations were obtained by centrifuging blood samples collected on liquemine Roche (heparin).

Thymic hormone in vivo assay - The thymic preparation was injected i.p. or subcutaneously on two consecutive days into mice thymectomized as adults 6 weeks previously. Twenty-four hours after the last injection, the spleen was collected and the ARFC assay performed. A control group of mice was injected with spleen extracts or another control preparation. The assay was considered as positive when the ARFC level was significantly lower in mice treated with thymic preparations than in untreated or control mice at the RBC/white cell ratio giving the highest ARFC values (usually 64 or 128).

RESULTS

Autologous rosettes in 4-6 week-old normal mice

Autologous rosettes were found in thymus, spleen, and blood of CBA mice at various levels (Table I), the thymus presenting the highest level. In all lymphoid organs, rosette numbers varied markedly with the erythrocyte/lymphocyte ratio, rosette values of the order of 2 per cent being obtained at highest ratios.

Autologous serum added to the cell mixture before rosette formation inhibited autologous rosette formation at dilutions less than 1/50. Fetal calf serum was also inhibitory, although only at still lower dilutions.

Variations with age

Fourteen to sixteen-month-old CBA mice were compared to 8-week-old mice of the same strain. The number of autologous rosettes was significantly higher in the spleen of the old mice. Similar results were obtained with thymocytes (Table I); the increase in autologous rosette numbers was then associated with a decrease in thymocyte number (110×10^6 versus 33×10^6 cells).

TABLE I

LEVEL OF AUTOLOGOUS ROSETTE-FORMING CELLS IN CBA/H AND NUDE MICE. ADULT THYMECTOMIZED (TX) AND TX IRRADIATED BONE MARROW RECONSTITUTED MICE WERE THYMECTOMIZED (AND EVENTUALLY IRRADIATED) AT THE AGE OF 6 WEEKS AND STUDIED 2 MONTHS LATER. ARFC PER 10^3 CELLS (MEANS $\pm$S.D.) ERYTHROCYTE/LYMPHOCYTE RATIO: 128.

	No. mice	*Thymus*	*Spleen*	*Peripheral blood*
Normal CBA/H 4–5 weeks	8	25 $\pm$4.5	10.8 $\pm$1.6	1.1 $\pm$0.1
Normal CBA/H 16 months	6	32.5 $\pm$4.1	24 $\pm$3.5	–
Adult Tx CBA/H 20 weeks	10	–	155 $\pm$23	2.1 $\pm$0.1
Nude mice	6	–	40 $\pm$7.5	–
Tx-irradiated bone-marrow reconstituted CBA/H mice	4	–	109 $\pm$12.8	–

Autologous rosettes in thymus deficiency states

The level of autologous rosettes was determined in several states of thymus deficiencies of varying degree. Adult thymectomized mice, which show only minor immunodeficiency, showed a marked increase in the number of spleen autologous rosettes. This effect was not immediate, appearing on day 7 and reaching its maximum at 12 weeks (Fig. 1). Differences with normal mice were best seen at highest erythrocyte: lymphocyte ratios. Thus, at a ratio of 128, the spleen autologous rosette level was 17.5 per cent $\pm$2.9 (S.D.) at 12 weeks

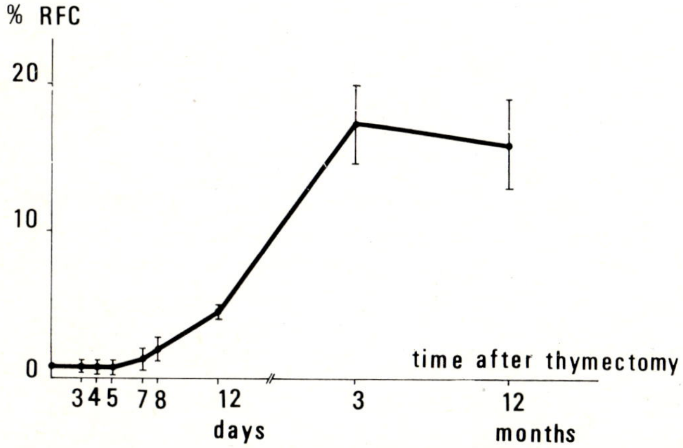

Fig. 1. Increase in the number of autologous rosette-forming cells after adult thymectomy performed at the age of 6 weeks. Four to eight mice were tested for each group (mean $\pm$S.D.).

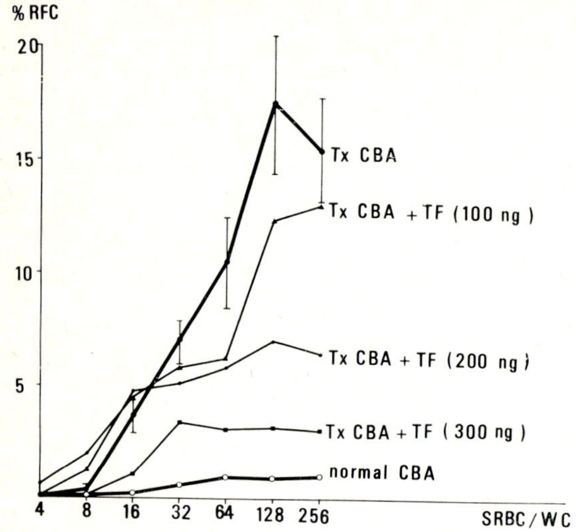

Fig. 2. Effects of subcutaneous injections of purified TF on autologous rosette formation in adult thymectomized CBA mice. Tests were performed 24 h after TF injection.

after thymectomy versus 1.08 per cent ±0.16 in normal mice, that is, a 17-fold difference.

Thymectomized-irradiated, bone marrow reconstituted, and 6-week-old nude mice showed higher values for spleen autologous rosettes than did normal mice of the same age (3-5-fold difference) (Table I). These values were lower, however, than those found in adult thymectomized mice, particularly in nude mice.

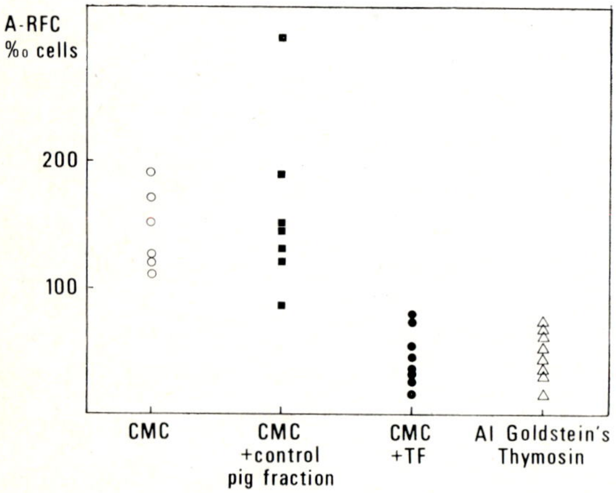

Fig. 3. Effects of TF and thymosin injection on ARFC level in adult thymectomized CBA mice. Tests were performed 24 h after the second of two TF injections. TF was given at a dosage of 500 ng (6 experiments) and thymosin at a dosage of 100 μg (4 experiments) or 1 mg (4 experiments). Each value represents the mean of ARFC evaluation in one mouse.

In vivo effects of thymic factor (TF)

Higher concentrations of thymectomized mouse serum than normal mouse serum were required to inhibit autologous rosette formation, suggesting a TF influence on ARFC. Purified circulating TF was tested *in vivo* by injecting it bound to carboxymethyl cellulose subcutaneously into adult thymectomized mice. Control mice received carboxymethyl cellulose alone. Almost complete correction of the abnormally high level of autologous rosettes was obtained at the highest TF dose (300 ng); a partial effect was obtained at lower doses (Fig. 2). A. L. Goldstein's thymosin also reduced the ARFC level when administered in two consecutive doses (of 100 g, or 1 mg). Fig. 3 gives the results obtained in several experiments with TF (500 ng) and thymosin (100 µg or 1 mg). Control experiments with mice injected with CMC alone, CMC+ control pig fraction, or A. L. Goldstein's spleen Fraction V (given at the same doses as active fractions) were totally negative.

DISCUSSION

Our data confirm Micklem's reports (1, 2) showing the existence of autologous erythrocyte-binding cells in mouse lymphoid organs. That these autologous rosettes are due to receptors for autoantigens is an attractive hypothesis which, however, remains to be proven. It is possible that the binding is not specific to any antigen, as is probably the binding of sheep red blood cells to human lymphocytes (7). The nature of the binding cell remains unclear, but most facts argue in favour of the ARFC being undifferentiated T cells (see ref. 8).

The decrease in autologous rosettes under the influence of circulating TF supports the hypothesis that T cell maturation is associated with a loss in the expression of self-recognition receptors. This data is also in keeping with the absence of circulating TF in the serum of adult NZB mice (4) and with Trainin's report that normal mouse serum prevents self-sensitization of lymphoid cells on reticuloepithelial cells, whereas thymectomized mouse serum does not have this property (9). The involvement of TF in the expression of self-recognition receptors is also suggested by the increase in autologous rosettes simultaneously with a decrease in serum TF level with ageing (10). The onset of autoimmune manifestations in adult thymectomized (11) and NZB (12) mice as well as in ageing mice (11, 13) is thus associated with high levels of autologous rosettes, probably thymus-dependent.

Finally, the autologous rosette *in vivo* assay for the evaluation of thymic hormones can be proposed as a reproducible and discriminative *in vivo* bioassay for thymic hormones. Its sensitivity is indicated by the positive results obtained with TF dosages as low as 200 ng. Its specificity seems good so far, since none of the few control preparations tested has ever been found positive. More data are needed, however, to confirm this important point.

REFERENCES

1. Micklem, H. S., Asfi, C. & Anderson, N. (1970) in *Developmental Aspects of antibody formation and structure* eds. J. Sterzl and I. Riha Prague Acad. Press p. 701.

2. Micklem, H. S. & Anderson, N. (1972) in *Third Lepetit Colloquium*. North Holland, Amsterdam p. 229.
3. Charreire, J. & Bach, J.-F. (1974) *Lancet* **11**, 229.
4. Bach, J. F., Dardenne, M. & Bach, M. A. (In press) *Ann. N.Y. Acad. Sci.*
5. Goldstein, A. L., Guha, A., Zatz, M. M., Hardy, M. A. & White, A. (1972) *Proc. Nat. Acad. Sci. (Washington)* **69**, 1800.
6. Dardenne, M. & Bach, J.-F. (This volume).
7. Bach, J.-F. (1973) *Transpl. Rev.* **16**, 196.
8. Bach, J.-F., Cantor, H., Roelants, G. & Stutman, O. (This volume).
9. Trainin, N., Carnaud, C. & Ilfeld, D. (1973) *Nature* **245**, 253.
10. Bach, J.-F. & Dardenne, M. (1973) *Immunology* **25**, 253.
11. Teague, P. O., Yunis, E. J., Rodey, G., Fish, A. J., Stutman, O. & Good, R. A. (1970) *Lab. Invest.* **22**, 121.
12. Howie, J. B. & Helyer, B. J. (1968) *Adv. Immunol.* **9**, 215.
13. Sutherland, J. C., Markham, R. V. & Mardiney, M. R. (1973) *Lab. Invest.* **29**, 111.

Biological Activity of Thymic Hormones

INDUCTION OF θ-POSITIVE CELLS BY THYMIC HORMONES. A CRITICAL EVALUATION

CATHERINE FOURNIER & JEAN-FRANÇOIS BACH

We reported in 1971 that thymic extracts converted a large proportion of bone marrow spontaneous θ-negative Rosette-Forming Cells (RFC) to θ-positive RFC (1). However, such θ conversion could not be demonstrated using a cytotoxic assay on unfractionated bone marrow cells. This failure was probably due to the low percentage of thymic-extract-sensitive cells, picked up by the rosette assay but diluted among other lymphoid cells. In other words, it is possible that the absolute increase in θ converted cells was not large enough to be detected by a cytotoxic assay: such an assay cannot accurately detect increases in θ-positive cells less than 10 per cent, particularly in cell mixtures initially containing a large number of θ-positive cells, e.g., 30-40 per cent for normal spleen cells. Fractionating spleen cells before studying the θ conversion, Komuro & Boyse showed that it was in fact possible to induce as much as 20 per cent θ-positive cells in normal spleen cells of low density, initially poor in θ positive cells (2). We have studied the effect of the purified circulating thymic factor in the Komuro's assay as well as an *in vivo* θ-conversion assay in nude mice. This latter assay was justified by the spontaneously low levels of θ positive cells in nude mice allowing the omission of BSA fractionation before studying TF conversion; the *in vivo* treatment avoiding, in addition, the use of the 90 min preincubation time with thymic hormones.

MATERIAL AND METHODS

1. *Cytotoxic assay*

Reagents Antitheta serum (AθS) was prepared by injecting 10^7 CBA thymocytes i.p. into AKR mice once weekly for 6 weeks. The antiserum specificity was checked: 1) by verifying the absence of cytotoxic activity on AKR thymocytes; 2) by comparing the number of θ-positive cells in normal thymus, spleen, and lymph nodes. Normal AKR mouse serum was used as a control. In some experiments, AθS prepared in A mice congenic at the θ locus (kindly donated by E. A. Boyse) was utilized and gave the same results as the conventional AθS batch.

INSERM U 25, Hôpital Necker, 161, rue de Sèvres, 75730 PARIS Cedex 15

As a complement source, guinea pig serum, stored at −70 °C and previously absorbed with mouse thymocytes and mouse red blood cells (1 h at 4 °C, 3 volumes of serum/1 volume of packed cells) was used.

Incubations The cell preparation was suspended in Hanks medium at a concentration of 6×10^6/ml. Plastic hemolysis tubes were filled with 0.1 ml of the cell suspension and 0.2 ml of AθS (diluted in Hanks' medium from 1/4 to 1/512). Complement was added after 15 min incubation at 37 °C. (0.1 ml of guinea pig serum diluted 1/2), and the final cell preparation was incubated for 60 more min at 37 °C after which the tubes were placed at 4 °C.

Cytotoxicity test. Expression of results

The percentage of dead cells was evaluated by adding 0.15 ml of 2 ‰ Trypan blue and counting Trypan blue stained cells. Results were expressed as cytotoxicity indexes with reference to the percentage of dead cells found in control tubes.

$$\text{Cytotoxic Index} = \frac{\%\ \text{dead cells} - \text{Control}}{100\% - \text{Control}} \times 100$$

The control values were evaluated as the average of 3-6 tubes. The percentage of dead cells utilized in the index calculation was the value of the plateau usually observed at high AθS concentrations. However, the highest AθS concentrations (1/4, 1/8) were not always those giving the highest cytotoxic values, probably because of a prozone effect. Experiments with background values over 25 per cent were discarded.

2. *In vitro* θ *conversion assay*

The technique utilized is essentially that described by Komuro & Boyse (2).

Mice - Normal CBA mice, aged 8-10 weeks, were obtained from the Centre d'Elevage des Animaux de Laboratoire (Orléans).

Spleen cells preparation - *BSA gradient* - Spleen cells were prepared by homogeneizing spleen pieces in a Potter homogeneizer. The cells were washed twice in Hanks medium and were suspended in a 35 per cent BSA solution in a volume of 1 ml at a concentration of 500×10^6 nucleated cells/ml. The BSA gradient was prepared by adding consecutively in 10 ml plastic tubes 1 ml samples of decreasing BSA concentration (29%, 26%, 23%, 10%); BSA was obtained from Sigma (Batch N° 102 C-0130). The tube was then centrifuged for 30 min at 10,000 rpm (12,000 g). Each layer was collected by gentle aspiration using a Pasteur pipette. The layers were designated as A, B, C, and D with increasing density. The cell pellet was discarded.

Experimental protocol - Spleen cells from A, B, C, or D layers were incubated with varying concentrations of purified TF at 37 °C for 90 min at the end of which they were resuspended in Hanks medium. The cytotoxic assay was then performed as described above. Purified TF was obtained from pig serum by ultrafiltration, G25 Sephadex filtration and carboxymethyl cellulose chromatography (3).

3. *In vivo Nude* θ *conversion assay*

Nude mice (nu/nu), aged 6-8 weeks, were obtained from the Centre d'Elevage des Animaux de Laboratoire (Orléans).

Nude mice were injected on two occasions subcutaneously with 500 ng of partially purified TF at 24 h intervals. In order to ensure a sufficient biological half-life, TF was bound to carboxy methyl cellulose (CMC) before the injection (3); TF binding to CMC was obtained by a simple incubation of the TF preparation at pH 6.3 (phosphate buffer, 0.02 M) with 40 mg of CMC for 30 min at 4 °C.

IN VIVO EFFECT OF TF ON THE NUMBER OF θ POSITIVE CELLS IN NUDE MICE

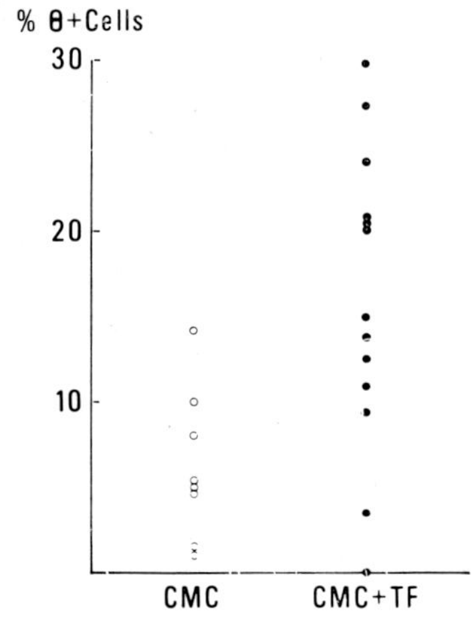

Spleen cells were collected 24 h after the 2 nd TF injection and were incubated for 1 h at 37 °C in Hank's medium before being tested in the cytotoxic assay described above. Control nude mice were injected with CMC alone or CMC incubated with a control pig serum fraction inactive in the rosette assay.

RESULTS

Effects of BSA fractionation

Cell layers obtained at different BSA densities showed significant differences in the percentage of θ-positive cells (Table I). The background of dead cells was always low, dead cells being excluded in the cell pellet. The A and B layers

TABLE I

BSA FRACTIONATION OF NORMAL SPLEEN CELLS (Aθs CYTOTOXIC INDEX AFTER INCUBATION WITH OR WITHOUT TF). A TYPICAL EXPERIMENT WITHOUT SPONTANEOUS INCREASE IN θ+CELLS AFTER INCUBATION

BSA cell layers	*Density*	*% cells recovered*	*% θ+cells after incubation without TF*	*% θ+cells after TF incubation*
A layer	10–23%	9,4%	5%∓2	22%∓2
B layer	23–26%	18%	19%∓3	26%∓3
C layer	26–29%	11,3%	32%∓3	34%∓3
D layer	29–35%	6,6%	61%∓3	59%∓4
Pellet		41,7%		
Initial suspension			31%±1.1	

were usually found to contain less than 15 per cent θ positive cells, in contrast to the C and D layers which contained more than 30 per cent of θ-positive cells. However, one should stress that the results were not totally consistent, since unexpected failures were observed in spite of identical conditions and constant use of the same BSA batch.

Effects of purified TF and of incubation without TF

When TF was added to the cell suspension in varying concentrations (from 10 to 200 ng/ml), a significant increase in the number of θ positive cells was noted (Table I). Interestingly, this θ conversion effect was less clear-cut at highest TF concentrations. However, the interpretation of these data was hampered by the observation of θ-conversion in experiments where no TF had been added (Table II); in some cases (8/17 experiments), AθS-incubated spleen cells

TABLE II

BSA FRACTIONATION OF NORMAL SPLEEN CELLS (Aθs CYTOTOXICITY INDEX BEFORE AND AFTER INCUBATION WITHOUT TF) FOUR TYPICAL EXPERIMENTS.

Initial suspension	34%∓3
A layer before incubation	9%∓2
A layer after incubation with TF	
Exp. 1	8.8%∓1
Exp. 2	10%∓2
Exp. 3	24.2%∓3
Exp. 4	18%∓2

showed a spontaneous increase in cell death without increase in the background values in the absence of AθS. In those cases, TF provided no further rise in percentages of θ-positive cells. This unexpected phenomenon was also seen when BSA or foetal calf serum was added during the incubation time, although with a lower incidence (3/8 experiments).

In vivo *experiments*

13 nude mice were injected with 500 ng TF and 8 mice with CMC alone. Fig. 1 shows that 6 out of the 13 TF treated mice showed a modest but significant increase in θ positivity. No effect was noted with CMC alone.

DISCUSSION

These data confirm the data recently reported by Komuro & Boyse (2) showing θ conversion of theta negative spleen cells *in vitro* (2) or *in vivo* (4) using our purified TF, which thus proves to be efficient in this assay at low concentrations (10 ng/ml) as are A. L. Goldstein's thymosin (4) and G. Goldstein's thymopoietin (5).

However, our data argue for some caution in the interpretation of this assay, since spontaneous θ conversion has been obtained when incubating spleen cells from the A and B layers of the BSA gradient in Hanks medium without TF. This spontaneous conversion was reduced but not suppressed by addition of foetal calf serum or of BSA. Similar data have been obtained in our laboratory using Ficoll fractionated spleen cells (6). This spontaneous θ conversion is probably associated with the cell fragility brought about by the 2 h incubation time preceding the AθS cytotoxic assay. It may be that the population of T cell precursors carrying a small amount of θ antigen detected only by the sensitive rosette inhibition (7) and immunofluorescence assays (8) and not by the less sensitive cytotoxic assay become detectable in the latter assay once becoming fragile. Fewer AθS molecules are then needed to effect cell killing.

The question is thus posed of the specificity of Komuro & Boyse's assay for the evaluation of thymic hormones. In fact, these authors have reported positivity in their assay of spleen, liver, and muscle extracts as well as that of endotoxin (4). It may well be that these products act nonspecifically, for example, by mere cell fragilization. The low concentrations reported to be active for thymopoietin (5) and TF (in this study) are reassuring but further investigation is needed to ascertain the specificity of the products in question. One may note, however, that these criticisms probably do not apply to the sheep cell rosette assay (1, 3, 9), since 1) in that case the incubation time is 75 min instead of 180 min without BSA fractionation, 2) serum from thymectomized mice does not show the activity presented by normal mouse serum (3, 9), and (3) the labile rosette phenomenon disappears before the nonspecific cell fragilization takes place. However, if the circulating thymic factor indeed has a specific θ conversion activity in comparison to nonthymic preparations, its mode of action in this assay remains open to question: unmasking of small amounts of θ antigen already present in the membrane? neosynthesis of θ antigen? cell metabolic changes rendering cells more "fragile"? In conclusion, in view of all these possibilities, it is important to rely "thymic hormone" definition of thymic preparations on parallel demonstration of biological activities other than θ conversion. This has been achieved for our circulating TF (3, 12) and for A. L. Goldstein's thymosin (13).

It is with the hope of minimizing cell fragility brought by BSA fractionation and *in vitro* TF treatment that *in vivo* TF treatment of nude mice has been attempted. Results obtained so far are encouraging, since no positive result was observed in the control mice. However, θ conversion was modest and especially was not regularly obtained, indicating on the whole a low sensitivity of the assay. Such low sensitivity is not unexpected in view of the difficulty in restoring T cell markers (9, 10, 3) and T cell function (10, 11) in nude mice with thymic humoral function in comparison to what is obtained in adult or neonatally thymectomized mice. Perhaps the best θ conversion cytotoxic assay for thymic hormones would consist in an *in vivo* assay in neonatally thymectomized mice treated as described above for nude mice.

REFERENCES

1. Bach, J. F., Dardenne, M., Goldstein, A. L., Guha, A. & White, A. (1971) *Proc. Nat. Acad. Sci.* **68**, 2734.
2. Komuro, K. & Boyse, E. A. (1973) *Lancet* **1**, 740.
3. Bach, J. F., Dardenne, M. & Bach, M. A. (In press) *Ann. N.Y. Acad. Sci.*
4. Scheid, M. P., Hoffmann, M. K., Komuro, K., Hammerling, U., Abbott, J., Boyse, E. A., Cohen, G. M., Hooper, J. A., Schulof, R. S. & Goldstein, A. L. (1973) *J. Exp. Med.* **138**, 1207.
5. Basch, R. S. & Goldstein, G. (In press) *Proc. Nat. Acad. Sci.* (Wash.)
6. Papiernik, M. & Fournier, C. Submitted to publication.
7. Bach, J. F. & Dardenne, M. (1973) *Cell. Immunol.* **6**, 694.
8. Loor, F. & Roelants, G. (1974) *Nature* **251**, 229.
9. Bach, J. F. & Dardenne, M. (1973) *Immunology* **25**, 353.
10. Bach, J. F., Cantor, H., Roelants, G. & Stutman, O., This volume.
11. Stutman, O., This volume.
12. Bach, J. F., Bach, M. A., Charreire, J., Dardenne, M., Fournier, C., Papiernik, M. & Pleau, J. M., This volume.
13. Goldstein, A. L. *et al.*, This volume.

Biological Activity of Thymic Hormones

MIXED LYMPHOCYTE REACTION BIOASSAY FOR THYMOSIN

GERALDINE H. COHEN & ALLAN L. GOLDSTEIN

INTRODUCTION

The mixed lymphocyte reaction (MLR) bioassay for thymosin is based on the observation of Cohen *et al.* (1) that bovine thymosin fraction 5 enhances *in vitro* the capacity of CBA/J thymocytes to respond against allogeneic mitomycin C-treated C57Bl/6J spleen cells, but not against syngeneic mitomycin C-treated spleen cells. Agents such as bovine serum albumin, human serum erythropoietin, and cyclic AMP do not similarly enhance this thymocyte MLR (1). In our hands, fractions prepared from other bovine tissues such as spleen contain some MLR-enhancing bioactivity, but the quantitation and dependence of such bioactivity on the presence of an intact thymus in the donor animal has yet to be determined.

TEST SAMPLE PREPARATION

The lyophilized, salt-free samples are suspended in pyrogen-free normal saline solution at a concentration of 2-10 mg protein/ml, neutralized to pH 7 with 0.1-0.2 N NaOH, and sterilized using a 0.22 μ pore size millipore filter. At protein concentrations >2 mg/ml, it is important to neutralize the sample before filtration, since thymic extracts have components which are insoluble below pH 7. The samples are aliquoted and stored frozen at −70 °C. Prior to each bioassay, the test sample is diluted with serum-free HRPMI (25 mM HEPES buffered RPMI-1640; Gibco, Grand Island, N.Y.) to the desired protein level which is four times the final concentration in the lymphocyte cultures described below. Thymosin fraction 5 is routinely diluted to 400 μg/ml and thus the final concentration in the bioassay system is 100 μg/ml.

ANIMALS

The animals used are 5-8 weeks old CBA/J male mice and 8-16 week old C57BL/6J male mice which are obtained from Jackson Laboratories, Bar Harbor, Maine.

Division of Biochemistry, University of Texas Medical Branch, Galveston, Texas 77550, U.S.A.

PREPARATION OF RESPONDER CBA/J THYMOCYTES

Aseptic technique is used throughout these procedures. Single cell suspensions are prepared at room temperature in a disposable plastic petri dish by mashing the thymus against a stainless steel mesh circular screen (100 wires/inch) using the flat end of a plastic disposable 1 cc syringe plunger. The screen is bathed in a few ml of cold Medium 199 with Hanks' salts (Med. 199) supplemented with 2 per cent heat-inactivated (56°, 30 min) human AB serum.

The cell suspension is washed with the same medium into a 15 ml conical plastic tube via a glass funnel lined with nylon monofilament cloth (15 μ pore size, NITEX HC-15). The tube is filled to the top with medium. From here on, the cell suspension is kept at 4°-10° unless otherwise indicated. The cell suspension is centrifuged at $200 \times g$ for 10 min, the supernatant medium is discarded, and the cell pellet is resuspended in fresh Med 199 by gentle refluxing with a pasteur pipet. After a second wash, the cell pellet is resuspended in HRPMI containing 6.67 per cent heat-inactivated human AB serum, fresh 2 mM L-glutamine, 100 units/ml penicillin and 100 μg/ml streptomycin. The cell density is measured with a Coulter Counter and the suspension is diluted to 10×10^6 cells/ml with the same medium.

TARGET SPLEEN CELLS

Cell suspensions are prepared from spleens of CBA/J and of C57Bl/6J mice as described above, except that the Med 199 is serum-free. After the first wash in Med 199, the cells are suspended in 17 ml of Med 199 ($10\text{-}20 \times 10^6$ cells/ml) containing 25 μg/ml mitomycin C (Sigma Chemical Co., St. Louis, Mo.) and incubated in 50 ml capped tubes (Falcon no. 2095) for 25 min at 37°. The cell suspensions are then diluted about three-fold with cold Med 199 and centrifuged at $200 \times g$. The supernatant is discarded and the cells are resuspended and washed once more in Med 199 and finally resuspended in HRPMI supplemented with 6.67 per cent heat-inactivated human AB serum. Cell density is adjusted to 8×10^6 cells/ml with the same medium.

MIXED LYMPHOCYTE REACTIONS

Quadruplicate cultures are prepared in microtiter trays (Limbro Chemical Co., New Haven, Conn.) with each flat bottom well containing a total volume of 0.2 ml HRPMI-1640, supplemented with 5 per cent heat-inactivated human AB serum, 2 mM fresh L-glutamine, 100 units/ml penicillin and 100 μg/ml streptomycin. The microtiter tray is turned on its side with the lettered border oriented towards the top. Using a Hamilton repeating syringe dispensor, each of the eight wells in a single horizontal row receives 50 μl of the test sample and then 100 μl (10×10^5 cells) of the thymocyte suspension. Each of the first four wells in the row receives 50 μl (4×10^5 cells) of the C57BL/6J spleen cell suspension, while each of the remaining four wells in the row receives 50 μl (4×10^5 cells) of the CBA/J spleen cell suspension. A sample is tested at several different dilutions, usually at 2- to 10-fold decrements. A row of eight wells is utilized for each concentration tested. Several dilutions of a standard preparation of bovine thymosin fraction 5 are included in every test run as a control for positive bioassay function. The lymphocyte cultures in one row of each tray receive the diluent medium alone instead of the test sample.

Cultures are maintained for 120 h in a humidified 5 per cent CO_2 atmosphere at 37 °C, and at 113 h, 1 μCi ^{3}H-thymidine (New England Nuclear Corp., Boston, Mass., 1.9 Ci/mmole specific radioactivity) is added to each well in a volume of 0.02 ml. Cultures are harvested with normal saline solution onto glass fiber filterpaper with a multiple automated sample harvester (MASH) according to the methods of Thurman *et al.* (2) and the radioactivity retained by the dried filter paper is measured by Liquifluor scintillation fluid (New England Nuclear Corp., Boston, Mass.) in a nuclear Chicago Scintillation Counter.

POSSIBLE PITFALLS

The first two washes of thymocytes in Med 199 (2 per cent human AB serum) are absolutely required to minimize lysis of thymocytes upon resuspension in HRPMI (6.67 per cent human AB serum). The "baseline" stimulation index (allogeneic cpm/syngeneic cpm) of cultures not containing thymosin under the conditions described above is usually about 1 to 2. The baseline stimulation index, however, can exceed this level as thymocyte numbers are increased, or if there is endotoxin contamination in the culture media, or possibly, as a result of physiological changes in the mice from time to time. Despite this increased baseline index (which should not exceed 5-10, for the purposes of bioassay), thymosin is capable of elevating the ^{3}H-thymidine cpm of allogeneic cultures to 3x-10x the cpm of control allogeneic cultures.

The capacity of thymocytes to respond in this MLR is highly stimulated by endotoxin (lipopolysaccharide). An increased thymocyte MLR is obtained with as little as 10 ng/ml endotoxin, but no increase is seen with 1 ng/ml or less of endotoxin. Therefore, test samples are routinely measured for endotoxin content using the Limulus lysate bioassay (4) and the samples are tested in the MLR bioassay at dilutions for which the endotoxin content has negligible effects.

Mercaptoethanol at concentrations above 10^{-7} M also increases the MLR bioassay and therefore should be removed if present in tissue fractions prior to bioassay.

DOSE-EFFECT CURVES

On comparing a fixed amount of protein of one sample to another, differences in the absolute cpm of allogeneic cultures may be obtained. We also measure the bioactivity as an endpoint titration, noting the lowest concentration at which the cpm of the test allogeneic cultures exceed those of the control (thymosin-free) allogeneic cultures, or, the cut-off concentrations after which further dilution no longer decreases or changes the cpm of the experimental allogeneic cultures.

POSSIBLE TARGET CELLS

We speculate that in the thymocyte MLR, thymosin facilitates and amplifies the antigen-driven differentiation of immature thymocytes (T_1 cells (3)) into immunocompetent T lymphocytes (T_2 cells (3)). This activity, however, does not preclude the possibility that thymosin may also act on a more primitive thymocyte precursor in the bone marrow.

ACKNOWLEDGEMENTS

This bioassay was developed with the aid of grants from the National Cancer Institute (CA 15419 and CA 14108) and the John Hartford Foundation, Inc.

REFERENCES

1. Cohen, G. H., Hooper, J. & Goldstein, A. L. (1975) *Annals of the New York Acad. Sci.* **249**, 145.
2. Thurman, G. B., Strong, D. M., Amed, A., Green, S. S., Sell, K. W., Hartman, R. J. & Bach, F. H. (1973) *Clin. Exp. Immunol.* **15**, 289.
3. Raff, M. C. & Cantor, H. (1971) In *Progress in Immunology* Ed. B. Amos, Academic Press, New York, p. 83.
4. Levin, J. & Bang, F. B. (1968) *Thromb. Diath. Haemorrh.* **19**, 186.

Biological Activity of Thymic Hormones

MITOGEN BIOASSAY FOR THYMOSIN: INCREASED MITOGENIC RESPONSIVENESS OF MURINE LYMPHOCYTES *IN VITRO* FOLLOWING *IN VIVO* TREATMENT WITH THYMOSIN

GARY B. THURMAN & ALLAN L. GOLDSTEIN

1. RATIONALE

The initial observation of increased lymph node lymphocyte responsivity to mitogens, and particularly Concanavalin A (Con A), following *in vivo* treatment with thymosin occurred while doing toxicity studies with thymosin prior to initiation of clinical trials. Normal C57BL/6J mice were given a range of doses (10 to 1000 mg/kg) of thymosin fraction 5 daily for 2 weeks. The lymphocytes from the lymph nodes and spleens were cultured with mitogens at the termination of the experiment. A marked increase in the Con A responsivity of the lymph node cells of the thymosin treated animals with increasing doses was noted. Subsequent experiments have indicated that *in vivo* treatment can markedly increase the responsivity of lymph node cells of aged C57BL/6J mice, $B6AF_1$, normal and aged mice, NZB and nude mice (1, 2), particularly to Con A and to a smaller extent PHA-P and PWM. The rationale for the bioassay is that by increasing the amount of thymosin in a mouse above normal, an increased rate of maturation should result causing a shift in the populations of cells in the peripheral lymphoid tissue. It is well known that, in contrast to spleen and lymph node cells, lymphocytes in the murine thymus respond well to Con A but not to PHA. An increase in the rate of peripheral maturation of immature cells (induced by hormone injection) should increase the percentage of Con A responsive cells in the peripheral lymphoid tissue (while not affecting the pokeweed mitogen or lipopolysaccharide response).

2. *IN VIVO* TREATMENT OF ANIMALS

A. *Preparation of thymosin for injection*

The purified hormone was prepared in saline at pH 7.0-7.4 and filter sterilized by filtration through a Millex disposable filter unit (0.22 μ, Millipore Corporation, Bedford, Mass.). It was diluted with sterile saline to the proper concentration, aliquoted at the proper volume, and frozen at −20 °C until just prior

Division of Biochemistry, University of Texas Medical Branch, Galveston, Texas 77550, U.S.A.

to injection. It was then rapidly thawed in warm water to ambient temperature.

B. *Treatment of animals*

The aliquoted hormone is generally injected intraperitoneally (i.p.) in a volume of about 0.5 ml. However, subcutaneous (s.c.) (footpad) injections have been more effective, but the difficulty in repeatedly doing s.c. injections in mice makes i.p. injections more convenient. Injections are continued every day for 14 days and on the 15th day the animals are sacrificed.

3. *IN VITRO* ASSAY OF LYMPHOCYTE RESPONSES

Animals were killed by cervical dislocation. Spleens and lymph nodes were removed using sterile precautions, placed in plastic petri dishes (1007, Falcon Plastics, Oxnard, Calif.) containing medium 199 (with 100 U/ml penicillin, 100 μg/ml streptomycin and 2 mM L-glutamine) and gently pressed through stainless steel mesh screens, 100 wires/inch (541-100 R, Cistron Corp. Elmsford, New York). Single suspensions were obtained by passage through 25 GA needles. The cells were washed once by centrifugation at $180 \times g$ in a Model PR-l Portable Refrigerated Centrifuge (Damon/IEC Division, Needham Heights, Mass.), the supernatant was drawn off and the cell pellet resuspended in RPM l-1640 (with 25 mM HEPES buffer, 100 U/ml penicillin, 100 μg/ml streptomycin and 2 mM L-glutamine) with 10 per cent fetal calf serum (Gibco, Grand Island, New York). The cells were counted using a Coulter Counter Model Z and suspended to give a concentration of 6×10^6 lymphocytes/ml. Cultures were prepared in flat bottom microtitre plates (IS-FB-96-TC, Linbro Chemical Co., Inc., New Haven, Conn.) by placing 0.10 ml of the cell suspension into each well using a Hamilton PB600-10 repeating dispenser with a Hamilton 1005 Syringe (Hamilton Company, Reno, Nevada). Control cultures received 0.10 ml of RPMI 1640, and the stimulated cultures received 0.10 ml of PHA-P, 0.1 per cent (3110-57, Difco, Detroit, Michigan), Con A, 2.5 μg/ml (234567, Calbiochem. La Jolla, Michigan), PWM, 2 per cent (536, Gibco, Grand Island, New York) or *E. coli* LPS, 100 μg/ml (3922-10, Difco, Detroit, Michigan) all made up in RPMI 1640. Cultures were pulsed by adding 1 μCi tritiated thymidine, 1.9 Ci/mM (Thymidine/methyl-^{3}H/, 2533-94, Schwarz/Mann, Orangeburg, New Jersey), in 0.02 ml of RPMI 1640 8 h before culture termination using a Hamilton PB600-1 repeating dispenser with a Hamilton 1001 Syringe. Cultures were harvested utilizing the Multiple Automated Sample Harvester (Microbiological Associates, Bethesda, Maryland). The resulting filter spots were dried and placed in 1 dram opticlear vials (60975 L, Kimble Glass Co., Toledo, Ohio) to which was added 3 ml of a scintillation cocktail (liquifluor in toluene, New England Nuclear, Boston, Mass.). The vials were stoppered, inserted in lidless polyethylene scintillation vials (600 1075, Packard Instrument Co., Inc., Downers Grove, Illinois) and the tritiated thymidine incorporation analyzed by scintillation spectrophotometry in a Packard 2450 Liquid Scintillation Spectrometer (Packard Instrument Co., Inc., Downers Grove, Illinois). Processing of the data and necessary statistical tests were performed on a Wang 720C Advanced Programming Calculator (Wang Labs, Tewksbury, Mass.).

A. *Possible pitfalls*

Lymph node cells from mice are very temperamental and are sometimes difficult to work with. Care should be taken to keep them as happy as possible and work them up quickly for culturing. Optimum culture conditions should be pre-established. An optimum treatment-time for *in vivo* injection of the hormone has not yet been established but from indications it seems that at least two weeks of treatment are necessary for good consistent results.

The strain of mouse one uses should give low responses to Con A so that the effect will be more pronounced. In normal, aged, and thymectomized CBA/J mice, the *in vivo* effect of hormone treatment has not been observed since these animals (even the thymectomized ones) respond quite well when their lymph-node cells are cultured with Con A. Enough animals should be used in each group so that there are sufficient lymph node cells for culturing.

4. The responses seen in thymosin treated nude mice have not always been consistent and not all nude mice within a given treatment group respond to the hormone treatment. The reason for the variability in nude mice is not well understood. It might reflect the general state of health of the animals or strain of nude mice used. Since at least 3 weeks is necessary for a thymic graft to instigate observable immunological reconstitution of nude mice, it might be better to use longer periods of treatment for these animals.

5. DOSE-EFFECT CURVES

It is desirable to run a dose-effect curve on every preparation of hormone being tested. Optimum concentrations often vary from batch to batch and optimum amounts should be established. Generally our dose-effect curves for thymosin fraction 5 begin at 1 μg per day for 14 days and range as high as 1 mg per day (For the toxicity test mentioned in (2) we used a high dose of 25 mg per day (1000 mg/kg).

6. SPECIFICITY AND POSSIBLE TARGET CELLS

Thus far in our experiments we have been unable to induce a similar response with endotoxin (LPS), ovalbumin, bovine serum albumine or 2-mercaptoethanol (2). Bovine brain fraction 5 has no effect but bovine spleen fraction 5 has demonstrated some ability to also cause increased Con A responses (to a lesser degree than thymosin).

The target cell for this effect could possibly be one of three types of cells:

(A) an immature lymphoid cell (pre-T cell), (B) a thymocyte or (C) a partially matured T cell having been to the thymus but now residing outside of the thymus gland (postthymic cell).

Thymosin injection may act to "short circuit" the normal maturational sequence in which a precursor-cell goes from the bone marrow to the thymus gland to undergo further maturation. Increased amounts of the hormone in the circulation caused by the injections may induce maturation of these bone marrow precursor cells without their going to the thymus gland. Their natural target organ after exposure to thymosin probably is the peripheral lymphoid tissue where these "virgin" T-cells are available for reacting against foreign substances.

A second possibility is that thymosin injections cause an increase of the rate of maturating of lymphocytes already in the thymus gland causing them to migrate to the peripheral lymphoid tissues at a higher rate than normally occurs. A third possibility is that a population of cells exists (probably in the spleen) that has been to the thymus but has not completed its maturation sufficiently to migrate to the peripheral tissue.

The fact that similar effects of thymosin treatment are seen in nude mice and thymectomized mice tends to favor the first possibility i.e. accelerating maturation of bone marrow derived precursor cells.

The authors wish to acknowledge the superb technical assistance of Margaret Freund, Barbara Simms and Beth Warlick.

These studies were supported by grants from the National Cancer Institute (CA 15408 and CA 14109) and from the John Hartford Foundation, Inc.

REFERENCES

1. Thurman, G. B., Silver, B. B., Hooper, J. A., Giovanella, B. C. & Goldstein, A. L. (1973) *Proceedings of the first international workshop on nude mice* Ed. J. Rygaard & C. O. Povlsen, p. 105.
2. Thurman, G. B., Ahmed, A., Strong, D. M., Gershwin, E., Steinberg, F. & Goldstein, A. L., (In press) *Transplantation Proceedings*.

Biological Activity of Thymic Hormones

TECHNICAL MANUAL
POPLITEAL LYMPH NODE ASSAY

D. W. VAN BEKKUM & S. KNAAN

INTRODUCTION

Among the most unequivocal of T cell functions is the capacity of lymphoid cell populations to induce a GvH reaction. Quantitative assays for GvH activity were introduced by Simonsen (1), who measured spleen and liver enlargement of newborn mice following the injection of test cells, by Elkins (2) who measured the increase of kidney weight of F_1 hybrid recipient rats, following subcapsular injection of parental test cells, and by Ford *et al.* (3) who employed the increase in popliteal lymph node weight of F_1 hybrid rats following injection of parental cells into the corresponding foot pad of the hind leg. Our experience with both the Simonsen assay and the Ford assay, made us explore the feasibility of using the latter one for assaying thymus hormone activity. We had employed the Simonsen assay previously in mice to measure the effects of injection with thymic hormone preparations on the GvH activity of spleen cells of neonatally thymectomized animals and had to abandon this approach, because the results were highly irreproducible, even when the thymectomized animals were restored with thymic implants.

The use of the popliteal lymph node (PLN) assay in rats seems to have the advantage of obtaining 2 points per animal, a rather wide dose-response range and little or no disturbance from loss of animals - which is a source of failures in the Simonsen assay. The disadvantage of the PLN assay for our present purpose is that for *in vivo* treatment of test cell donors, a relatively large amount of active hormone preparation is needed. Such a disadvantage obviously does not hold for experiments employing *in vitro* incubation of test cells with hormone preparations. However, we have not so far obtained any consistently positive reaction by incubating lymphoid cells from thymectomized donor rats with hormone preparations, so that this type of experiment is not described here. We shall instead briefly describe the method we employed to investigate the ability of injection of thymic preparations to restore the GvH reactivity of lymphoid cells from neonatally thymectomized rats. As shown in Table I, cells from the spleen, the lymph nodes and the peripheral blood from neonatally thymectomized animals show a clear-cut decreased response in the PLN assay as compared to the cells from intact animals.

Radiobiological Institute - T.N.O., Rijswijk (Z.H.), The Netherlands

TABLE I

EFFECT OF NEONATAL THYMECTOMY ON ABILITY OF LYMPHOID CELLS TO INDUCE POPLITEAL LYMPH NODE WEIGHT INCREASE

Donor	*Spleen* *(20×10^6)*	*Lymph nodes* *(5×10^6)*	*Peripheral blood* *(0.2 ml)*
Intact	26 (4)	16 (3)	19 (3)
Thymect.	6 (3)	7 (2)	6 (2)

Donors WAG/Rij rats
Recipients (BN $\times$ WAG) F_1 rats
Figures in the body of the table represent average of PLN weights in mg. Number of experiments between brackets. In each experiment 6–8 popliteal lymph nodes were measured per assay point.

Technique

Animals: Eight to ten-weeks-old WAG/Rij rats are used as donors. They are newborn-thymectomized or intact. Recipients are (BN/Rij $\times$ WAG/Rij) F_1 hybrids of the same sex as the donors and 6 weeks of age; 3-4 recipients are used for each test group. Test cells are injected s.c. in each of the foot pads of the hind legs. Recipients are sacrificed after 7 days. Popliteal lymph nodes are dissected out, cleaned from adhering tissue and weighed to 0.1 of a mg.

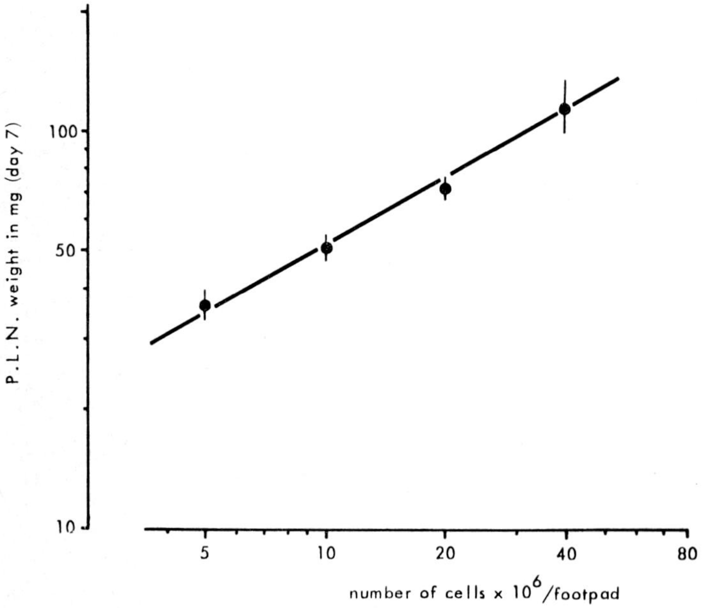

Fig. 1. The increase of lymph node weight with time after injection of 0.3 ml of peripheral blood of WAG/Rij rats into the foot pad of (BN $\times$ WAG) F_1 recipients. (R. L. Marquet, Rijswijk, unpublished results).

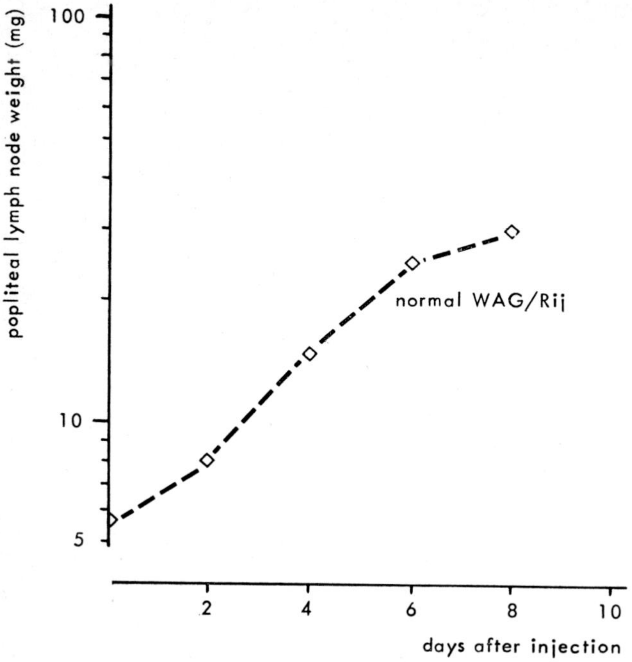

Fig. 2. The relation between lymph node response and the number of spleen cells injected into the foot pad. Vertical bars represent S.E. Each point represents the mean of 10 measurements on day 7 after inoculation.

The test cells are collected and administered as follows: Peripheral blood is collected from the tail in a heparinized syringe and 0.2 ml is injected into each foot pad. Nucleated cell counts are made on parallel samples.

Spleen cell suspensions are prepared in RPMI 1640; 2-3 spleens are pooled. The suspension is washed once, counted and brought to the proper dilution. 20×10^6 cells/0.2 ml are injected into the hind foot pads of the recipient rat. For preparation of the lymph node cell suspension, mesenteric, axillar, inguinal, cervical and submandibular lymph nodes from 2-3 animals are usually pooled. The cells are suspended in RPMI 1640+10 per cent FBS, washed and counted. 5×10^6 cells are injected in a volume of 0.2 ml into each footpad. As a positive control, cells from intact animals are employed, as negative controls either F_1 hybrid cells or RPMI solutions.

It was previously found (4) that the increase in lymph node weight plateaus off after the 6th day (Fig. 1) so that the 7th day is the earliest time of obtaining stable results. Fig. 2 shows that a linear relationship is obtained between the number of cells injected and node weight on a double log scale, in accordance with the data published by Ford *et al.* (3).

The assay of the thymic hormone

Newborn-thymectomized and intact WAG/Rij ♀♀ (3 animals/test group) are injected i.p. in 3 successive days with different thymic and control preparations. On the 4th day, animals are sacrificed and peripheral blood, spleen and lymph nodes of each test group are pooled, suspended, counted and injected into the foot pads of 6-week-old F_1 hybrid recipients.

So far, consistent restoration of the GvH reactivity of the cells of the thymectomized animals has not been achieved by administration of thymus hormone preparations for this short period. Perhaps the dose of hormone has been too low (1 mg of protein/rat/day for both the thymosin fraction 5 and THF). A more prolonged treatment of the rats by daily injections e.g. for 2 or 3 weeks yielded inconclusive results because cells from thymectomized animals treated with control solutions, including physiological saline, were found to give positive reactions occasionally.

Further exploration of the usefulness of the PLN assay for thymic hormone monitoring has to await experiments with larger doses of hormone preparations and the elucidation of the question concerning the specificity of the response.

REFERENCES

1. Simonsen, M. (1962) *Prog. in Allergy* **6**, 349.
2. Elkins, W. L. (1964) *J. Exp. Med.* **120**, 329.
3. Ford, W. L., Burr, W. & Simonsen, M. *Transplantation* **10**, no. 3, 258.
4. Marquet, R. L. & van Bekkum, D. W. (1973) *Transpl. Proc. vol.* **V**, no. 1, 631.
5. Dorsch, Susan E. & Roser, Bruch (1974) *Ajebak* **52** (Pt 2) 253.
6. Yoshida, Y. & Osmond, D. G. (1971) *Transplantation* vol. **12**, no. 2.

LIST OF PARTICIPANTS

Astaldi, A., Central Laboratory of the Blood Transfusion Center, The Netherlands Red Cross, Amsterdam, The Netherlands
Astaldi, G., Central Laboratory of the Blood Transfusion Center, The Netherlands Red Cross, Amsterdam, The Netherlands
Bach, J.-F., Hôpital Necker, Paris, France
Bach, M. A., Hôpital Necker, Paris, France
Bakker, W., Pathology Anatomy Laboratory, State University, Groningen, The Netherlands
Bakkeren, J. A. J. M., Department of Pediatrics, Radboud Hospital, Nijmegen, The Netherlands
Balner, H., Primate Center TNO, Rijswijk, The Netherlands
Bekkum, D. W. van, Radiobiological Institute TNO, Rijswijk, The Netherlands
Benner, R., Department of Cell Biology and Histology 2, Erasmus University, Rotterdam, The Netherlands
Bentvelzen, P., Radiobiological Institute TNO, Rijswijk, The Netherlands
Berg, R. J. van den, Organon n.v., Oss, The Netherlands
Betel, I., Radiobiological Institute TNO, Rijswijk, The Netherlands
Bierling, R., Pharma-Research Center, Bayer Ltd., Wuppertal, Germany
Blankwater, M.-J., Institute for Experimental Gerontology TNO, Rijswijk, The Netherlands
Blijham G. H., Histology Laboratory, State University, Groningen, The Netherlands
Bolhuis, R. L. H., Institute for Experimental Gerontology TNO, Rijswijk, The Netherlands
Bogaerts, W. J. C., Medical-Biological Laboratory RVO-TNO, Rijswijk, The Netherlands
Brocades-Zaalberg, O., Medical-Biological Laboratory RVO-TNO, Rijswijk, The Netherlands
Broek, A. A. van den, Histology Laboratory, State University, Groningen, The Netherlands
Buurman, W. A., Department of Cell Biology and Histology 2, Erasmus University, Rotterdam, The Netherlands
Cantor, H., Division of Tumor Immunology, Harvard Medical School, Boston, Massachusets, U.S.A.
Carnaud, J., Tumor Biology Department, Karolinksa Institute, Stockholm, Sweden
Charreire, J., Hôpital Necker, Paris, France
Cohen, G., Division of Biochemistry, University of Texas Medical Branch, Galveston, Texas, U.S.A.
Cybulski, L., Department of General Surgery, University of Cracov, Cracov, Poland
Dardenne, M., Hôpital Necker, Paris, France
Dooren, L. J., Department of Pediatrics, Academic Hospital, Leiden, The Netherlands
Dijk, H. van, Department of Microbiology, Academic Hospital, Utrecht, The Netherlands
Elferink, B. G., Blood Bank, Academic Hospital, Leiden, The Netherlands
Es, L. A. van, Department of Renal Diseases, Academic Hospital, Leiden, The Netherlands
Eijsvoogel, V. P., Central Laboratory of the Blood Transfusion Center, The Netherlands Red Cross, Amsterdam, The Netherlands
Ford, A. C., Radiobiological Institute TNO, Rijswijk, The Netherlands
Fournie, G., Laboratoire d'Immunopathology Rénale, Centre d'Hemodialyse Periodique, Toulouse, France
Fournier, C., Hôpital Necker, Paris, France
Furth, R. van, Department of Microbial Diseases, Academic Hospital, Leiden, The Netherlands
Gagnerault, M. C., Hôpital Necker, Paris, France
Gastkemper, M., Histology Laboratory, State University, Groningen, The Netherlands
Gerver, J. A. M., Department of Electronmicroscopy, Free University, Amsterdam, The Netherlands
Gisler, R. H., Research Department, Pharmaceuticals Division, CIBA-GEIGY Ltd., Basel, Switzerland
Goldstein, A. L., Division of Biochemistry, University of Texas Medical Branch, Galveston, Texas, U.S.A.

Grollé, P. F., Blood Bank, Academic Hospital, Leiden, The Netherlands
Habu, S., Department of Zoology, University College, London, England
Hardy, M. A., Department of Surgery, Bronx, New York, U.S.A.
Harten, J. J. van der, Institute for Pathology, Free University, Amsterdam, The Netherlands
Hensen, E., Blood Bank, Academic Hospital, Leiden, The Netherlands
Hess, M. W., Institute for Pathology, University of Bern, Switzerland
Hoebeke, Janssen Pharmaceutica, Beerse, Belgium
Hoefsmit, E. C. M., Department of Electronmicroscopy, Free University, Amsterdam, The Netherlands
Hollander, C. F., Institute for Experimental Gerontology TNO, Rijswijk, The Netherlands
Hollander, F. C., Organon n.v., Oss, The Netherlands
Hondius-Boldingh, W., Organon n.v., Oss, The Netherlands
Hijmans, W., Institute for Experimental Gerontology TNO, Rijswijk, The Netherlands
Incefy, G. S., Memorial Sloan-Kettering Cancer Center, New York, New York, U.S.A.
Jonker, M., Blood Bank, Academic Hospital, Leiden, The Netherlands
Jordan, R., Department of Anatomy. The University of Newcastle-upon-Tyne, Newcastle-upon-Tyne, England
Kacaki, J., Organon n.v., Oss, The Netherlands
Kater, L., Division of Immunopathology, University Hospital, Utrecht, The Netherlands
Kindred, B., Basel Institute for Immunology, Basel, Switzerland
Kook, A., Department of Cell Biology, The Weizmann Institute of Science, Rehovot, Israel
Kreeftenberg, J. G., State Institute for Public Health, Bilthoven, The Netherlands
Kruisbeek, A. M., Institute for Experimental Gerontology TNO, Rijswijk, The Netherlands
Kruisinga, R. J. H., Netherlands Society of Gerontology, Wassenaar, The Netherlands
Lalleman, E., Hôpital Necker, Paris, France
Langevoort, H. L., Histology Laboratory, Free University, Amsterdam, The Netherlands
Leerling, M., State Institute for Public Health, Bilthoven, The Netherlands
Leeuw, J. H. S., Department of Electronmicroscopy, Free University, Amsterdam, The Netherlands
Levey, R. H., Department of Surgery, Harvard Medical School, Boston, Massachusets, U.S.A.
Levy, A., Department of Cell Biology, The Weizmann Institute of Science, Rehovot, Israel
Löwenberg, B., Radiobiological Institute TNO, Rijswijk, The Netherlands
Lubbe, F. H., Medical-Biological Laboratory TNO, Rijswijk, The Netherlands
Lucas, C. J., Central Laboratory of the Blood Transfusion Center, The Netherlands Red Cross, Amsterdam, The Netherlands
Luckey, T. D., Department of Biochemistry, University of Missouri, Columbia, Missouri, U.S.A.
Maat, B., Radiobiological Institute TNO, Rijswijk, The Netherlands
Matsuzaki, F., 3rd Department of Internal Medicine, University of Tokyo, Tokyo, Japan
Muiswinkel, W. B. van, Department of Cell Biology and Histology 2, Erasmus University, Rotterdam, The Netherlands
Mul, N. A. J., Department of Immunology, Academic Hospital, Utrecht, The Netherlands
Nieuwenhuis, P., Histology Laboratory, State University, Groningen, The Netherlands
Nieuwerkerk, H. T. M., Radiobiological Institute TNO, Rijswijk, The Netherlands
Ohsawa, N., 3rd Department of Internal Medicine, University of Tokyo, Tokyo, Japan
Pelt, F. van, Institute for Experimental Gerontology TNO, Rijswijk, The Netherlands
Putte, L. B. A. van der, Department of Rheumatology, Academic Hospital, Leiden, The Netherlands
Putten, L. M. van, Radiobiological Institute TNO, Rijswijk, The Netherlands
Radl, J., Institute for Experimental Gerontology TNO, Rijswijk, The Netherlands
Reerink-Brongers, E. E., Central Laboratory of the Blood Transfusion Center, The Netherlands Red Cross, Amsterdam, The Netherlands
Reymond, J. F., Immunology Laboratory, University Hospital, Zürich, Switzerland
Roelants, G., Basel Institute for Immunology, Basel, Switzerland
Rood, J. J. van, Department of Immunohaematology, Academic Hospital, Leiden, The Netherlands
Rothbarth, Ph. H., Wilhelmina Children Hospital, Utrecht, The Netherlands
Rotter, V., Department of Cell Biology, The Weizmann Institute of Science, Rehovot, Israel

Ruitenberg, E. J., State Institute for Public Health, Bilthoven, The Netherlands
Rygaard, J., University Hospital, Copenhagen, Denmark
Rijke, E. O., Wilhelmina Children Hospital, Utrecht, The Netherlands
Schellekens, P. Th. A., Central Laboratory of the Blood Transfusion Center, The Netherlands Red Cross, Amsterdam, The Netherlands
Schjerven, L., Animal Department, State Hospital, Oslo, Norway
Schuit, H. R. E., Institute for Experimental Gerontology TNO, Rijswijk, The Netherlands
Schuurs, A. H. W. M., Organon n.v., Oss, The Netherlands
Singh, U., Department of Anatomy, The University of Newcastle-upon-Tyne, Newcastle-upon-Tyne, England
Skotnicki, A. B., Haematological Clinic, Medical Academy of Cracow, Cracov, Poland
Small, M., Department of Cell Biology, The Weizman Institute of Science, Rehovot, Israel
Smits, S. P., Lichtenberg Hospital, Amersfoort, The Netherlands
Snyder, J., Hoffmann-La Roche, Kings and Nutley, New Jersey, U.S.A.
Sousa, M. de, Department of Bacteriology and Immunology, Western Infirmary, Glasgow, United Kingdom
Splinter, T. A. W., Central Laboratory of the Blood Transfusion Center, The Netherlands Red Cross, Amsterdam, The Netherlands
Stutman, O., Department of Cellular Immunobiology, Section Sloan-Kettering Institute, New York, New York, U.S.A.
Swart, A. C. W., Institute for Experimental Gerontology TNO, Rijswijk, The Netherlands
Sybesma, J. P. H. B., Department of Haematology, Academic Hospital, Utrecht, The Netherlands
Tamaoki, N., Department of Pathology, Tokai University, Kanagawa, Japan
Thurman, G., Division of Biochemistry, University of Texas Medical Branch, Galveston, Texas, U.S.A.
Touraine, J. L., Hôpital Edouard Herriot, Lyon, France
Trainin, N., Department of Cell Biology, The Weizmann Institute of Science, Rehovot, Israel
Tweel, J. G. van den, Department of Immunohaematology, Academic Hospital, Leiden, The Netherlands
Umiel, T., Department of Cell Biology, The Weizmann Institute of Science, Rehovot, Israel
Veldhuizen, R. W., Institute for Pathology, Free University, Amsterdam, The Netherlands
Vlek, L. F. M., Laboratory of Renal Diseases, Academic Hospital, Leiden, The Netherlands
Vrede, M. S., Division of Immunopathology, University Hospital, Utrecht, The Netherlands
Waarde, D. van, Department of Microbial Diseases, Academic Hospital, Leiden, The Netherlands
Warren-Johnson, H. S., Fibiger-Laboratory, Copenhagen, Denmark
White, A., Department of Biochemistry, Stanford University School of Medicine, Stanford California, U.S.A.
Willers, A., Department of Microbiology, Academic Hospital, Utrecht, The Netherlands
Woesik, L. van, Blood Bank, Academic Hospital, Leiden, The Netherlands
Woody, J., Department of Zoology, University College, London, England
Zipori, D., Department of Cell Biology, The Weizmann Institute of Science, Rehovot, Israel